WOMEN'S HEALTH
handbook

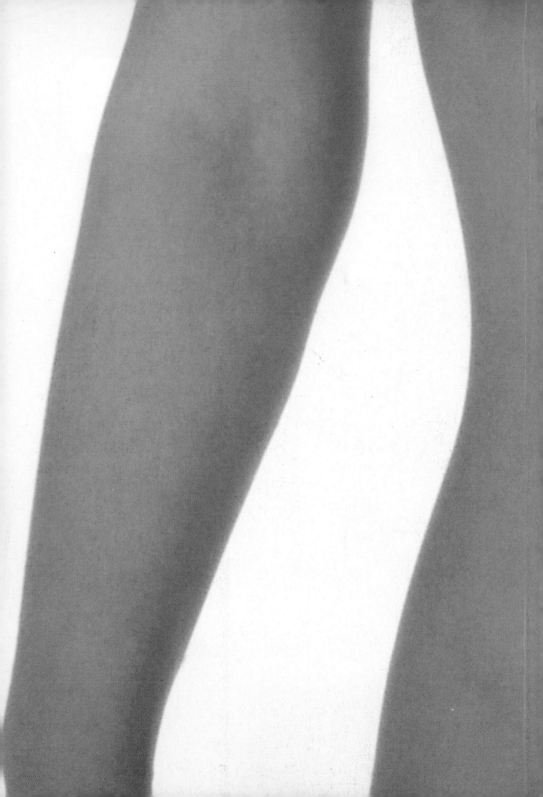

Dr. **miriam stoppard**

WOMEN'S HEALTH
handbook

A Dorling Kindersley Book

Dorling 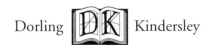 Kindersley

LONDON, NEW YORK, DELHI, MUNICH, MELBOURNE

Editorial and Design: Julie Whitaker and Brian Rust

Senior Managing Editor: Corinne Roberts
Senior Managing Art Editor: Lynne Brown
Senior Editor: Julia North
Senior Art Editor: Karen Ward
Production: Maryann Rogers

First published in Great Britain in 2001 by
Dorling Kindersley Limited, 80 Strand, London WC2 ORL
A Penguin Company

2 4 6 8 10 9 7 5 3 1

Copyright © 2001
Dorling Kindersley Limited, London
Text copyright © 2001 Miriam Stoppard

Material in this publication was previously published by
Dorling Kindersley in *Well Woman, HRT, Healthy Sex,
Breast Health* and *Natural Menopause.*
Copyright © 1998 Dorling Kindersley Limited, London
Text copyright © 1998 Miriam Stoppard
(*Natural Menopause, Well Woman, Breast Health, Healthy Sex*).
Copyright © 1999 Dorling Kindersley Limited, London
Text copyright © 1999 Miriam Stoppard (*HRT*).

A CIP catalogue record for this book is available
from the British Library.

ISBN 07513 1434 X

Reproduced by Colourscan, Singapore
Printed in Singapore by Star Standard Industries (PTE) Ltd

This edition published for Index Books Ltd 2002

ABOUT THE AUTHOR

DR. MIRIAM STOPPARD has been at the forefront of the revolution in health information since she began her writing and broadcasting career in the early 1970s. Since that time, Dr. Stoppard has become well-known to millions all over the world as one of the leading authorities on women's health, relationships and sexual well-being, as well as parenting, baby and child care.

Her blend of medical training and direct experience of the problems of ordinary people have made her uniquely qualified as a writer on popular health issues. More importantly, Dr. Stoppard is also a parent herself – with two sons of her own as well as four step-children.

Dr. Stoppard's first book for Dorling Kindersley – *Everywoman's Lifeguide* – was published in 1982. Since then she has published over 40 DK titles, of which 30 have also been published in the USA.

As she has said, her main aim is to give her readers "the confidence to follow their own instincts", and her approach applies equally to couples facing parenthood for the first time or, as in this book, to women facing up to the menopause, seeking guidance on breast health or trying to enhance their sex life.

Developed and informed by the experience of more than 30 years of communication, Dr. Miriam Stoppard's ideas and approach remain totally fresh and up-to-date. In 1998, she was made a Fellow of the Royal College of Physicians in recognition of her work in promoting health issues, a thoroughly deserved honour that will be endorsed by everyone who has benefited from her practical and sympathetic approach.

Contents

SECTION 1
WELL WOMAN

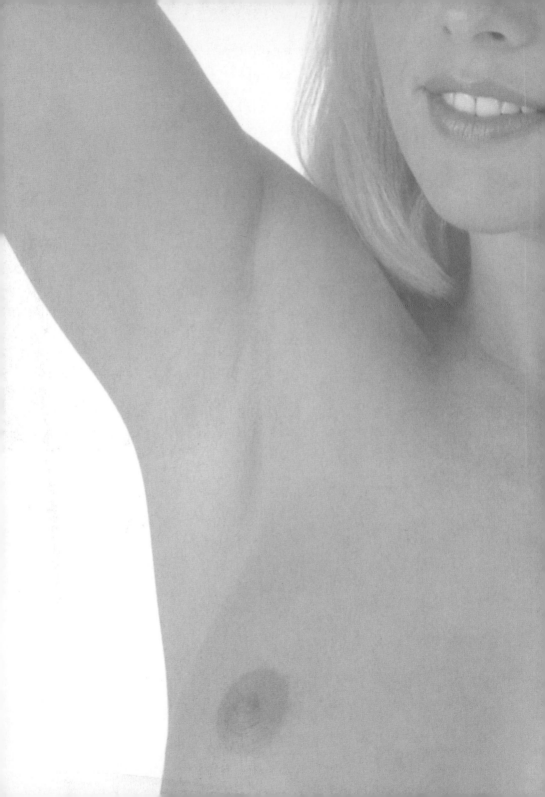

1

WELL WOMAN

INTRODUCTION

ALTHOUGH MANY MEDICAL conditions affect both men and women, there are aspects of women's health that are unique to them. The complicated chemistry of the female hormones, and the position of the reproductive organs deep within the abdomen, mean that many women may experience some imbalance or health complication in this area at some point in their lives.

The good news is that medical research has dramatically improved our understanding of how women's bodies work, and how problems can be prevented or eliminated at an early stage. Understanding the function of hormones has enabled drugs to be developed that can often avoid the more invasive treatments which were a necessity in the past. Screening, diagnostic tests and microsurgery mean that potential medical conditions can now be detected or ruled out early on, providing for reassurance or prompt treatment.

In the excitment of rapid scientific advances, there was a tendency for doctors sometimes to overwhelm women with their superior knowledge, leaving them feeling bewildered and no longer in control of their bodies. Nowadays, however, it is widely recognized that women have the right to know what is happening to them, what is possible and what is not, and why certain treatments are recommended and what they involve. This section is designed to lead you through conditions and diseases that are particular to women, and the procedures likely to be used to diagnose and treat them.

Maintaining health – being a well woman – means being aware when something is amiss, taking advantage of screening and being informed – so that if you need treatment you can have confidence in what is being offered by your doctor, and what it means for the future.

1

HEALTHY FEMALE BODY

Millions of years of evolution have gone into adapting the female body to perform its biological functions efficiently. In this chapter, the major physical changes we undergo as we grow older are explored in detail, beginning with menstruation, leading on to fertility and conception, and finally to the menopause. All are explained clearly, and the various ways of dealing with them are set out. Knowledge is power, and understanding what is happening to you at these different stages in your life can help you make informed decisions about how you want to live.

THE FEMALE BODY

We start being female from the moment of conception, when an X sperm fertilizes the female egg. After just a few weeks of development in the uterus, an embryo's female characteristics are visible. Even at this stage, the female genitals – the labia, clitoris, vagina and primitive uterus – are all present, and the ovaries already contain a lifetime's supply of eggs, many in excess of those to be shed monthly from puberty to the menopause.

THE BEGINNING OF FERTILITY

At puberty, the potent female hormones, oestrogen and progesterone, begin to create a cycle of fertility. Every month the ovaries

MILESTONES IN DEVELOPMENT

From babyhood, the differences in body shape between boys and girls are noticeable. Girls tend to have more rounded buttocks and their angled thigh bones make another obvious difference. At about nine or ten the pelvic bones begin to grow, and more fat is deposited on the thighs, hips and breasts. By 12, nipples have budded and pubic hair sprouts. By about 18, bone growth is completed and adult height is reached. The next time of change is the period known as the climacteric, between the onset and ending of menopause symptoms. At the menopause, the ovaries run out of eggs, oestrogen and progesterone hormones stop being released and periods cease.

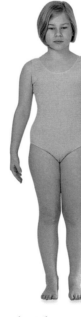
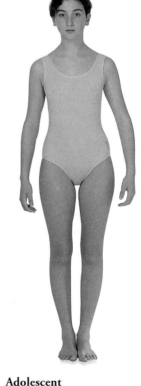

Young child
Even from a very young age, a girl's body is more rounded than a boy's.

Prepubertal
From 9–10, girls start to grow rapidly and their pelvic bones become more developed.

Adolescent
At 14, most girls are sexually mature, but they have not yet reached adult height.

release an egg, which travels down one of the two Fallopian tubes that connect the ovaries with the uterus. If the egg is not fertilized, it is eventually expelled from the body during menstruation.

This very complicated combination of hormones and biology is created solely to enable us to become pregnant and give birth, thus ensuring the continuation of our species. If the egg *is* fertilized by sperm, pregnancy results.

PREGNANCY AND BIRTH

Pregnancy is divided into three distinct stages, called trimesters, each one lasting about three months. During the first trimester, your body starts to make the adjustments that will enable you to carry the baby to term: heart and breathing rates increase, the uterus thickens and grows and the size and weight of your breasts increase. In the second and third trimesters, nipples enlarge and darken, the heart works twice as hard as that of a non-pregnant woman and the uterus continues to expand outwards to accommodate the fetus; during the last few weeks of pregnancy, walking becomes uncomfortable and hands and feet may swell.

On or about the 40th week of pregnancy, you will go into labour and give birth, an event like no other you will ever experience. No one knows precisely how labour starts, but there is increasing evidence to show that the baby plays a major role. The onset of labour is triggered by the secretion of hormones, one of which is produced by the baby. The uterus responds by starting to contract regularly at shorter and shorter intervals and with increasing force until the baby is expelled from the womb.

Within about six weeks of the birth of the baby, the uterus should have shrunk back to its normal pre-pregnancy size — from about 1kg (2lbs) at the end of the pregnancy to about 50g (2oz) — and within several weeks after that, menstruation will usually recommence. The cycle of fertility has begun all over again.

LIMITING FERTILITY

We are fertile for well over 30 years and are theoretically capable of many pregnancies. Much ingenuity, therefore, has always gone into evolving ways to limit the effects of such fertility. Until this century, however, methods were hit or miss, depending on a mixture of avoidance of sex at what was believed to be the "crucial" time of the month (the calendar method), or on the man withdrawing before ejaculating (coitus interruptus).

Nowadays, of course, we have the ability to manipulate our fertility much more accurately through various artificial methods of contraception, including oral, intrauterine or barrier devices. For both men and women, this ability has probably been one of the most significant developments in history: it has allowed us to control the size of our families; for us as women, it has also meant freedom to decide not just when, but if, we wish to become mothers.

THE END OF FERTILITY

The great milestone of middle age is the menopause. In the years leading up to it, our body prepares us for the end of fertility: periods can become irregular, sometimes heavy, and we may not ovulate every month.

Just as the beginning of menstruation brings about significant changes to our body, so does the end. The symptoms that signal the passing of our reproductive years include hot flushes, sweating, fragile bones and dryness of the vagina; lowering oestrogen levels can not only lead to a redistribution of body fat but also make us more susceptible to illnesses, such as heart disease and osteoporosis. But the advent of HRT and other alleviants, and a greater understanding of the part diet and exercise can play in maintaining health, has meant that such discomfort and pain can now be minimized. What was once referred to ominously as *the* change of life can be thankfully demoted to being merely one of many changes in a busy, enjoyable and productive life.

MENSTRUATION

The medical term for the beginning of menstruation is the menarche. The advent of the menarche (usually about the age of 12 in developed countries) means that a girl is entering her fertile life. Cyclical female hormone production starts and ovulation each month is a possibility, although few girls ovulate consistently in their first year or two of menstruation.

HORMONAL EFFECTS

Hormone production is not smooth in the beginning and may result in peaks and troughs, explaining why a teenage girl can become rebellious, moody, confused and mixed up. It also leads to the maturing of a girl's body and the appearance of adult characteristics, such as breasts and pubic hair.

The regular production of female hormones results in various changes in our bodies throughout the month. In the first half of the cycle, oestrogen is produced, which makes the skin bloom and raises our mood so that we feel that we can tackle anything. It also affects the appearance of vaginal discharge prior to ovulation; at this time of the month it is thin, clear and runny, with very little smell.

After ovulation, progesterone begins to show its effects. Vaginal secretions become thicker, opaque, more rubbery and definitely have a fishy odour. The breasts enlarge, become heavy and tender, and towards menstruation the nipples may tingle and feel sore. This is perfectly normal and the effects subside on or before the beginning of bleeding. Progesterone can cause acne-like spots on the face at this time of the month, and very few of us escape without having one or two of these at some point in our lives. They should disappear when menstruation starts.

MENSTRUAL PROBLEMS

Most of the time, monthly periods follow a predictable pattern. For most women some of the time, however, problems can and do occur, particularly during the early years of menstruation and in the premenopausal years, as the body prepares itself for menstruation to cease. Disorders can range from **premenstrual syndrome** (which about 75 percent of us suffer from at one time or another in our lives) to painful periods (**dysmenorrhoea**). Common menstrual problems are described in chapter 3.

THE REPRODUCTIVE ORGANS

The reproductive glands in women are the two ovaries. From puberty they release the ova (eggs), and manufacture the sex hormones, oestrogen and progesterone. Oestrogen influences the development of female body shape, enlargement of the breasts and the menstrual cycle. Each month an egg is released by the ovaries and travels down one of the two Fallopian tubes to the uterus, a hollow structure in the centre of the pelvis; if the egg is not fertilized, menstruation occurs.

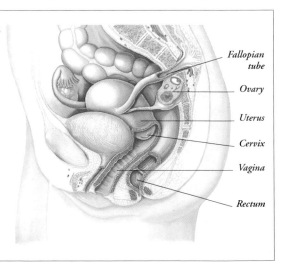

Fallopian tube

Ovary

Uterus

Cervix

Vagina

Rectum

THE MENSTRUAL CYCLE

The average cycle is about 28 days, but a cycle can be as long as 33 or as short as 26 days. It is counted from the first day of bleeding to the last day before the next period.

Days 1–13

At the beginning of the cycle, levels of the female hormones – oestrogen and progesterone – are low. Then the pituitary gland (which masterminds the production and distribution of hormones in the body) secretes follicle-stimulating hormone (FSH). This stimulates the ovary to start to grow egg follicles which, in their turn, secrete oestrogen. Oestrogen levels rise, encouraging the lining of the uterus (the endometrium) to thicken and prepare for a possible pregnancy.

Day 14 Ovulation

When oestrogen levels peak, this stimulates production of yet more FSH and another hormone, called luteinizing hormone (LH). This causes the follicle to burst, releasing the ripe egg. This is ovulation.

Days 15–28

The egg starts to move down the Fallopian tube and the follicle matures into a corpus luteum (small mass of yellow tissue), which secretes large amounts of progesterone in the second half of the month. Three days prior to menstruation, the corpus luteum begins to age, and progesterone levels fall. If unfertilized, the egg is absorbed and the endometrium is shed. Menstruation has begun.

MENSTRUAL HYGIENE

Menstruation is no longer the taboo subject it once was. When I was young, it was said that young girls shouldn't wash their hair or bathe during menstruation because the blood might go to the brain. This is nonsense, and the general rule should be to bathe as often as you want to, or at least use the bidet if you have one, so that you feel comfortable. Wash yourself with ordinary soap and water.

For protection, some girls prefer to use sanitary towels and these are ideal to begin with, but you might also want to consider tampons which can be more comfortable, hygienic and discreet. Quite a good way to experiment with tampons is to try them at the same time as a friend. I remember doing so with one of my college friends as we stood in adjacent toilets and gave running commentaries to each other on our progress. If you do use tampons, don't forget about them; they should be changed every four to six hours.

MENSTRUATION AND SEX

To protect you from sexually transmitted diseases, it is best to use a condom when having intercourse with any new partner, but it is even more important during menstruation. This is because blood-borne viruses such as HIV (which causes AIDS), hepatitis B and hepatitis C are transmitted more easily by unprotected sex during menstruation than at any other time of the month.

SEE ALSO:
Dysmenorrhoea
Menstrual Problems
Premenstrual Syndrome
Vaginal Discharge

FERTILITY AND CONCEPTION

Fertility is the term generally used to describe the ability to have a baby; conception is the first step to pregnancy.

During sexual intercourse, millions of sperm are released into the vagina. At ovulation, an egg is released from the ovary and begins to travel down the Fallopian tube towards the uterus. The mucus at the cervix becomes thinner to enable sperm to travel up through the cervix and uterus towards the egg. Only an extremely small proportion of the sperm originally ejaculated reaches the Fallopian tubes, however. They cluster round the egg until one actually penetrates its outer shell when fertilization takes place. The rest then drop off and die.

Conception is the implantation of the fertilized egg in the uterus. The ovaries increase their levels of female hormones to prepare the lining of the uterus to support the pregnancy until the placenta can take over. It is this increased level of hormone production that can cause early symptoms of pregnancy such as morning sickness, giddiness, fainting, tingling in the breasts and a desire to pass urine frequently. If conception does not occur, hormone production diminishes, thus triggering the monthly menstrual period.

GAUGING FERTILITY

A woman's fertility depends on several events but the most crucial one is that even someone who ovulates regularly is fertile for only about three days each month.

A woman's age is a significant factor in determining her fertility: she reaches her peak at about the age of 24 (in fact, at exactly the same age as a man reaches his peak). Eggs decline in quality with increasing age. There is a definite decline after about the age of 30 and it is very rare, though not impossible, for a woman to conceive after the age of 50. Even with normal fertilization, however, the uterine environment during the premenopausal years may be much less favourable and the egg will have less chance of survival.

THE TIMING OF INTERCOURSE

To ensure fertilization, intercourse must occur within a day or so of ovulation – you can confirm that ovulation has taken place with an ovulation kit, or by checking your vaginal discharge.

Sperm can survive within a woman's body for between two and three days after intercourse takes place; an egg is only viable for about two days following ovulation. During an average 28-day cycle, therefore, the fertile period is a comparatively short one. Although every woman's pattern is slightly different, you are much more likely to conceive in the middle of your cycle and much less likely to conceive very early in the cycle or within the last few days before your period.

If you menstruate regularly, there are ways to confirm when you ovulate. The

HOW GENES DETERMINE SEX

Each ovum (egg) and each sperm consists of 23 chromosomes; 22 of these pair with each other and on fertilization make up the genetic material of the future child. The 23rd chromosome determines a child's sex, and is X (female) or Y (male). The father produces X and Y sperm, while a woman's eggs are always X. If an X sperm unites with the egg, the child will be female; if a Y sperm unites with it, the child will be male.

The other chromosomes contain genetic material such as hair and eye colour; the tendency to inherit certain diseases, such as cystic fibrosis, and conditions such as colour blindness, are also carried in the genes.

BEGINNING OF LIFE

Cell division

Once the egg is fertilized, it quickly divides, first into two cells, then four, then eight and so on. These early cells are called totipotential cells, because they could develop into any part of the body.

TWO CELLS   FOUR CELLS   EIGHT CELLS   BLASTOCYST

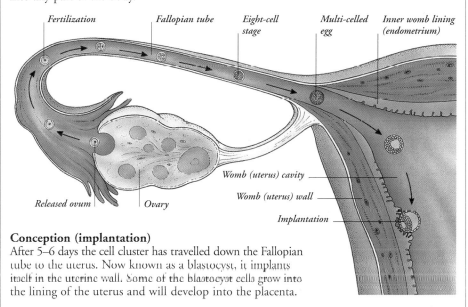

Fertilization   *Fallopian tube*   *Eight-cell stage*   *Multi-celled egg*   *Inner womb lining (endometrium)*

Womb (uterus) cavity

Womb (uterus) wall

Released ovum   *Ovary*

Implantation

Conception (implantation)

After 5–6 days the cell cluster has travelled down the Fallopian tube to the uterus. Now known as a blastocyst, it implants itself in the uterine wall. Some of the blastocyst cells grow into the lining of the uterus and will develop into the placenta.

easiest way is the temperature method and examining your cervical mucus. In the temperature method, take your temperature first thing in the morning throughout the month; when it stays up 0.2°C (0.4°F) three days in a row, and there is no other possible cause, this usually indicates ovulation. With the mucus method, you should examine your mucus regularly throughout the cycle: it should become slippery and clear, and you should feel "wet", two or three days prior to ovulation. An ovulation kit available from pharmacies is the most accurate method.

It isn't true that conception is more likely if you have intercourse very frequently; in fact, the opposite may be true – the more often a man ejaculates, the fewer sperm are contained in his ejaculate each time. If you are keen to become pregnant, therefore, it may be a good idea to abstain from sex for a few days prior to ovulation to build up the numbers of sperm, or at least to confine it to alternate days.

SEE ALSO:
Fertility Problems
Menopause
Menstrual Problems
Menstruation

CONTRACEPTION

If you need your contraceptive method to be nearly 100 percent effective without resorting to sterilization, there are two choices. You can use the combined contraceptive pill or the progesterone intrauterine device, which prevents conception and the implantation of the fertilized egg.

The next most effective means is what is called the "mini-pill" (progesterone-only pill) and the IUD (intrauterine device), followed by the various barrier methods.

WHAT METHOD IS BEST FOR ME?

The best method for you is the one that is most effective, but effectiveness can be judged by two criteria: theoretical and actual. Invariably, the latter has a higher failure rate because of the human element.

The least effective, largely because of human error, are the so-called "natural" methods, the ones that rely on determining safe periods and abstaining from intercourse during that time. As all the medical complications of pregnancy outweigh those of the combined pill, getting pregnant is always more risky than taking the pill. Contraceptives with the greatest risk are those with the highest failure rate.

Your choice of birth control will probably change during your fertile years. No one method is ideal for this length of time, punctuated as it may be by planned pregnancies and changes in sexual partners. You need to think about all the forms of contraception and match them to your personality, sexual practice and stage in life.

NATURAL METHODS

These methods include the oldest forms of contraception and consist of periodic abstinence, breastfeeding and withdrawal.

PERIODIC ABSTINENCE

Abstaining from intercourse during the time of ovulation is based on calculations using the calendar, plus the rise and fall of the woman's body temperature and the appearance of vaginal secretions. Using these indicators, you can decide to abstain from penetrative sex during ovulation.

A home ovulation test kit is the best method of detecting ovulation but there are older methods. The first is the calendar or rhythm method, which requires you to chart your cycle and abstain from intercourse during your fertile days.

The sympto-thermal method involves taking your temperature and observing the consistency and colour of your vaginal secretions. By taking your temperature with a very accurate thermometer at the same time every day (preferably first thing in the morning), you should be able to notice a rise of a fraction of a degree during the second half of your cycle, providing you are not suffering from an infection.

The second part of the routine is known as the Billings method. Your vaginal secretions also change during your cycle. Immediately after menstruation, you will be comparatively dry. Then, as the mucus builds up, you may notice it becoming thick, cloudy and sticky. This changes to clear, stretchy and abundant at the time of ovulation, when you should avoid intercourse.

WHAT ARE THE RISKS?

These methods are hopeless for women with irregular cycles and have a high failure rate. They require a strong commitment from both partners. Although there are no risks to health, there may be to relationships and, with a comparatively high failure rate, problems of unwanted pregnancy. The techniques need at least six months to become established and for you to be clear about what is normal for you.

BREASTFEEDING

Breastfeeding over a 24-hour period of time changes the levels of hormones and prevents ovulation. However, it is not a

BARRIER DEVICES

Condoms

Condoms are plastic sheaths which create a physical barrier to prevent sperm from reaching the ovum. They must be used with spermicides as well.

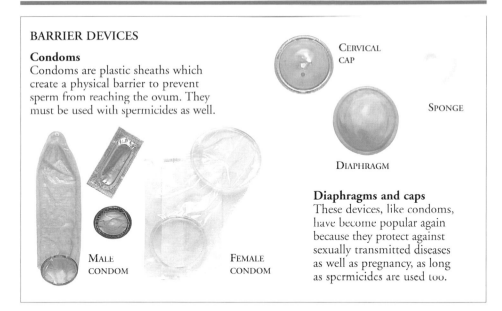

CERVICAL CAP

SPONGE

DIAPHRAGM

MALE CONDOM

FEMALE CONDOM

Diaphragms and caps

These devices, like condoms, have become popular again because they protect against sexually transmitted diseases as well as pregnancy, as long as spermicides are used too.

reliable means of birth control and becomes particularly unreliable once the 24-hour feeding regime is reduced. Just because you don't have a period during breastfeeding does not mean that you are not producing eggs and you must make sure, therefore, that you use some form of contraception, such as the mini-pill.

WITHDRAWAL

This is another ancient method with a very high failure rate, where the penis is withdrawn just before ejaculation. It doesn't require discussion about methods with doctors and at clinics and requires no financial outlay, but it also leaves much of the responsibility with the man.

BARRIER METHODS

These methods physically block the sperm from reaching the ovum or they chemically inactivate them.

MALE CONDOM

The condom is a latex rubber or plastic sheath that is placed over the erect penis before penetration. It should be lubricated and freed from air so that it doesn't burst inside the vagina. It works by preventing the sperm from entering the vagina.

The condom has been available for many years, and can be bought in a variety of retail outlets. It is widely used even where another form of contraception is used because of the danger of sexually transmitted diseases, especially AIDS. I would therefore advise all women who have not been engaged in monogamous relationships for over five years to insist on using male or female condoms.

FEMALE CONDOM

The female condom is designed to line the inside of the vagina. It consists of a lubricated plastic sheath with an anchoring ring to keep it in place within the vagina and an outer ring that holds the sheath open to allow insertion of the penis.

It allows a woman to control the method of contraception as well as providing good protection against sexually transmitted diseases, but has the disadvantage of being slightly awkward to insert. It is as effective as the male condom in preventing pregnancy.

CONTRACEPTION: CONTINUED

DIAPHRAGM AND CERVICAL CAP

The diaphragm, a dome of rubber with a coiled metal spring in its rim, is made in different sizes, depending on a woman's internal shape and size. It fits diagonally across the vagina and is used with a spermicidal agent; it must be left in place for six hours after intercourse.

The cervical cap is smaller and more rigid and fits over the cervix, where it is held in place by suction. Like the diaphragm, it must be fitted to size and used in conjunction with a spermicide. The diaphragm and cap work by preventing sperm reaching the cervix. They must be refitted regularly, because of childbirth or weight gain or loss.

CONTRACEPTIVE SPONGE

This is an old form of contraception now updated with contemporary materials. These days it is usually made of polyurethane foam and is impregnated with spermicide. The sponge is moistened with water to activate the spermicide and left in place for six hours after intercourse.

SPERMICIDES

The use of a spermicide is essential with these barrier methods to ensure their effectiveness. Spermicides are not effective on their own as they must be at the cervix, not just somewhere in the vagina. They come in many forms, including aerosols, pessaries, foams, film and creams. Some need to be inserted 15 minutes before intercourse, and a spermicide should not be washed away for at least six hours afterwards. Spermicides seem to be an added protection against contracting sexually transmitted diseases.

HORMONAL METHODS

These methods use hormones to suppress ovulation. They interfere with the cervical mucus, making it thick and impenetrable to sperm, and thin the uterine lining so that conception cannot occur. Forms include the combined pill, the low-dose mini-pill, hormonal injections and implants. The post-coital pill also contains hormones.

The *combined pill* uses synthetic progestogen and oestrogen to suppress ovulation. It must be taken for the full course of either 21 or 28 days to be effective. The *low-dose mini-pill* contains progestogen only. It is slightly less reliable because ovulation may occur. Oestrogen is implicated in some of the side-effects of the combined pill because of its effect on the circulatory system.

Injectable contraceptives contain only progestogens and are administered every two or three months. They are ideal for women who have difficulty remembering to take the pill regularly. *Implants* are also available, usually inserted under the skin of the upper arm, remaining active for five years. Both these methods are relatively free from side-effects. The return to fertility can sometimes be slow after an injectable contraceptive, but is usually quite soon after an implant is removed. There may be some breakthrough bleeding.

HORMONAL CONTRACEPTION

Advantages
- The most effective method
- Regulates menstruation and reduces pain and bleeding
- Reduces the effects of PMT
- Reduces the incidence of benign cysts and ovarian cancers, and protects against brittle bones (osteoporosis)

Disadvantages
- Slightly increased risk of thrombosis in women using this method
- Occasional breakthrough bleeding with some forms
- It requires motivation to take the mini-pill at the same time every day

POST-COITAL METHODS

There are two means of preventing conception after unprotected sex and they must be started within 1–5 days after intercourse, but they are not recommended as a routine form of birth control.

The hormonal method involves a short high-dose course of the combined pill. It is not entirely clear how this method works in preventing pregnancy. For women who cannot take the high-dose pill, a copper-bearing IUD can be inserted within five days of unprotected intercourse; this prevents a possible pregnancy.

WHAT ARE THE RISKS?

A pill containing oestrogen may not be suitable for you if you are overweight; if you smoke; are over 35; suffer from diabetes, high blood pressure, a heart condition, deep-vein thrombosis or migraine.

INTRAUTERINE DEVICE

This is a plastic or copper-containing device inserted into the uterus and left there. It probably works by slowing the sperm passing through the womb or by preventing the fertilized egg from

INTRAUTERINE DEVICES

Advantages
• One of the most reliable methods (second only to hormonal contraception)
• No need to remember to take pills every day
• Do not interfere with ovulation or breastfeeding

Disadvantages
• Can be expelled without the wearer being aware of it
• Copper-containing devices are known to cause occasional complications in some women
• May increase pain and bleeding during menstruation

implanting in the uterine lining. An IUD is immediately effective in preventing pregnancy and does not interfere with breastfeeding or your natural hormonal balance. There are many different shapes and sizes of IUDs. Most have a tail for easy removal and as a quick check that they are still in place.

PROGESTERONE INTRAUTERINE DEVICE

The progesterone IUD is similar to other IUDs in that it sits in the uterus. However, because it contains a progesterone hormone it actively prevents the lining of the uterus from increasing in thickness and causes the mucus in the cervix to remain thick. It also acts as a physical barrier to conception by being present in the uterus. In some women it will also suppress ovulation. Overall, it is an excellent contraceptive, lasting for a minimum of three years.

RISKS AND DISADVANTAGES

IUDs are not suitable for young women who have not had children. IUDs have been implicated in cases of perforation of the uterus, septic abortion, **pelvic inflammatory disease** and **ectopic pregnancy**. They may increase bleeding and pain during menstruation, so they are not suitable for women with heavy periods. Expulsion of the devices is not uncommon and they are painful to insert in some cases.

Disadvantages of the progesterone IUD include possible risk of **ovarian cysts** and a shorter lifespan than some of the other copper-containing IUDs.

SEE ALSO:
Ectopic Pregnancy
Fertility and Conception
Menstruation
Ovarian Cysts
Pelvic Inflammatory Disease

MENOPAUSE

Strictly speaking, menopause is your last menstrual period, but you only become aware of this in retrospect, when you've not had a period for a year. The average age of the menopause in this country is 51, although it is not unusual to experience it during your early 40s or mid-50s.

STAGES OF THE MENOPAUSE

The menopause is also known as the "climacteric". It encompasses three distinct stages: *premenopause,* the beginning of the climacteric (usually the early 40s) when periods may become heavy or irregular; *perimenopause,* the stage (usually a few years) on either side of your last period when physical symptoms such as hot flushes begin and periods become more irregular; and *postmenopause,* which encompasses the rest of your life, after your periods stop.

CAN I PREDICT MY MENOPAUSE?

Most periods stop gradually. A few years before the menopause, they may become irregular: you have them for several months then skip a month or two, then start again, with the interval between periods becoming longer and longer until eventually they stop completely. If you are over 50 and have not had a period for over six months, you have probably reached the menopause.

There is no way that you can predict when your last period will be. The age when you first menstruated could be significant, and the earlier you start, the later you finish. The age at which your mother experienced menopause may also affect when you have yours, although this is difficult to prove. Whether you took the oral contraceptive pill and the age at which you had your first and last child do *not* affect the timing.

It seems most likely that each one of us has our own inbuilt biological clock that dictates both when we start to menstruate and when we stop, although a variety of physical factors including diet, smoking and obesity can either slow the clock down or speed it up.

PREMATURE MENOPAUSE

A premature natural menopause is a menopause that occurs before the age of 35. It is very rare – it affects less than one percent of women.

Surgical removal of the ovaries (oophorectomy) is the most common cause of premature menopause and is carried out for a variety of reasons, such as a ruptured **ectopic pregnancy** or **ovarian cancer**. It is usually done as part of a total **hysterectomy**, which entails removal of both the ovaries, the Fallopian tubes and the uterus. Other factors that can cause an artificial menopause include radiation therapy (for stomach and pelvic cancers and, rarely, mumps).

For both natural and artificial early menopause, hormone replacement therapy is given immediately to offset possible problems arising from the earlier-than-usual loss of oestrogen.

LATE MENOPAUSE

Anyone still menstruating after the age of 55 is considered to have a late menopause. Late menopause can have health consequences, too, since your body is exposed to oestrogen for longer than normal, which, theoretically, carries a slightly increased risk of uterine and breast cancer. You can protect yourself against this risk by making sure that you receive regular mammograms and pelvic examinations.

WHAT HAPPENS DURING THE CLIMACTERIC?

Many women experience the symptoms of oestrogen deficiency during the time that menstruation begins to decline. Periods become less and less frequent and then menstruation finally stops. Old-fashioned phrases like the "change of life" imply that

SYMPTOMS

Non-physical symptoms include:
- *Depression*
- *Irritability*
- *Tearfulness and inability to cope*
- *Loss of libido*
- *Insomnia*

Physical symptoms include:
- *Hot flushes*
- *Night sweats*
- *Itchiness of the perineum – vaginitis*
- *Pain during intercourse*
- *Fatigue and lack of energy*
- *Aches and pains as a result of softening bones*

the menopause means an unavoidable decline in life. This is not so. In fact, most women find that life improves.

WHAT CAUSES MENOPAUSAL SYMPTOMS?

The decline in monthly periods is only a symptom of a parallel decline in the production of female hormones, particularly oestrogen, by your body. What started at puberty with a first period and a change in your physical shape, now wanes as ovarian activity falls off and you fail to ovulate. Nearly all the symptoms of the menopause can be explained by these decreasing levels of oestrogen in your blood.

SHOULD I SEE THE DOCTOR?

Three out of four menopausal women have symptoms that are worth treating and that should be treated. Don't grin and bear it. Decide to have the menopause you want, and seek medical advice and treatment. Don't ignore self-help remedies, there are lots to try (see overleaf).

By far the most common menopausal symptoms are hot flushes, night sweats and vaginal dryness; these can lead to other symptoms, such as insomnia and reduced sexual desire.

However, if any of the symptoms trouble you, make sure that you see your doctor right away. It is never normal to have frequent heavy or painful periods nor to pass blood clots during the menopause, so do consult your doctor if you experience these symptoms.

WHAT WILL THE DOCTOR DO?

By far the majority of women manage to cope with the menopause reasonably easily. Because of the unsympathetic attitude of some male doctors, however, many women view it as something to be suffered and not worth treating. This is not so. Hormone replacement therapy can replace the oestrogen deficiency so that the symptoms disappear. HRT is more than 90 percent effective. If you feel your doctor isn't being very helpful or sympathetic, or won't let you try hormone replacement therapy, go to another doctor.

HORMONE REPLACEMENT

Hormone replacement therapy (HRT) is the most effective way to relieve menopausal symptoms. It works essentially by replacing the hormones that the body loses: oestrogen and progesterone.

HRT is available as tablets, patches, implants and creams or pessaries. The first three are usually prescribed in a combined oestrogen-progestogen (a synthetic form of progesterone) form, and all women who take them will have a monthly bleed when the progestogen phase of the course stops. Women who have had a total hysterectomy will be prescribed oestrogen-only HRT.

Tablets are taken every day; skin patches need to be changed every three or four days, while implants are inserted by your doctor and need to be renewed every six months. Vaginal creams or pessaries only have a local effect and will not alleviate problems such as hot flushes and brittle bones.

MENOPAUSE: CONTINUED

With the end of the protective effects of female hormones, women are at equal risk with men from heart disease. Plenty of exercise and a low-fat diet with healthy combinations of foods will help to keep this problem at bay. Some emotional problems cannot be treated with hormone therapy alone and your doctor may prescribe tranquillizers and counselling to get you through the roughest patch.

ARE THERE NATURAL REMEDIES?

You don't always have to rely on medical doctors. Complementary therapies, such as homeopathy, aromatherapy, herbalism, yoga and massage, all offer treatments for menopausal symptoms.

Homeopathic remedies

Many women consult homeopathic practitioners to relieve menopausal symptoms. Remedies – administered in minute doses – include *Lachesia* for hot flushes; *Pulsatilla* for insomnia, premenstrual syndrome and joint pain; *Sepia* for dry vagina, thinning hair and prolapse; *Sulphur* for itchy vulva and skin; *Bryonia* for PMS and breast pain; and *Belladonna* for night sweats.

Aromatherapy remedies

Essential oils from certain flowers and plants are also believed to relieve symptoms. Oils from cypress, geranium and rose are recommended for heavy periods; avocado and wheatgerm for dry skin; juniper, lavender and rosemary for muscle and joint pain; lavender and peppermint for headaches; basil for fatigue; neroli and lavender for insomnia; lemon grass for premenstrual syndrome; and clary sage and rose for depression.

Guidelines for taking herbs

If you're interested in herbal remedies, consult a trained herbalist, but also bear the following points in mind:

- Always use herbs in moderation.
- Stop using them if you experience any side-effects.
- Assess each herb's efficacy over a week or so.
- Start by taking a herb in tea form. Increase the amount from half a cup a day to several cups over a period of a week.
- If you're taking medication, check with your doctor before taking a herbal remedy.
- Don't defer seeking medical advice because you are taking a herbal remedy.

WHAT CAN I DO?

A good diet is as important in maintaining health during and after the menopause as at any other time of your life. In particular, calcium levels and vitamin D need to be kept up after the menopause to avoid thinning and softening of the bones – a condition that can lead to osteoporosis.

Never view yourself as over the hill. Keep up your self-respect and self-assurance with your work, or retrain or get involved in voluntary activities. This is often the time in your life when your children leave home, adding extra stress when you may be least capable of coping with it.

On the other hand, many women experience a new lease of life once they are freed of reproductive responsibilities. We hear all the time about women who really come into their own in middle age. Those women who have a positive view of the menopause suffer fewer symptoms less seriously. Remember that it marks the end of one phase of your life and the beginning of another. It should not be a time for sadness and regret; in fact, it should be a time for looking forward to enjoying new interests and experiences.

SEE ALSO:
Cervical Smear
Ectopic Pregnancy
Hysterectomy
Ovarian Cancer

2

GENITAL PROBLEMS

Just because a woman's genitalia are less exposed

than a man's does not mean that they are

necessarily better protected. Problems can and

do occur from minor ailments, such as pruritis

vulvae or thrush, to much more serious diseases,

such as cervical cancer. These conditions and the other

common problems that can affect this area of the

body are described in detail in the pages that follow,

with the emphasis on self-help where possible;

practical advice is also given about seeking medical

assistance, when this is more appropriate.

PRURITIS VULVAE

Pruritis vulvae is the name given to an intense itching around the genital organs and rectum, when no obvious cause can be found. The itch often leads to scratching to relieve the irritation, and the cycle becomes difficult to break. If you end up scratching repeatedly for several days, the condition may become chronic, causing a thickening of the vulval skin.

There are no dangers directly associated with pruritis vulvae itself, but if white patches of abnormal skin (leukoplakia) develop in the irritated area, there is a slightly increased risk of developing cancer of the vulva.

SYMPTOMS

- *Intense itchiness of the vulva*
- *Urgent need to scratch*
- *Sensitive skin in the vulval area*
- *Dryness and scaling*
- *Scalding and burning when passing urine – scratching causes minute tears, and urine irritates these abrasions*

WHAT CAUSES IT?

The most common cause of pruritis vulvae is an increasing or decreasing supply of the female hormones, oestrogen and progesterone. For this reason, pregnant women and young girls approaching puberty, both of whom have increasing levels, are susceptible, while in older women, it is a direct consequence of the menopause, where the supply of hormones decreases.

Other possible causes include diabetes, and an allergy to talcum powder, vaginal deodorants or to nylon tights.

If none of these factors apply, the reason for the itching could be emotional – anxiety about a sexual involvement, perhaps, or even a lack of confidence in relationships.

When the itching is accompanied by a thick discharge, the cause could be a vaginal infection such as **thrush**.

SHOULD I SEE THE DOCTOR?

If the itching persists and you are unable to resist scratching, see your doctor as soon as possible. If you try the self-help measures suggested below, and there is no improvement in a week or so, see your doctor.

WHAT WILL THE DOCTOR DO?

- For any skin symptoms, your doctor may suggest a course of antihistamine pills to reduce the itching sensation, and a mild sleeping pill, particularly if the itchiness is more severe during the night and causes bouts of insomnia.
- Your doctor may recommend a steroid or hormone cream to be applied to the affected area to relieve irritation.
- If you are over 45, your doctor may suggest that you have some form of HRT, such as oestrogen pessaries or creams, to alleviate the problem.

WHAT CAN I DO?

- If the genital area is dry, use an emollient cream to keep the skin well lubricated.
- Cut down on soap when washing the area, and avoid hot baths; these overheat the skin, which sets up the itchiness. Have a shower instead.
- Avoid possible irritants, such as scented soaps, douches, talcum powder, vaginal deodorants and bath oils, and wear pants made from cotton or natural fibres. Wash with warm water after passing urine.
- Use a lubricant, such as a water-soluble jelly, during sex.
- Never put antiseptics in the bath water.

SEE ALSO:
Menopause
Painful Intercourse
Thrush
Vaginal Discharge

VAGINAL DISCHARGE

The vagina is kept clean and moist by secretions (discharge) from its lining, and in menstruating women they change their character during each monthly cycle due to the influence of fluctuating hormones. In the first half of the cycle, under the influence of oestrogen, the vaginal discharge is clear, thin and stretchy. After ovulation, it becomes thick, opaque and rubbery. This change denotes ovulation.

The hormonal changes that occur during pregnancy also affect your discharge and it becomes thick and white.

The amount of vaginal secretions increases with sexual excitement to lubricate the vagina in preparation for sexual intercourse.

Abnormal vaginal discharge is different in colour, consistency and smell from normal discharge and there may be other symptoms, such as soreness and itching. In general terms, any symptoms that accompany abnormal vaginal discharge, such as burning, a rash and bleeding, should be investigated as soon as possible.

If you cannot make a diagnosis from the information given below, see your doctor.

NATURE OF THE DISCHARGE	PROBABLE CAUSE
There is an increase in your normal secretions	You may be pregnant, have just started taking the contraceptive pill or have recently had an IUD fitted. This is normal and nothing to worry about (see **Contraception**).
It is thick and white and your vulva is itchy	This could be **thrush**, a fungal infection of the vagina. Thrush is more common during pregnancy and if you are taking antibiotic medication for any reason.
The discharge is greenish/yellow and has an unpleasant smell	This could be **trichomoniasis**, or perhaps you have forgotten to remove a tampon or your diaphragm.
You notice a slight discharge, and your sexual partner has sores on his genitals	This could be a cervical infection, possibly due to a sexually transmitted disease such as **gonorrhoea.**
The discharge is brown, like blood, and usually follows intercourse	This is probably cervical erosion; see your doctor.
The discharge is spotted with blood, either mid-period or following intercourse	This could be a polyp on the cervix; see your doctor.

THRUSH

This is a common infection caused by a fungus, *Candida albicans,* that lives in the digestive tract and is generally kept under control by other bacteria.

If thrush appears in the mouth it is known as oral thrush. If you attempt to wipe away the creamy-yellow or white patches in the mouth, red sore patches are left.

The presence of *Candida albicans* in the vagina often causes a thick "cottage cheese" discharge and itchiness. It is referred to as a vaginal yeast infection.

SYMPTOMS

- *For vaginal thrush, a thick white curdy discharge with soreness and irritation of the vulva*
- *Red rash around the anus which can extend down to the thighs*
- *Urine may burn or irritate the area*
- *Pain during sexual intercourse*
- *For oral thrush, creamy-yellow or white patches inside the mouth that adhere to the mucous membrane*

WHAT CAUSES IT?

For thrush to infect a woman, the conditions in her vagina need to be unbalanced, as the vagina is usually too acid for thrush to thrive. But in some circumstances the acid levels may be lowered; for example, vaginal deodorants can destroy the natural bacteria that prevent the overgrowth of the fungus. A course of antibiotics also alters the natural balance; resistance is low after illness anyway. Diabetics are often affected as are women with altered hormonal levels (during pregnancy and premenstrually) and women who are on the contraceptive pill.

SHOULD I SEE THE DOCTOR?

See your doctor immediately after you notice the symptoms of thrush, and refrain from sexual intercourse until you have received treatment.

WHAT WILL THE DOCTOR DO?

- Your doctor may take a swab of discharge to check that the initial diagnosis is accurate and what treatment is appropriate.
- In most cases of vaginal thrush, he will prescribe antifungal pessaries and soothing ointment, such as clotrimazole (Canestan), immediately to give you relief from the symptoms. Treatment can take from a day to two weeks. He will also recommend similar treatment for your partner or partners, to prevent reinfection.

WHAT CAN I DO?

- Take the complete course of treatment and return to your doctor if the infection recurs.
- Try not to scratch because the fungus can be spread by hand. Constant scratching will also cause toughening of the skin.
- Some women gain short-term relief by applying natural yoghurt to the genital area. Leave it for at least two hours – you can insert it on a tampon to prevent it from leaking out.
- Don't apply anything containing a local anaesthetic. It may bring instant relief but it may cause a local allergy too.
- The thrush fungus likes warm, moist conditions, so folds of fat around your groin may be a reason for recurrent vaginal thrush. You may be able to reduce this recurrence by losing weight.
- Always wipe your anus from the front to the back to prevent infection from stools entering your vagina.
- Wear natural fibres – cotton or silk – next to your genital area. Avoid nylon tights and panties as they don't "breathe" and they give the fungus warm conditions for growth.

SEE ALSO:
Painful Intercourse
Pruritis Vulvae
Trichomoniasis
Vaginal Discharge

TRICHOMONIASIS

Trichomoniasis is an infection caused by a very small one-celled organism (*Trichomonas vaginalis*), which affects the vagina, cervix, urethra and bladder. The symptoms are similar to those of **thrush**, except that the discharge is green and has an offensive smell. It is contagious, and is usually transmitted sexually, although it can occasionally be caught indirectly from items such as damp towels. The most common time of infection is just after a menstrual period.

SYMPTOMS

- *Offensive-smelling, yellowish-green, bubbly vaginal discharge*
- *Itching of the vagina and perineum (the area between the legs behind the genitals and in front of the anus)*
- *Burning sensation when urine is passed*
- *Symptoms of cystitis if the bladder is affected*

SHOULD I SEE THE DOCTOR?

If you suspect you may be infected, see your doctor as soon as possible for an accurate diagnosis, and refrain from sexual inter-course until you are given the all-clear. Let your partner know as soon as possible that you may have a sexually transmitted infection and that treatment might be necessary for him too.

WHAT WILL THE DOCTOR DO?

- Your doctor will probably take a swab of the discharge for laboratory analysis. This is important because the drugs used to cure trichomoniasis are strong and should not be overprescribed, and also because some other sexually transmitted disease may be diagnosed too. Give your doctor full details of your medical history.
- Normal treatment is by antibacterial drugs of the metronidazole family, such as Flagyl. These drugs can sometimes produce side-effects, such as nausea and abdominal pain, and they should not be taken by pregnant or breastfeeding women. A normal course of antibacterial drug treatment will last between five and ten days.

WHAT CAN I DO?

- Take the full course of pills as prescribed and do not take alcohol while you are taking them. If a second course is necessary, you should have a blood count first to check that your blood is normal.
- As with other vaginal infections, practise good hygiene and avoid vaginal deodorants, douches and tampons.
- Wear natural fibres, such as cotton or silk, next to your skin.
- Don't have sexual intercourse until you are clear of the infection.
- Provide the names and addresses of your sexual partners so that they can be identified and have treatment too.

SEE ALSO:
Cystitis
Sexually Transmitted Diseases
Thrush

CERVICAL CANCER

Cancer of the cervix is the second most common female cancer (breast cancer is the first). It is becoming more common, particularly among young women.

Each year about one-quarter of women with cervical cancer die, despite the fact that precancerous changes can be detected by regular smear tests and treated. As the condition has no early symptoms it can only be detected by routine **cervical smear** screening. Women's groups and concerned medical practitioners constantly lobby politicians, both to improve the screening facilities available and to co-ordinate a more efficient call-up system to catch those women who are most at risk because they don't have regular smear tests.

Cervical cancer has a pre-invasive stage during which time it may grow but not spread. As this pre-invasive stage may last for several years, any woman who has regular smear tests should be identified early enough for the cancer to be totally removed by simply taking out the tissue from the cervix.

SYMPTOMS

- *In its early precancerous stages (CIN I and II), there are no symptoms*
- *By CIN III or Stage 1, ulceration of the cervix can be seen on vaginal examination using a speculum*
- *By stage 1 or 2, inter-menstrual bleeding, spotting after intercourse or after the menopause*
- *Offensive vaginal discharge*

WHAT CAUSES IT?

It is thought that sexual activity plays a part in causing cancer of the cervix because the lining cells of the cervix are vulnerable in adolescence. Frequent intercourse during this time, especially with several different partners, may initiate the cancer process.

The inference is that there is a carcinogenic component in seminal fluid. This may account for the higher incidence of cancer among young women, as sexual intercourse is occurring earlier in women's lives. This is backed up by looking at certain religious groups such as Orthodox Jewish and Moslem women. Cervical cancer is much rarer among these women, probably because their men are circumcised and extramarital intercourse is less common. Women whose mothers took DES (a drug to prevent recurrent miscarriages) in pregnancy are among others with a particularly high risk.

WHAT IS THE MEDICAL TREATMENT?

- All stages of CIN (cervical intrapithelial neoplasia) should be treated, although some doctors adopt a "wait and see" approach, involving repeat smear tests for early CIN and changes thought to be due to infection with **genital warts**.
- Treatment of CIN involves performing a **colposcopy** usually in the outpatient department, when the cervix is viewed with a special microscope. Areas with abnormal cells may be identified and, if necessary, a biopsy may be taken to examine the tissue.
- Following a colposcopy a woman will either be reassured and a follow-up smear arranged, or treated further.

WHAT IS THE SURGICAL TREATMENT?

- Surgical treatment of CIN involves removing the precancerous tissue under a local anaesthetic with a laser, or freezing or burning away the tissue with an electric current (LLETZ – large loop excision of the transformation zone).
- Occasionally, a general anaesthetic is required for a **cone biopsy**. This may be done with a scalpel or a laser beam. After the tissue is examined microscopically, doctors decide if you require any further treatment.

• The treatment of full-blown cancer of the cervix depends on the stage that the disease is at. Treatment may involve either surgery or radiotherapy, or both. As a general rule, however, radiotherapy is more often used for older women and surgery for younger, fitter patients, irrespective of the stage of the disease.

• Surgery involves removing affected tissue. A radical (Wertheim's) **hysterectomy** is most often performed. This involves removing the uterus and the surrounding tissue, including some lymph nodes.

• If retaining your fertility is important, trachylectomy, or removal of the cervix, may be performed, though this is rare.

• If there is a recurrence of the cancer following radiotherapy, major surgery involving removal of the bladder or bowel may be necessary.

HOW IS RADIOTHERAPHY USED?

Nearly half the cases of cervical cancer are treated with radiotherapy. The aim is to give a fatal dose of radiation to the centre of

STAGES OF CERVICAL PRECANCER AND CANCER

For precancer
• The mildest stage, known as mild dysplasia or CIN I
• More severe inflammation called moderate dysplasia or CIN II
• Severe dysplasia, with or without non-invasive carcinoma in situ, or CIN III

For cancer
• Stage 1: Cancer confined to the cervix
• Stage 2: Cancer extends beyond the cervix to involve the upper third of the vagina and/or lateral tissue immediately surrounding the cervix
• Stage 3: Cancer extends to the lower third of the vagina and/or pelvic side wall
• Stage 4: Cancer extends beyond the pelvis and/or involves the bladder or rectum

the cancer. Radiation also kills those parts of the growth that were invading other areas. It is very interesting to note that comparing women who had radiotherapy with those who had radical surgery, after five years the survival rate was about the same, so it's worth discussing the options fully with your doctor.

WHAT CAN I DO?

• You will be required to have regular checks over the next five years or so to make sure the cancer spread has been stopped.

• You will almost certainly not be able to have any more children and, if you had your ovaries removed, you will go through a premature menopause. If this causes you to suffer unpleasant symptoms, see your doctor for treatment.

• If you maintain regular appointments for smear tests, any cancer will be caught at a time when chances of a cure are high. Even if cancerous cells are found, you should take an interest in the disease and co-operate with your medical advisers as much as possible to fight it. Cancer cures do depend to a certain extent on the determination of the sufferer to beat the disease.

SEE ALSO:
Cervical Smear
Colposcopy
Cone Biopsy
Genital Warts
Hysterectomy
Sexually Transmitted Diseases

CYSTITIS

Cystitis is an inflammation of the bladder, which may be the result of an infection or bruising after athletic sex.

The most common symptom is a frequent urge to urinate, with only a small flow occurring each time; this is nearly always accompanied by severe pain, which worsens when urination is completed. Other symptoms that may occur include smelly or blood-stained urine, fever, occasional chills and lower abdominal pain.

Many of the symptoms of cystitis can apply to unrelated problems and other vaginal diseases. For instance, a strong yellow- to orange-coloured urine, even one with a strong smell, is not necessarily indicative of cystitis, or indeed any other infection. It is just as likely to be a symptom of dehydration, either due to vomiting or sweating profusely, or simply because you have not drunk enough fluid. Occasionally, food such as asparagus, if eaten in large quantities, can also cause urine to change colour.

Cystitis is very common, annoying and inconvenient, but it does not endanger general health. Most women have it at some time in their lives. It is particularly common during pregnancy: in the first few months, when the urethra relaxes under the influence of the hormone progesterone, and infections spread more easily, and later on when the pressure of the enlarging uterus may cause a small amount of urine to remain in the bladder after urination. This becomes stagnant and the lack of flow may encourage bacteria to multiply, which results in cystitis.

WHAT CAUSES IT?

The commonest infecting organism is *E.coli,* a bacterium that normally lives in the bowel and around the anus and only causes problems when it spreads up the urethra into the bladder. Women are more prone to cystitis than men because their urethra is shorter than that of men.

The type of cystitis known as "honeymoon cystitis" is caused by unusual amounts of frequent, strenuous sexual intercourse, which can cause bruising of the urethra.

Occasionally, infection can be caused by the use of antiseptics in bath water, or by the over-zealous use of vaginal deodorants or douches.

As women get older and reach the menopause, a shortage of oestrogen and progesterone can lead to the thinning of all genital organs and the perineum (the area between the genitals and the anus), and in some unexplained way this can contribute to a menopausal type of cystitis. **Prolapse** of the front of the vaginal wall may also be a cause because of poor urinary flow and stagnating urine.

If a woman needs an indwelling catheter, as she might after an operation or if she suffers from incontinence due to a disease such as multiple sclerosis, for example, then an infection may occur. This rarely happens, however, as long as the catheter is inserted and removed correctly using a sterile technique.

SYMPTOMS

- *The urgent need to pass urine frequently though only a small amount may be passed each time*
- *A severe dragging-down pain, usually in the front of the abdomen but quite often radiating up the flanks and to the back*
- *A burning or stinging sensation while passing urine*
- *A severe pain on passing urine*
- *The passage of blood in the urine which may be pink, red or simply streaked with blood*
- *The urge to get up several times in the night to empty your bladder even though there may be very little urine present*

Contrary to popular belief, dirty toilet habits do not *per se* cause cystitis, although you should always wipe yourself from the front to the back.

SHOULD I SEE THE DOCTOR?

If the self-help measures listed below don't bring relief, seek help from your doctor as soon as possible.

WHAT WILL THE DOCTOR DO?

• Your doctor may take a urine specimen to confirm which bacterium is causing your symptoms so that he can gauge its sensitivity to a range of antibiotic drugs, the normal treatment for cystitis.

• As soon as the specimen has been analyzed, he can start you on a course of antibiotics, usually a penicillin derivative. It's absolutely essential that you take the full course of treatment even if your symptoms subside completely within 24 hours (they often do; some sufferers report complete relief after about only two hours). If you do not do so, the infecting organisms may become resistant to antibiotics and your cystitis can become chronic. If this happens, it can be exceedingly difficult to eradicate.

• If your cystitis does not respond to treatment, your doctor may recommend a full hospital investigation to see whether or not there is any predisposing internal cause.

• If investigation shows no trace of a bacterium, you may be suffering from an irritable bladder, which is often caused by emotional factors.

WHAT CAN I DO?

• Drink plenty of fluids at the first sign of the symptoms. It's important to get urine flowing fast to flush out the bladder, so try to drink the equivalent of a glass of water every half hour.

• Make your urine alkaline by adding a little bicarbonate of soda to your drinks. You will find that alkalinizing your urine eases bladder pain quite considerably.

• For pain relief, take paracetamol every four hours. A warm pad or wrapped-up hot water bottle on the front of the abdomen may also help.

• Drink cranberry juice, which is a urinary antiseptic.

TO PREVENT A RECURRENCE

• Drink plenty of water at all times.

• At the first symptom, increase your water intake and alkalinize your urine by adding a little bicarbonate of soda to your drinks. (Don't continue this for too long; you could have unpleasant side-effects, such as wind.)

• If you are having sex frequently, "cover" it by drinking a lot of fluid and keeping the urine flowing. Pass urine before and after sexual intercourse.

• Use tampons instead of sanitary towels as they are less likely to allow the bacteria to thrive; some women find, however, that tampons irritate the bladder further.

• If you suspect that wearing a diaphragm is a contributory cause, ask about another form of contraception.

• Wear cotton panties or cotton liners.

• Don't use antiseptics in the bath water, and don't use vaginal douches or deodorants.

• Don't be obsessive about washing your perineum with soap and water. Using a bidet after moving your bowels is a good idea so that you avoid contamination of the vagina and urethra from the rectum.

• Depending on the drugs prescribed by your doctor, you can help them be more effective by adjusting the acidity or alkalinity of your urine. Ask your doctor what your antibiotic is. For example, tetracycline will be more effective if your urine is acidic, so drink plenty of cranberry juice while you are taking it.

PROLAPSE

Another name for prolapse is "pelvic relaxation". Vaginal wall prolapse occurs when the pelvic muscles become weakened and allow one or several pelvic organs to drop down the vagina. Pelvic organs, including the bladder, rectum and urethra, can prolapse into the vagina, but the most commonly affected organ is the uterus. The vaginal wall is pushed down by the unsupported and descending uterus and, depending on the severity, the cervix may protrude from the vulva.

If the rectum bulges into the back of the vaginal wall, it is called a *rectocele*; when the urethra bulges into the front of the vaginal wall this is known as a *urethrocele*; while if the bladder drops into the front of the vaginal wall, it is called a *cystocele*.

Prolapse tends to occur in older women, and is much more common in those who have had children.

WHAT CAUSES IT?

Pelvic floor muscles can weaken with age, but prolapse is nearly always caused by earlier injury to the pelvic floor muscles, cervix or supporting tissue of the uterus during labour, especially if you had a rapid delivery, were allowed to go on too long in labour or if your babies were large.

SYMPTOMS

- *Severe backache*
- *Intense pain during sexual intercourse or inability to achieve orgasm if the vagina is slack*
- *Stress incontinence*
- *For uterine prolapse, a dragging down feeling in the pelvis*
- *For urethrocele, frequency of urination*
- *For cystocele, frequency of urination and cystitis-type symptoms of pain and burning when passing urine*
- *For rectocele, discomfort on moving the bowels, difficulty in defecating*

SHOULD I SEE THE DOCTOR?

If your prolapse is accompanied by severe backache or pelvic discomfort, you should consult your doctor as soon as possible.

WHAT WILL THE DOCTOR DO?

- Your doctor will give you an internal pelvic examination to confirm a prolapse and to determine which type you have.
- He or she will ask you about your deliveries, for example if your babies were larger than normal, and if the second stage of labour lasted a long time.
- Being overweight can cause the prolapse to be more troublesome, so your doctor will advise you to lose excess weight.
- If you have a severe prolapse, your doctor may recommend surgery. This is rarely absolutely necessary, but will improve your quality of life by maintaining urinary continence and improving sexual enjoyment.
- For mild prolapse a doctor will recommend pelvic floor exercises (see opposite). For older women who are too frail for surgery, there are vaginal rings to help support the vaginal walls or uterus. You may be fitted with a ring or sponge pessary that is placed high in the vagina; these, however, can erode internal tissues so should not be worn for long periods.

SURGICAL TREATMENT

- Surgery is carried out to improve a woman's quality of life. If there are any reasons why surgery may not be a good idea, for example due to extreme frailty, it is best avoided and non-surgical methods employed to control the symptoms. Very rarely an anterior repair may result in urinary incontinence, and a posterior repair may sometimes result in uncomfortable or painful intercourse.
- Most prolapse repairs are performed through the vagina and involve a general anaesthetic. Occasionally the operation may be performed under an epidural anaesthetic,

PELVIC FLOOR MUSCLES

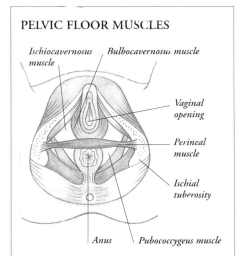

Ischiocavernosus muscle
Bulbocavernosus muscle
Vaginal opening
Perineal muscle
Ischial tuberosity
Anus
Pubococcygeus muscle

Pelvic floor muscles
Supporting the bowel, bladder and uterus, these muscles can become stretched during pregnancy owing to the weight of the fetus.

PELVIC FLOOR EXERCISES

You should do this routine at least five or six times a day. If you find it difficult to set aside time specifically for it, then do it when urinating. If you are pregnant, you should only do these exercises as a test occasionally; it is not good practice to do them all the time.

- First, identify the muscles you are going to use. The easiest way to do this is to stop the flow of urine in midstream when you next empty your bladder.
- Now, draw up these muscles in the same way or as if you were holding a tampon in place, hold for a count of five – and relax.
- Repeat this process at least five times or as often as you can – more if you have just had a baby.
- After a while, you could repeat the process as above, but hold for a longer count before relaxing.

especially if the patient is old and infirm.

- The repair involves making an incision in the wall of the vagina and strengthening the tissues that have become weakened using buttressing sutures (stitches). Any excess or stretched tissue is removed from the vaginal walls and the incision is closed using stitches that are absorbed by the body.
- Following the operation, the vagina is packed with gauze, which remains in place for one or two days. A catheter is inserted into the bladder during the operation to help drain urine. It is common to have some discharge from the vagina for a few days following surgery.
- You will probably stay in hospital for five to seven days. An outpatient appointment is usually made six weeks later, after which sexual intercourse can be resumed if there are no problems.
- For difficult-to-treat or recurrent prolapse an abdominal operation is occasionally carried out to strengthen the walls of the vagina.

WHAT CAN I DO?

- If you suffer from backache, try to avoid standing for long periods at a time. Wear a tight girdle to counteract any dragging feeling you may have in your pelvis
- If you are having difficulty with sexual intercourse, you and your partner may need to explore alternative ways of achieving sexual pleasure.
- Wear panty liners if you are troubled by leakage of urine (stress incontinence). If the leakage becomes worse, see your doctor.
- The most important preventative treatment is being conscientious about doing pelvic floor exercises regularly during pregnancy and especially after the birth of your baby, whether you have stitches or not.

SEE ALSO:
Cystitis
Hysterectomy
Incontinence
Painful Intercourse

INCONTINENCE

Incontinence is the involuntary leakage of urine when you are unable to control your bladder. Many women suffer from occasional bouts of incontinence from their middle twenties onwards, particularly if they have borne children, and most older women suffer from it from time to time to a greater or lesser degree.

SYMPTOMS

- *Inability to control your bladder, particularly when you exert pressure on the abdominal muscles*
- *Frequency of urination, even when your bladder is not full*
- *Urgency, even when your bladder is not full*

WHAT CAUSES IT?

There are three major causes of incontinence in women. In the aftermath of pregnancy, the pelvic and perineal tissues can become so stretched that a **prolapse** of the vaginal wall occurs. If even a very small part of the urethra or bladder accompanies the prolapse, this nearly always leads to urinary symptoms of some kind or other, whether it is urgency, hesitancy, frequency and/or pain.

As a woman becomes older, the exit valve from the bladder can weaken slightly. (This is not uncommon during pregnancy, in fact, but goes away after the birth.)

Urine may also leak away when pressure inside the abdominal cavity is increased when, for example, we sneeze, cough, strain to open our bowels or lift a heavy weight. This is called stress incontinence.

If the muscles of the bladder wall become over-sensitive to the presence of urine in the bladder, they respond by contracting uncontrollably and trying to empty the bladder even when there are only small quantities of urine present. This is sometimes called irritable bladder.

SHOULD I SEE THE DOCTOR?

You should seek help as soon as the symptoms of incontinence appear. The earlier it is treated, the less likely it is that weaknesses will persist and the condition become chronic. Both stress incontinence and irritable bladder can be treated successfully.

WHAT WILL THE DOCTOR DO?

- Your doctor will take a midstream urine sample to check whether there is any urinary tract infection, such as **cystitis**, present. He may also refer you for a special X-ray of your bladder.
- He will advise you to strengthen your pelvic floor muscles by doing a series of exercises. Since obesity weakens the pelvic floor, if you are overweight you may be advised to consult a dietitian, or to exercise in order to reduce your weight.
- Recommended treatment for prolapse involves wearing a special ring or sponge in your vagina during the day.
- If treatment for stress incontinence fails to work, your doctor will advise you to have a surgical operation to tighten up your pelvic floor muscles.
- If you are suffering from an irritable bladder, he may encourage you to hold on to urine for as long as possible to strengthen the bladder muscles, or he may suggest a drug to relax them. If neither of these work, he may advise a surgical operation to stretch the urethra.

WHAT CAN I DO?

Try to practise pelvic floor exercises regularly to regain muscle, and therefore, bladder control.

SEE ALSO:
Cystitis
Prolapse

3

MENSTRUAL PROBLEMS

Menstruation is a normal part of a woman's life. Most women menstruate for well over 30 years, from their early teens to their late 40s or early 50s. Most of the time, periods occur in a regular pattern and are trouble-free, but many women experience complaints at some point. The most common disorders are painful periods (dysmenorrhoea) and premenstrual syndrome. Less common but potentially more serious conditions include vaginal bleeding between periods and amenorrhoea (no periods); all these and more are detailed here, with the accent on what can be done to cure or alleviate them.

PREMENSTRUAL SYNDROME

More widely known as PMS, this disorder affects about 75 percent of all women emotionally, mentally and physically in the days prior to menstruation. The most common symptoms are irritability, depression, tiredness and fluid retention.

SYMPTOMS

- *Fluid retention – with heavy breasts, thickened waistline, puffy face, hands and feet, causing headaches and pain especially in the breasts and abdomen*
- *Changes in mood – irritability, bad temper, tearfulness*
- *Depression, often leading to suicidal feelings and violence towards oneself and others*

WHAT CAUSES IT?

The exact cause is still not known but it is likely that the symptoms are in some way linked with falling levels of the female hormones, oestrogen and progesterone, in the days just prior to menstruation.

SHOULD I SEE THE DOCTOR?

If your symptoms are severe enough to disturb your normal life every month and self-help measures don't alleviate them, contact your doctor as soon as possible.

WHAT WILL THE DOCTOR DO?

- Your doctor will question you about the symptoms and possibly ask you to record them over several months.
- He may suggest progesterone therapy, probably in pessary or suppository form, on a trial basis. This can help some women, although there is no convincing evidence to suggest that all women would benefit from it. Treatment should start four days before you expect symptoms.
- If you suffer from fluid retention, he may offer you a diuretic drug. These are taken for about ten days before your period.

- Your doctor may offer antidepressant drugs or suggest that you take the oral contraceptive pill, both of which are known to help symptoms in some women.

WHAT CAN I DO?

- Keep a diary of when your symptoms occur so that you can start the treatment that works for you at the appropriate time.
- Eat little and often to keep your strength up and, if you are constipated, eat plenty of high fibre foods.
- If you are prescribed a diuretic, you will urinate much more often and possibly flush important minerals out of your system, so watch your diet by increasing your intake of foods rich in minerals such as potassium (fruit, seafood, nuts and beans) and by taking extra amounts of vitamins C and B, either in your diet or as supplements.
- To help prevent fluid retention, cut salt out of your diet as far as you can. Salt absorbs water and therefore increases the possibility of retention.
- Get plenty of rest to prevent exhaustion, and try to limit stressful situations if this is at all possible.
- Talk about your feelings to anyone who will listen, and make sure your close family knows to what extent you are affected.
- Try evening primrose oil, which has been shown to benefit some women.
- For pain such as that associated with **dysmenorrhoea**, try aspirin, which will inhibit prostaglandin production. Excessive prostaglandin is believed to be the cause of the contraction-like pains experienced during menstruation.
- Exercise, such as swimming and walking, deep breathing and relaxation techniques can all be helpful in bringing relief from tension and insomnia.

SEE ALSO:
Dysmenorrhoea

AMENORRHOEA

Amenorrhoea is the medical term for an absence of menstrual periods. It is described as *primary* if they have never started, and *secondary*, when normal menstruation is interrupted for four months or more. Amenorrhoea does not necessarily mean you are ill; it does usually mean that you are not producing eggs and so cannot conceive.

SYMPTOMS

- *For primary amenorrhoea, a failure to start menstruation and pubertal development – no development of sexual characteristics such as body hair, breasts and pelvic broadening*
- *For secondary amenorrhoea, periods stop suddenly or gradually cease with each successive month until the flow dries up*

WHAT CAUSES IT?

Primary amenorrhoea is usually due to late onset of puberty, although it can also be caused by a disorder of the reproductive or hormonal system. The commonest reason for secondary amenorrhoea is pregnancy. If the hormonal balance is interrupted for any other reason, however, periods may stop. So, for example, many women who breastfeed find that their periods do not start again until they wean their babies.

More seriously, amenorrhoea can be a side-effect of being grossly underweight, such as with anorexia nervosa. This will be suspected if your weight is as much as 12kg (26lbs) below average for your height and frame. Stress, chronic ailments such as thyroid disease, and long-term medication with drugs such as tranquillizers and anti-depressants can also cause amenorrhoea, as can excessive physical training.

Amenorrhoea is, of course, a permanent condition after the menopause, or if you undergo a **hysterectomy** with removal of your ovaries.

SHOULD I SEE THE DOCTOR?

The tendency to start menstruation late may be inherited, so if your mother started her periods late, don't worry if you aren't developing at the same rate as your friends. However, if you are 16 and have not yet menstruated, contact your doctor to check that there is no abnormality. If your periods suddenly stop, pregnancy could be the cause, so do a pregnancy test first before contacting him. See your doctor if your periods have been absent for six months and you are not pregnant or menopausal.

WHAT WILL THE DOCTOR DO?

- If you have never had a period, your doctor will probably give you a physical examination and take a blood sample to measure the level of pituitary hormones. (The pituitary hormones include those responsible for menstruation.)
- With secondary amenorrhoea, once pregnancy is excluded, you should receive a full medical examination by a specialist, and if you are taking any long-term medications, these should be checked and stopped if necessary.
- Your doctor may arrange for you to have an X-ray to make sure that your pituitary gland is healthy.
- If you are not ovulating, and not pregnant, he may suggest that you take a course of fertility drugs or pituitary hormones.

WHAT CAN I DO?

- The lack of periods is not dangerous and in most cases there is no cause for alarm; be patient and they will start up naturally.
- You may need to change your lifestyle to correct any dietary or physical problems, if these are the cause.

SEE ALSO:
Hysterectomy
Menopause

ABNORMAL BLEEDING

All women bleed from the vagina during menstruation. Any change in your normal cycle, however, or bleeding between periods should be treated with suspicion.

If you notice any bloody discharge during pregnancy, call your doctor, lie down and wait. The cause will depend on whether you are in early or late pregnancy.

If you are postmenopausal, and you know that your periods have definitely stopped, remember that vaginal bleeding is not normal unless you are taking combined oestrogen-progestogen HRT.

If you are unable to make a diagnosis from the information listed here, consult your doctor.

NATURE OF THE BLEEDING	PROBABLE CAUSE
Irregular bleeding, particularly if you are younger than 15 and older than 45	Irregular bleeding can be the result of hormonal changes. An occasional irregularity may not be cause for concern, but see your doctor if the cycle hasn't settled down after two months.
Your periods become unusually heavy	This is known as **menorrhagia**. You may suffer from anaemia if you lose a lot of blood every month. See your doctor.
Bleeding following intercourse	This could be cervical erosion. Make an appointment with your doctor for a **cervical smear** test.
Bleeding during pregnancy	This might be a **miscarriage**, or if there is severe abdominal pain, an **ectopic pregnancy**. Call the doctor immediately.
Bleeding is only spotting, and you're on the pill	This may be breakthrough bleeding. If it is bothersome, see your doctor; you may want to change your method of contraception.
Breakthrough bleeding after you have had an IUD fitted	See your doctor or go to the family planning clinic.
Excessive bleeding during the menopausal years	During the menopause, your periods may change in character, but if they are heavy, see your doctor immediately.

DYSMENORRHOEA

Dysmenorrhoea is the medical name for menstrual periods accompanied by cramps and pain. There are two different types: *primary*, which is painful periods experienced within three years of the onset of menstruation and in which there is no underlying disease to account for it; and *secondary*, which is a symptom of an underlying gynaecological disease such as **endometriosis** or **fibroids**.

SYMPTOMS

- *Violent abdominal cramps lasting up to three days*
- *Diarrhoea*
- *Frequency of urination*
- *Sweating*
- *Pelvic soreness with the pain radiating down into the upper thighs and into the back*
- *Abdominal distension*
- *Backache*
- *Nausea and vomiting*

WHAT CAUSES IT?

About a third of all menstruating women will experience some pain with their periods. Women who have primary dysmenorrhoea produce excessive quantities of the hormone prostaglandin at the time of menstruation and are extremely sensitive to it. Prostaglandin is one of the hormones released during labour and is in part responsible for the uterine contractions. Dysmenorrhoea can therefore be seen as a mini-labour with the prostaglandin causing uterine muscle to go into spasm, producing cramp-like pain.

SHOULD I SEE THE DOCTOR?

If you have recently begun to menstruate, visit your doctor if painkillers in moderate quantities are not sufficient to dull the pain and you need to spend at least a day in bed each month. If you have been menstruating for three years and the blood flow and pain increase, visit your doctor to confirm that there is no underlying disorder responsible.

WHAT WILL THE DOCTOR DO?

- Some doctors may imply that the pain is psychosomatic, but it isn't. Don't be put off from consulting your doctor by the hope that the pain will pass as you get older or if you have children.
- Insist on a trial of anti-prostaglandin drugs, which should be taken just prior to, and for the first two to three days of menstruation. The contraceptive pill is often prescribed to relieve dysmenorrhoea because it inhibits egg production and alters hormonal balance, and is a highly effective treatment. The progesterone IUD also helps dysmenorrhoea.
- If you have developed painful periods after several years of predictable menstrual characteristics, your doctor will examine you and recommend treatment according to the diagnosis.

WHAT CAN I DO?

- Experiment with herbal teas such as mint or camomile that reduce spasmodic pain.
- Relaxation or special yoga-type exercises can also help to relieve the pain; hot-water bottles, hot baths and bedrest can all bring relief.
- Non-steroidal anti-inflammatory drugs and aspirin impede the production of prostaglandins and are, therefore, the best painkillers to take.

SEE ALSO:
Contraception
Endometriosis
Fibroids

MENORRHAGIA

Menorrhagia is the term used to describe menstruation when blood flow is unusually heavy. It can be a single bout of flooding, a period that goes on for a long time (say, for more than seven days) or very frequent periods so that the blood loss in any given month is excessive. On average only about 60ml (2 floz) of blood is lost during a single period, but sufferers from menorrhagia can lose up to a third more than this.

SYMPTOMS

- *Blood flow during menstruation so rapid and excessive that several sanitary pads must be worn at the same time*
- *Pallor, fatigue and breathlessness indicating anaemia*

WHAT CAUSES IT?

Menorrhagia may be triggered by an imbalance of oestrogen and progesterone, which causes the lining of the womb (endometrium) to thicken, with a consequently heavier blood loss as the lining is shed during menstruation. It is common in women approaching the **menopause**. The recent fitting of an IUD can cause heavier periods for a few months afterwards, and **fibroids** may also cause heavy bleeding because they increase the inner surface of the womb and its lining.

If an excessive rate of flow continues over several days and throughout several periods, anaemia may develop which, if left untreated, could become severe.

SHOULD I SEE THE DOCTOR?

If your periods change and become longer or much heavier than they were, see your doctor to check for the underlying cause.

WHAT WILL THE DOCTOR DO?

- Your doctor will examine you for any abnormality of the uterus, such as fibroids, and for signs of anaemia.

- He may give you a blood test to determine if you are anaemic; if you are, this will be treated with iron supplements.
- If you have an IUD fitted, your doctor may remove it or fit another device if it is not right for you; a progesterone-carrying intrauterine device can be highly effective, for instance.
- If there is no disease of the uterus, he will recommend hormone therapy aimed at preventing build-up of endometrial tissue prior to menstruation. This is often the combined contraceptive pill unless you are already on it or it is unsuitable for you, in which case another drug will be prescribed.
- If fibroids or some other cause is suspected, you will be given a **hysteroscopy** to scrape out the uterine lining.
- If the menorrhagia is grossly debilitating, your doctor may suggest a **hysterectomy**. You should not agree to have this operation without the fullest discussion with your gynaecologist, and then only after careful consideration.

WHAT CAN I DO?

- If you have just one period with heavy bleeding, rest if you can and use extra-absorbant sanitary pads with tampons to minimize embarrassment.
- Increase the iron content in your diet; liver, egg yolks and dark green leafy vegetables are all rich in iron. To improve the absorption of iron supplements, take them with drinks rich in vitamin C, such as orange juice. Cooking in iron pots also helps increase the iron content of food.

SEE ALSO:
Contraception
Endometriosis
Fibroids
Hysterectomy
Hysteroscopy
Menopause

PELVIC PROBLEMS

Most of the time our reproductive system functions smoothly but, particularly during the later years of menstruation, problems can occur. Some of the conditions described in the previous chapter, for example, can be symptoms of pelvic problems such as endometriosis and fibroids, while a small percentage of women have ovary problems, from cysts to cancer. All of these can be serious, but help is available and the most important thing is to make the most appropriate decisions about your treatment. The information given on the following pages will enable you to make an informed choice.

ENDOMETRIOSIS

This is a very common condition, defined as the presence of cells from the lining of the uterus at other sites in the pelvis. The principal route of spread is via the Fallopian tubes, with implantation of deposits on the ovaries, bowel, bladder or in the pelvis. The deposits respond to the cyclical changes of the ovarian hormones, so bleeding occurs at the site of implantation when you are menstruating, but the blood cannot escape. The repeated bleeds can cause menstrual pain and painful sexual intercourse as well as generalized pelvic tenderness. Adhesions may form, interfering with ovulation and possibly conception.

SYMPTOMS

- *Heavy or abnormal bleeding*
- *Severe abdominal and pelvic pain, often leading to painful intercourse*
- *Severe cramping pain, starting before the period is due and continuing during menstruation, after which it gradually eases*
- *Occasional urinary or bowel pain, including diarrhoea*
- *Fertility problems: difficulty in conceiving a baby*

SHOULD I SEE THE DOCTOR?

If you are in your late twenties and have been unable to conceive, or if you suffer very painful periods or pain deep in your pelvis during intercourse, you should see your doctor as soon as possible. If you have never suffered from **dysmenorrhoea** (painful periods) before, it is very unlikely to develop in your late twenties without a major reason.

WHAT WILL THE DOCTOR DO?

- Medical treatment of endometriosis is usually only offered to women who are not trying to conceive; it has not been shown to improve fertility rates.

- The drugs used to treat endometriosis suppress ovulation and menstruation, thus permitting the disease to regress. The drugs include the continuous use of high dose oestrogens and/or progestogens or drugs to suppress ovarian-stimulating hormones. All these treatments are contraceptive.
- For women wishing to conceive, surgical treatment, usually laparoscopic, includes diathermy or laser vaporization of the endometriosis deposits, and adhesiolysis (removal of adhesions).
- In vitro fertilization (IVF) should be offered straightaway to women trying to conceive who have dense, widespread adhesions that are not amenable to, or recur after, surgery.
- Radical surgery with removal of the uterus and ovaries may be necessary in older patients with advanced disease.

WHAT CAN I DO?

Join a self-help group where you can share your experience with other women and discuss the latest treatments and side-effects of the hormone treatment.

SEE ALSO:
Dysmenorrhoea
Fertility Problems
Hysterectomy
Laparoscopy
Menstrual Problems
Painful Intercourse

FIBROIDS

These are benign tumours in the muscle lining the uterine wall. They vary in size and number; they can be anything from the size of a pea to as large as a tennis ball. About one woman in five develops fibroids by the time she is 45 years old.

There is often no reason for concern because the fibroids may never grow large enough to distort the uterus and present symptoms to alarm you. However, if you are having difficulty in conceiving, they may be interfering with your fertility by blocking the Fallopian tubes. Large fibroids cause the muscular coating of the uterus to feel lumpy and bumpy to the doctor when he examines your abdomen during routine pelvic examinations.

SYMPTOMS

- *About a quarter of women have no symptoms at all*
- *Very heavy or abnormal menstrual bleeding*
- *Swelling and a feeling of heaviness in the abdomen*
- *Discomfort or pain during intercourse*
- *Pressure on the bladder and bowel, leading to urinary problems and backache*

SHOULD I SEE THE DOCTOR?

If you are having difficulty in conceiving, if you have increasing pain or bleeding with your periods or if you have any other change in your normal menstrual cycle, see your doctor at once.

WHAT WILL THE DOCTOR DO?

- Your doctor will first perform a routine pelvic examination and question you about any symptoms you may have experienced.
- If he feels that your condition warrants it, he may then refer you to a gynaecologist for further investigation and tests, which will probably include an **ultrasound scan** of your uterus, a **hysteroscopy** or **laparoscopy**.

WHAT IS THE TREATMENT?

- Fibroids are treated according to the seriousness of the symptoms and whether you wish to conceive. Once you are past childbearing days, the fibroids usually shrink and disappear anyway.
- If you want children and the fibroids are numerous, your doctor may suggest a **myomectomy**. This removes the fibroids from the uterine lining and leaves the uterus intact and back in its usual shape.
- If the symptoms are difficult and you have already completed your family, a **hysterectomy** might be advised. This should be considered as a last resort and only after two opinions and discussion with your doctors.
- Anti-oestrogen hormone treatments may be given. These make fibroids shrink, but can only be given for a period of six months because of the risk of osteoporosis, and are only given before a myomectomy.

WHAT CAN I DO?

- Fibroids are the commonest reason for hysterectomy operations in the United States, so be on your guard against an unnecessary operation of such a radical nature. If you are suffering from profound anaemia, or have unbearable symptoms, obviously you should consider it, otherwise look for alternatives.
- There is a high incidence of **uterine cancer** in women who suffer from benign fibroids, so any unusual bleeding or other irregularity in your menstrual pattern should be investigated immediately.

SEE ALSO:
Hysterectomy
Hysteroscopy
Laparoscopy
Menstruation
Myomectomy
Ultrasound Scan
Uterine Cancer

OVARIAN CYSTS

A cyst is a fluid-filled sac. Ovarian cysts are nearly always benign and a significant proportion of women suffer from them. Benign cysts may be subdivided into two major categories.

Functional cysts are merely large cysts that occur normally in a woman's monthly cycle. They do not usually cause any problems, but there may be several and they may be present in both ovaries. They rarely grow larger than about 6–8cm (2–3in) in diameter and commonly shrink back to normal size spontaneously.

They are usually detected on routine **ultrasound** screening or **pelvic examination**. Very occasionally a functional cyst may cause the ovary to twist so causing severe abdominal pain. A cyst may also leak, releasing a jelly-like material into the abdominal cavity.

The second type of benign ovarian cyst is called a *dermoid cyst*. These are most commonly found in women in their thirties. Dermoid cysts are also benign and occasionally they may be present in both ovaries. They do not usually cause any problems unless they cause the ovary to twist or if the cyst leaks.

Dermoid cysts contain immature cells that are capable of growing into various types of tissue, and it is therefore not uncommon for dermoid cysts to contain bone, teeth and hair.

Polycystic ovaries create a specific syndrome in women who experience the condition, and this is discussed in detail in the box opposite.

SYMPTOMS

- *Pain during intercourse*
- *Painful, heavy periods*
- *If a cyst twists or ruptures, it results in severe abdominal pain, nausea and fever*
- *Urinary problems due to pressure on the bladder*

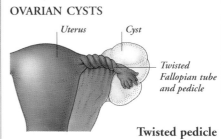

OVARIAN CYSTS

Uterus   Cyst

Twisted Fallopian tube and pedicle

Twisted pedicle

If the stalk, or pedicle, of a cyst becomes twisted, it cuts off its blood supply and causes sudden, severe abdominal pain.

SHOULD I SEE THE DOCTOR?

While ovarian cysts are small, they produce few symptoms. Many disappear on their own and you may never even know you had them. As they get larger, however, they may cause pain and discomfort and may also affect your menstrual cycle; the severe pain of a twisted ovary requires an emergency operation, so see your doctor as soon as possible if you suffer any of the symptoms detailed in the box on the left.

WHAT WILL THE DOCTOR DO?

- Your doctor will examine you both externally and internally in order to assess the size of the ovarian cyst. Further tests will be arranged depending on what your doctor finds, and on your age.
- These tests will probably include an ultrasound examination of your ovaries, plus blood tests and X-rays.
- Laparoscopic surgery may be attempted to help diagnose the type of cyst present and, in younger women, to remove the cyst if it is benign.
- In older women, those in whom the cyst is too large to be removed by **laparoscopy**, or if there is a suspicion of malignancy, an abdominal operation will be performed. Both ovaries are always examined and checked during surgery.

POLYCYSTIC OVARIAN SYNDROME

Polycystic ovaries are benign cysts of the ovary found in 15–20 percent of women. Women with polycystic ovarian syndrome may have other symptoms, which include a tendency to obesity, excessive body hair and acne. The ovary seems to produce an excessive amount of male hormones. The condition may cause fertility problems and sufferers may have irregular periods.

What causes it?

The exact cause is not known. There may be a hormonal imbalance, but whether this is a cause or consequence of the syndrome remains to be worked out fully.

What will the doctor do?

Polycystic ovaries are often discovered because of one of the complaints listed above. The doctor will examine you internally and will probably arrange an ultrasound examination of your ovaries and blood tests to confirm the diagnosis. You may be given the pill to stimulate a normal monthly period and combat the excessive male hormones. Fertility treatment could be necessary if you are having some difficulty in conceiving.

What can I do?

Discuss the symptoms fully with your doctor so you understand the nature of all the treatments that are offered to you.

What is the outlook?

The outlook for women with polycystic ovaries depends on the severity of the problems encountered. Currently available treatments provide good control of the majority of symptoms.

WHAT HAPPENS DURING SURGERY?

• Benign ovarian cysts may be punctured and their contents carefully sucked out through the laparoscope.
• If the cyst is too large or if there is suspicion of a malignancy, the type of abdominal operation will depend on the appearance of the cyst and your age.
• In younger women, the benign cyst will be removed and the ovary conserved if possible. In older women with a benign cyst the whole ovary will be removed. Women in their middle forties onwards are usually offered the option to have both ovaries and their womb removed.
• If both ovaries are removed you will be offered hormone replacement therapy to prevent menopausal symptoms.

WHAT CAN I DO?

Discuss all of the possibilities with your doctor before you agree to have an operation. Ask him whether it will be absolutely necessary to have both ovaries removed and about taking HRT (hormone replacement therapy).

WHAT IS THE OUTLOOK?

There is an excellent outlook for benign cysts. Even if it is necessary to remove both ovaries, the possibility of HRT means that you will have few of the problems associated with the menopause.

SEE ALSO:
Hysterectomy
Laparoscopy
Menstrual Problems
Menopause
Ovarian Cancer
Pelvic Examination
Ultrasound Scan

OVARIAN CANCER

Rarely, ovarian cysts may be malignant. They tend to occur in childless women over the age of 35. Unfortunately, malignant cysts do not usually cause any symptoms until they have grown to a large size, by which time they may be very difficult to treat effectively.

WHAT CAUSES IT?

There are many theories about what causes malignant ovarian cysts to develop. They are more common in older women and in women who have not had any children. They are less common in women who have used the oral contraceptive pill and HRT for a number of years, and in those women who had a late start to their periods and an early menopause.

"Resting" the ovary – that is, periods in a woman's life when ovulation is suppressed, for example during pregnancy or while on the pill – may protect a woman against the development of ovarian cancer. Genetic factors have been shown to be important in the development of ovarian cancer.

SYMPTOMS

- *Abdominal pain*
- *Swelling of the abdomen*
- *A hard lump in the abdomen*
- *If the cyst is large, pressure on the bladder can cause frequent urination*
- *Occasional breathlessness if the tumour puts pressure on the diaphragm*

SHOULD I SEE THE DOCTOR?

Some families carry a gene called BRCA1 that increases the likelihood of both ovarian and breast cancer. Genetic tests for this gene are now available to help identify those women at risk of developing ovarian and breast cancer.

If you have a strong history of ovarian or breast cancer in your family, it is important to tell your doctor.

WHAT WILL THE DOCTOR DO?

- Malignant cysts need more thorough surgery than benign ovarian cysts, depending on the type of tumour found. The doctor will attempt to remove the whole tumour and any deposits.
- Minimal surgery involves the removal of both ovaries and the Fallopian tubes as well as the uterus.
- If the disease has already spread beyond the reproductive organs, much more extensive surgery will be necessary, involving the removal of other organs such as the bowel and bladder.

WHAT IS THE OUTLOOK?

- If a malignancy is found, further treatment may well be necessary. Chemotherapy will be started to help shrink the tumour. Drugs containing platinum are commonly used to treat ovarian cancer, but radiotherapy has not been found to be effective for it.
- Further surgery may well be performed to find out if the chemotherapy has worked or to remove any recurrences.
- The outlook in the longer term depends on the stage of the disease and the type of malignant cell present in the ovary.

SEE ALSO:
Hysterectomy
Laparoscopy
Menstrual Problems
Ovarian Cysts
Ultrasound Scan

UTERINE CANCER

This rare cancer results from a malignant growth in the lining of the uterus, the endometrium. It is sometimes known as endometrial cancer. Cervical cancer can also sometimes be referred to as uterine cancer as the cervix is part of the uterus. Precancerous forms of the disease may exist for many years before the condition becomes malignant.

This cancer is more common in older women (less than five percent of sufferers are under 40), in those who used DES during pregnancy (or whose mothers' did) and in those of the higher socio-economic groups. There has been a lot of controversy during recent years about the incidence of uterine cancer among women who take hormone replacement therapy (HRT) for menopausal symptoms. Good medical practice demands a regular three-monthly bleed induced with 14 days of progestogen or the insertion of a progesterone IUD.

SYMPTOMS

- *Abnormal vaginal bleeding, between periods or after intercourse*
- *Heavy or prolonged periods*
- *Postmenopausal bleeding*
- *Cramping pain in the lower abdomen*
- *Pressure in the lower abdomen*
- *Frequency of urination due to pressure of the tumour on the bladder*

SHOULD I SEE THE DOCTOR?

If you have any change in your normal menstrual pattern or if you have any post-menopausal vaginal bleeding, consult your doctor immediately.

WHAT WILL THE DOCTOR DO ?

- If your doctor suspects that you have a growth in your uterus, the only effective way to check whether there is any malignancy is to undergo a **D&C** (dilatation and curettage) investigation.

- If the uterine lining has some cancerous cells, your doctor will recommend a total hysterectomy with removal of the ovaries and Fallopian tubes as well as the uterus. This is nearly always combined with four to six weeks of radiotherapy.
- If the growth is advanced, an extended total **hysterectomy** will be performed to remove the top of the vagina and the glands of the pelvis too.

WHAT IS THE OUTLOOK?

The news is good. The overall cure rate is as high as 90 percent when the cancer is localized to the lining of the womb itself. If the spread is beyond the lining and the muscles of the uterus, the figure after five years is reduced to a 40 percent cure rate.

SEE ALSO:
Abnormal Bleeding
Cervical Cancer
D&C
Fibroids
Hysterectomy
Hysteroscopy
Menstrual Problems

PELVIC INFLAMMATORY DISEASE

This is a general term used to describe grumbling inflammation of any of the pelvic organs – the uterus, Fallopian tubes or ovaries. Irrevocable scarring of the Fallopian tubes and ovaries is the most serious complication because it causes sterility. Others include scarring and **painful intercourse** (dyspareunia). At one time, the commonest cause of this disease was tuberculosis. Now it is **chlamydia**. There is some evidence that the use of intrauterine contraceptive devices may be a contributing factor.

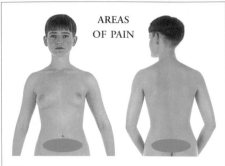

AREAS OF PAIN

Pelvic pain
The most common symptoms of PID are abdominal pain and backache, both of which can cause acute discomfort.

SYMPTOMS

- *Abdominal pain*
- *Back pain*
- *Persistent menstrual-like cramps*
- *Vaginal spotting of blood*
- *Tiredness*
- *Pain during and after intercourse*
- *Foul-smelling vaginal discharge*
- *Flu type symptoms of fever and chills*
- *Sub-fertility or infertility*

SHOULD I SEE THE DOCTOR?

PID must be treated early to prevent long-term problems. The symptoms can be those of an acute infection with fever, nausea, discomfort and pain, which should alert you to the fact that there is something wrong. A chronic infection may only cause recurrent mild pain and sometimes backache. But both forms must be investigated. Don't wait for it to go away, see your doctor as soon as possible. If you have an IUD, go to your clinic immediately.

WHAT WILL THE DOCTOR DO?

- You will be examined and tested to identify the organism causing the infection. Your doctor will probably prescribe antibiotics and bedrest. Eat well and don't have sexual intercourse during the course of treatment. If antibiotics are not suitable for you, you may have to have more treatment.

- If PID develops into a chronic infection, it can be difficult to eradicate. You may need investigative laparoscopy to confirm the diagnosis. In severe cases, for a long-term infection, **hysterectomy** can be the only course of action, although you should go through any alternatives fully before agreeing to this operation.

WHAT CAN I DO?

- Don't let any vaginal discharge continue for any length of time without full investigation and treatment. Because PID can recur, have a full check-up to confirm that your infection has been completely eradicated.
- If you suspect that you or your partner may have a venereal disease, go to a sexually transmitted diseases clinic right away.

SEE ALSO:
Chlamydia
Contraception
Ectopic Pregnancy
Fertility Problems
Hysterectomy
Laparoscopy
Miscarriage
Painful Intercourse

SEXUAL PROBLEMS

A fulfilling sex life should be a basic part of
human existence. For some people, however,
things aren't that simple at least some of the time,
as various problems occur that prevent them
from enjoying their relationships to the full.
Basic complaints, such as painful intercourse,
lack of sex drive and vaginismus (vaginal spasms
that can prevent intercourse) are described here,
with the accent firmly on what can be done to
cure or alleviate them, so that your lovemaking
can improve or resume.

PAINFUL INTERCOURSE

Any type of pain or discomfort during sexual intercourse, whether because of a local genital problem or pain deep in the pelvis, can be described as dyspareunia. It can vary from mild discomfort or tightness to an exquisite pain that prevents intercourse altogether. Psychological factors are by far the most common cause. Inhibitions about the sexual act, resentment, anger, fear or shame – and anticipating that sex will be unsuccessful – are all causes of disturbed psychological attitudes affecting sex.

SYMPTOMS

- *Pain during intercourse; either externally or deep in the pelvis during penetration*
- *Lack of desire or inclination for sex*
- *Involuntary closing of the legs and vagina to prevent penetration (vaginismus)*
- *Dryness in the vagina*

ARE THERE PHYSICAL REASONS?

There are several medical conditions that must be eliminated first. These include vaginal infections, PID (**pelvic inflammatory disease**), **endometriosis**, **prolapsed uterus**, urinary tract infection, irritation of the vulva (**pruritis vulvae**), hormonal deficiency at the **menopause** or after childbirth causing dryness in the vagina, and painful perineal scars after an episiotomy.

SHOULD I SEE THE DOCTOR?

If you experience physical pain during intercourse or for some reason you are reluctant to permit your partner to penetrate your vagina, see your doctor.

WHAT WILL THE DOCTOR DO?

- Your doctor will examine you to check for any underlying disorder. If you have an infection, antibiotics should clear it up. If the discomfort is the result of poor stitching after childbirth, your doctor may advise you to wait another couple of weeks, or to have the area restitched. This depends on how recently you have given birth.
- If your problem is not a physical one, your doctor will refer you to a psycho-sexual counsellor, who will try to uncover the reasons for your fear of sexual intercourse. However, if your relationship is no longer a loving one, sex counselling will not help. It is not possible to heal a broken relationship with sex and you should admit this from the outset.

WHAT CAN I DO?

- Don't keep quiet about your expectations and preferences. You have to take responsibility for your own pleasure. Try to discuss this with your partner and try not to feel guilty about ordinary sexual practices. The only prerequisite for good sex is loving your partner, and if you do, most of your sexual problems should be resolved.
- If your problem has a physical cause, find other ways of showing affection.
- Forget labels. No woman is frigid. If you label yourself or are labelled frigid, you may become anxious and lose hope.
- Remember also that even if you are aroused by your partner, unless you have sufficient clitoral stimulation and your vagina lubricates sufficiently to make penetration easy and comfortable, you won't experience good sex. You may find you need to use a lubricating jelly.

SEE ALSO:
Cystitis
Endometriosis
Menopause
Pelvic Inflammatory Disease
Prolapse
Pruritis Vulvae
Vaginismus

LACK OF SEX DRIVE

Problems with intercourse and lack of interest can stem from both physical and emotional factors. It can become a chronic problem and failure to discuss it will have an effect on your relationships, and your image of yourself as a woman.

WHAT CAUSES IT?

Physical causes of lack of desire include diabetes, neurological disorders like multiple sclerosis, pain during intercourse, and taking certain drugs such as alcohol or barbiturates. Removal of the ovaries (as part of a **hysterectomy)** depletes the supply of testosterone, the male hormone, which is now known to be responsible for sex drive in women. An underactive thyroid gland reduces sex drive.

Some symptoms that make sex uncomfortable and painful relate to sexually transmitted diseases, so check to see whether your partner has had intercourse with anyone else recently.

Fear is the commonest cause of loss of desire. A woman may be fearful of letting herself go both physically and emotionally. She may have ambivalent feelings about intercourse, stemming from some incident in early life. These feelings will inevitably be transferred onto her partners. She may use her reluctance to punish herself; wanting to enjoy sex but hating herself for doing so. She may be angry with her partner or lovemaking may be rather predictable. Pregnancy is often a fear if **contraception** isn't discussed and practised.

WHAT CAN I DO?

• Professional counselling is often the answer, particularly if there is friction in a relationship. A psycho-sexual counsellor will try to uncover the reasons for your fear, although if your relationship is no longer a loving one, sex counselling will not help. A broken relationship cannot be helped with sex and this needs to be admitted by both partners at the outset of any therapy.

• Many women prefer to attend sex clinics where women are treated on their own by counselling, followed by masturbation training. The view is that a woman must be able to excite herself before she is able to be excited by anyone else.

• Psycho-sexual counselling is normally carried out at a specialist clinic, where trained counsellors conduct physical and psychological tests. The types of problem that would be dealt with by a counsellor are nearly always looked upon as something couples have to explore together, requiring frank discussion.

• If you feel that psycho-sexual counselling will be useful for you, the first step you have to take is to admit that you have a problem, and this will mean you have to overcome many inhibitions.

WHAT WILL THE COUNSELLOR DO?

• Depending on the particular problem, you will be given advice about relaxing and losing your anxieties. The counsellor will encourage you to go back to the beginning and find out how your body responds to sexual contact.

• She will suggest that you to return to the simplest exploration of your partner's body through touch without sexual response. She will also teach you to concentrate on feelings and experiences, but to forget about orgasm for the time being.

• She will ask you to refrain from sexual intercourse for a few days or weeks.

• Later she will advise you to go on to enjoy touching, fondling and caressing each other, then to orgasm without intercourse and finally to orgasm during intercourse.

SEE ALSO:
Contraception
Menopause
Pruritis Vulvae
Sexual Problems

VAGINISMUS

This is an involuntary spasm of the muscles around the entrance to the vagina, causing the opening almost to close whenever an attempt is made to insert something, such as a speculum, tampon or penis, into the vagina. The spasm can be so great that it prevents intercourse or makes penetration extremely painful. Sexual drive and arousal are usually normal until penetration itself is attempted. The pelvic floor muscles then tighten up, virtually closing the vaginal entrance, and a sufferer will arch her back and close her legs.

SYMPTOMS

- *Intense pain and difficulty during intercourse*
- *Involuntary closing of the vagina; the thighs often close tightly too*
- *Acute fear of penetration of any kind*

WHAT CAUSES IT?

Vaginismus usually occurs in anxiety prone individuals who have never been able to insert a tampon or a finger into the vagina because of the anticipation that this will be painful. In some women, a contributing factor may be underlying guilt or fear associated with the sexual act, due to a restrictive upbringing or an inadequate sex education. Vaginismus can also occur when a woman is in sexual disharmony with her partner. Disharmony is often the result of a partner liking the idea of something that the other is repelled by. There can also be difficulty if the role a woman wants to play – active or passive – is at odds with her partner's likes and dislikes. Vaginismus may also result after a shocking experience, such as rape.

SHOULD I SEE THE DOCTOR?

If you find you are unable to enjoy sex, see your doctor and talk it over. Don't let it fester because it may cause disenchantment with the sex act altogether.

WHAT WILL THE DOCTOR DO?

- Your doctor will first of all examine you to rule out the possibility of any anatomical abnormalities that could cause pain that results in spasm.
- He may then put you in touch with a psycho-sexual counsellor or marriage guidance clinic where counselling for this kind of problem is undertaken. You may also like to make contact with a self-help group.
- Many women who experience vaginismus are not familiar with their sex organs. Some therapists work by helping you familiarize yourself with your genitalia. By learning that the insertion of your own finger or a speculum into your vagina is not painful, you may gain confidence about allowing penetration by your partner's penis.

WHAT CAN I DO?

- Vaginismus is an uncommon result of sexual problems but be reassured, most problems don't stem from you or your inadequacy. You are not abnormal.
- Look at your sexual relationship, see where the disharmony lies and discuss it with your partner. The commonest problem is when you feel something is distasteful. Perhaps oral sex, anal intercourse or too frequent lovemaking upsets you.
- Talk about your likes and dislikes with your partner. If he understands, you should both acknowledge that neither of you is abnormal for wanting it, or for not wanting it, and that it is not selfish to refuse, although it is selfish to insist on something that either partner finds distasteful.

SEE ALSO:
Painful Intercourse
Pruritis Vulvae
Sexual Problems

SEXUALLY TRANSMITTED DISEASES

There is nothing more frightening than suffering from an infection passed on by a partner, even when that infection is relatively minor, such as genital herpes or warts. There are, unfortunately, also more serious problems that can be transmitted sexually and which need urgent treatment. These range from the serious, such as gonorrhoea, to the terrifying, such as AIDS. In the pages that follow, each complaint is described in detail to help recognition, and the various options available are outlined.

GENITAL HERPES

This is a common viral disease transmitted during sexual intercourse when the virus is active in the surface layers of the skin around the genitals. Millions of people are infected with the virus but probably only a quarter experience symptoms.

Herpes is caused by the herpes simplex II virus. The virus is transmitted through exposed raw areas of skin and is more common in women because their genital areas are warmer and more moist than men's. Herpes is highly contagious; there is a high chance of catching it if either partner has an active blister; it can also be caught from people who don't have symptoms. The symptoms appear between three and twenty days after sexual contact with an infected partner.

Today herpes is considered incurable but manageable; once in the body the virus stays there although treatment can clear the symptoms or suppress activity. The waxing and waning course of the disease can cause the sufferer much psychological misery as well as physical pain.

SYMPTOMS

- *For a primary attack, many women sufferers have no symptoms*
- *The skin on the vulva feels sensitive to the touch, ticklish, even numb*
- *Blisters appear within a few hours, enlarge, burst and become painful ulcers within two or three days*
- *The ulcers form scabs and take 14–21 days to disappear*
- *Pain on urination*
- *There may be a raised temperature and swollen glands in the groin*

SHOULD I SEE THE DOCTOR?

See your doctor immediately if you feel numb or sensitive in the genital area, if blisters appear or if you have had sexual relations with anyone with the herpes virus.

WHAT WILL THE DOCTOR DO?

- There is no cure for genital herpes but new oral antiviral treatments, if taken early enough, are often effective both in limiting the blisters and shortening the attack. Idoxuridine, in an ointment or liquid cream, is still successful for some.
- Other remedies include daily douches with providone iodine solution, or painting the blisters with gentian violet. Your doctor may also prescribe an antibiotic.
- It is possible to transmit the virus to a new-born baby during delivery. If you have an attack when your baby is due, your doctor may suggest a Caesarean.

WHAT CAN I DO?

- A long soak in a tepid bath can help, as can cold packs applied directly to the labia and vulva. Do not use ice cubes.
- About 50 percent of herpes sufferers have another attack, so try to recognize the early warning signs and treat them at once. The initial attack is usually the most severe.
- Irritation of the vagina from other causes is known to trigger attacks, so can stress, fever, cold, periods and tight-fitting clothes.
- To avoid the virus do not have sex with someone who is infected, and do not have sex if you have the active disease. Condoms must always be worn for penetrative sex.
- Prevent recurrences with lots of rest and a balanced diet. Manage stress by learning relaxation exercises or yoga. Many sufferers feel unclean and stigmatized; try to overcome this feeling through counselling.
- As there is a greater risk of **cervical cancer** in women who have had herpes, it is very important to have regular **cervical smears**.

SEE ALSO:
Cervical Cancer
Cervical Smear
Genital Problems

GENITAL WARTS

Genital warts are the commonest sexually transmitted disease. They are small, benign lumps of skin that appear on the vulva and anus, inside the vagina and on the cervix.

WHAT CAUSES THEM?

Genital warts are caused by the same virus that causes warts on other parts of the body. The virus is called HPV or the human papilloma virus, and can be spread through personal and sexual contact. It is possible to transfer the virus from one part of the body to the genital region, although this is rare.

Genital warts are most often transmitted sexually. It may take several months after infection before a wart becomes visible in the genital region.

SYMPTOMS

- *The appearance of a single raised, soft wart, or a group of warts, in and around the entrance of the vagina and the anus*
- *A cluster of tiny, itchy lumps on the perineal skin (the area between the genitals and the anus), on the labia or inside the vagina, including right up to the cervix*

SHOULD I SEE THE DOCTOR?

Genital warts do not usually cause any symptoms. However, left untreated they may grow and spread. There is also the risk that they may be transmitted to a new sexual partner. Perhaps the most serious consequence of infection with HPV is the increased risk of developing **cervical cancer** that untreated infection brings. The diagnosis of genital warts is made on the basis of the examination your doctor makes.

WHAT WILL THE DOCTOR DO?

- Treatment of genital warts depends on their location. After examining you thoroughly and perhaps screening you for other sexually transmitted diseases, the doctor may treat you with a special lotion called podophyllin which you will be asked to apply to the warts, carefully avoiding any healthy skin surrounding the warts. If the warts are in a difficult location, it is sometimes best for medical staff to apply the lotion for you to prevent damage to the surrounding skin.
- If podophyllin does not succeed in clearing the warts after a few weeks, stronger agents such as trichloroacetic acid could be used. Occasionally the genital warts may be frozen off with liquid nitrogen and, rarely, a laser may be used to burn them away.
- If you haven't had a **cervical smear** recently, your doctor will take one, and may arrange a **colposcopy** to make sure your cervix is free from infection.
- Apart from the increased risk of an abnormal smear test, there are very few other complications of infection with the HPV virus.

WHAT CAN I DO?

- As soon as you notice any abnormal area of skin in or around your genital area, it is best to see your doctor.
- Having a regular smear test will also protect you from the dangers of untreated infection with HPV. You must ask your doctor to explain all the treatments he suggests to you.
- Try and persuade your sexual partner to see his doctor or attend a genito-urinary clinic to check for genital warts.

SEE ALSO:
Cervical Cancer
Cervical Smear
Colposcopy

CHLAMYDIA

Any sexually active woman runs the risk of getting chlamydia, especially with multiple partners. Women with untreated infections risk losing their fertility, hence the alarm now caused by this once little-known disorder. Although easy to treat, chlamydia is difficult to diagnose because symptoms are usually slow to develop, mild or non-existent. But as long as there is awareness of the possibility of the disease, modern tests and treatments can eradicate it before any serious consequences develop.

Theoretically, chlamydia infects the linings of the vagina, the mouth, the eyes, the urinary tract or the rectum, but in women the infection is usually confined to the cervix, leading to an offensive yellow-coloured discharge. About a third of cases can go on to **pelvic inflammatory disease**, which damages the Fallopian tubes and causes infertility.

Chlamydia may also be responsible for **ectopic pregnancy**, which is potentially life-threatening and could result in infertility due to tubal blockage or scarring. During childbirth an infected woman may infect her baby, who will have conjunctivitis and, rarely, develop pneumonia.

SYMPTOMS
- *Most women sufferers have no real symptoms*
- *Once it gains a hold, there can be unusual discharge*
- *Abdominal pain, particularly during sexual intercourse*
- *Fever*

SHOULD I SEE THE DOCTOR?

If you have any symptoms of unusual discharge or, more likely, your sexual partner has these symptoms, go to see your doctor as soon as possible, or go to the nearest sexually transmitted diseases clinic. It is very important to treat this disease as early as possible.

WHAT WILL THE DOCTOR DO?

At one time it was necessary to take a specimen of the vaginal secretions in order to culture chlamydia in a laboratory. This meant waiting at least 48 hours for the result of the tests. However, new laboratory tests have been devised that can give results in 30–60 minutes, thus permitting immediate treatment.

WHAT IS THE TREATMENT?

- Chlamydia is simply and completely cured with a course of antibiotics. It is essential to take the medication exactly as prescribed and to complete the full course. Do not stop taking the tablets because the symptoms disappear; the chlamydia could return. It is essential that your partner is treated at the same time.
- What was once diagnosed as non-specific urethritis was probably chlamydia.
- If the diagnosis is wrongly stated as **gonorrhoea**, the treatment given will not cure the chlamydia. Therefore, as many people with gonorrhoea also have chlamydia, and penicillin is not adequate, tetracyclines or sulphonamides are used.

WHAT CAN I DO?

- If you have many sexual contacts, all of them must be informed of the infection, and screened and treated if necessary.
- To prevent re-infection use barrier contraceptives such as condoms and diaphragms with spermicidal creams.

SEE ALSO:
Contraception
Ectopic Pregnancy
Fertility Problems
Pelvic Inflammatory Disease
Vaginal Discharge

GONORRHOEA

This is a common venereal disease that is caused by the bacterium *Neisseria gonorrhoeae*. It can affect both men and women, and in five out of every six women infected by the bacterium there are no symptoms, which makes it more dangerous. The most serious aspect of this disease is that if it remains untreated during the incubation period (usually between about two and ten days), it progresses to the chronic form that sets up inflammation in the pelvis. If the ovaries and Fallopian tubes are affected, they may become blocked and the scarring may cause infertility.

The risk of contracting gonorrhoea seems to become higher if you are using the contraceptive pill – the infection seems to spread more quickly. The most common way many women suspect they may have become infected, is if they notice the recognizable symptoms of the disease in their male partners.

SYMPTOMS

- *There may be vaginal discharge with pain and a burning sensation when passing urine*
- *The entire perineum (the area between the genitals and the anus) may be sore, and inflammation of the rectum causes pain when passing a stool*
- *A sore throat if the bacterium has been passed there during oral sex*
- *Penile discharge in your partner*

SHOULD I SEE THE DOCTOR?

If you suspect that you have gonorrhoea, go to your doctor or to a sexually transmitted disease clinic and don't have any sexual contact with anyone until you are clear.

WHAT WILL THE DOCTOR DO?

- Diagnosis of gonorrhoea can be difficult, so your doctor will take some samples of the secretions from your urethra, cervix and rectum and send them to a laboratory for further investigation. There is no reliable blood test.
- Special STD clinics give the best results, so even if you have a negative test and you know or think you may have had intercourse with someone with gonorrhoea, insist on more tests or treatment.

WHAT IS THE TREATMENT?

- Penicillin is the mainstay of treatment and may be given in a slow-release injectable form which requires only the one injection, making treatment easy. If the organism is resistant, ciprofloxacin can be given.
- You should then have a full gynaecological examination to make sure the disease hasn't caused **pelvic inflammatory disease**. Have a repeat gonorrhoea culture to ascertain that the infection is gone.
- Gonorrhoea can mask the symptoms of other sexually transmitted diseases, so you should be tested for **syphilis** too.

WHAT CAN I DO?

- If you discover you have gonorrhoea, give the names of your sexual contacts so that they can get treatment before they infect others. Stop all sexual activity until you have been treated.
- You would be wise to have an IUD removed. You can have a new one fitted when you are clear of infection.
- As with all sexually transmitted diseases, gonorrhoea is most common in young people under 25 who have many sexual partners. Using condoms will decrease the probability of you getting an infection or being re-infected.
- Check that your partner is not a carrier, as he could re-infect you even after you have been successfully treated.

SEE ALSO:
Pelvic Inflammatory Disease
Syphilis

SYPHILIS

Two or three hundred years ago syphilis was the medical scourge of the time in very much the same way that **AIDS** is now. It is a venereal disease that infected large numbers of people of both sexes. Syphilis has a very long history and produces severe symptoms; even as recently as the 1930s, it was fatal for many.

With the discovery of penicillin, syphilis has been almost completely eradicated except in a few underdeveloped and under-privileged communities. Syphilis is caused by a bacterium, *Treponema pallidum*, and can be transmitted from person-to-person through sexual contact.

SYMPTOMS

- *For primary syphilis, a "chancre" or sore on the vulva and swollen glands in the groin*
- *For secondary syphilis, a rash, which can cover most of the body*
- *For tertiary syphilis, widespread problems, including blindness, brain damage and paralysis*

SHOULD I SEE THE DOCTOR?

Primary and secondary syphilis can be treated and cured completely with a single course of penicillin. It is therefore a great tragedy if the disease goes undiagnosed. If you suspect that you may have contracted syphilis, seek confidential medical attention immediately. Unfortunately, once the disease has destroyed certain tissues, such as joints, it is impossible to cure.

WHAT WILL THE DOCTOR DO?

- The diagnosis will be made after a blood test and taking samples from the sore or rash. Treatment involves a course of antibiotic injections.
- You should also have regular blood tests for at least two years after contracting syphilis to ensure the disease has been eradicated.

WHAT CAN I DO?

- Avoid casual sexual contacts.
- If you discover a genital or any other kind of sore that you can't account for, have a medical check-up.
- If you suspect that you may have caught a venereal disease, go along to your sexually transmitted diseases clinic for a blood test.
- You can help eradicate the disease if you give the names of all your sexual partners to your doctor or the clinic so they can be traced and treated. Because the disease can be cured, it is imperative that all partners are treated, otherwise the risks remain. This information is always kept confidential.

SEE ALSO:
Chlamydia
Gonorrhoea
HIV/AIDS

HIV/AIDS

AIDS stands for "acquired immune deficiency syndrome". It is caused by the human immunodeficiency virus (HIV). There are two types of HIV, type 1 and type 2; infection with either form can lead to AIDS, although HIV-2 seems to be a less aggressive form of the virus.

While HIV is infectious, it is not as contagious as some other viruses such as the common cold or influenza. It cannot, for example, be caught simply by touching and normal social contact, and is not spread by coughs and sneezes.

It is usually transmitted by the mixing of body fluids – mainly blood, semen and vaginal secretions. The most common route of transmission is through sexual intercourse but it may also be passed on via blood transfusions and the sharing of needles by intravenous drug users.

The virus is also found in saliva and tears, although the concentration of viral particles is too low to be infectious. HIV affects all racial and social groups, as well as both heterosexuals and homosexuals.

AIDS weakens the body's natural immune system to such an extent that it is unable to fight off opportunistic infections or control cancerous growths. AIDS sufferers often succumb to diseases that rarely cause any illness in the general population.

SYMPTOMS

- *Marked weight loss over a relatively short period of time*
- *Enlarged lymph glands*
- *Many HIV sufferers have infections such as pneumonia, oral thrush, herpes simplex infections or shingles*
- *Cancers, such as Kaposi's sarcoma and lymphoma, and opportunistic auto-immune diseases*
- *Dementia-like syndrome when brain and nervous system are affected*

HOW CAN I TELL IF I AM HIV POSITIVE?

The body's response to infection with HIV is to produce antibodies, though they may take up to three months to appear. You would only be identified as HIV positive when antibodies are detected in your blood. For that reason, if you take an AIDS test too soon after possible exposure, it can be negative. It is usually recommended that you take a test about six months after you suspect infection may have taken place.

An HIV-positive person does not necessarily have AIDS, which may take up to ten years to develop, during which time he or she may remain well. It is therefore possible for people to be unaware they are HIV positive and to pass on the virus unknowingly.

WHERE DID HIV COME FROM?

There are many theories about how the virus first entered the human population HIV probably arose as a variant of a virus affecting African monkeys and apes. It was able to cross over to infect the human population of Africa, from where it spread to the rest of the world. Although it originally affected the homosexual community in the West, heterosexual transmission is now the main form of transmission worldwide.

HOW CAN I PREVENT IT?

- The main route of HIV infection is through sex. It may be passed through both vaginal and anal intercourse. Sexual transmission may be prevented, however, by the use of good quality condoms. Spermicides actually kill the AIDS virus so they must always be used.
- Theoretically, sexual intercourse with only one infected individual is enough to pass on the HIV virus. As it is impossible to tell whether an individual is HIV positive from his or her appearance, precautions must be used with all new sexual partners.

HIV/AIDS: CONTINUED

• Intravenous drug users can pass on the virus by sharing needles and syringes, so sharing needles should always be avoided.

• HIV has also been transmitted through infected blood products; the major group to be infected in this way were haemophiliacs. Thankfully, however, all blood products are now screened for HIV in most developed countries.

• Transmission from an HIV-positive mother to her baby may also occur during pregnancy, birth or breastfeeding.

WOMEN AND HIV

Women need to be assertive in order to protect themselves from HIV. The practice of "safe sex" should be compulsory for everyone until such time as you are able to confirm that your partner is HIV negative. As it can take up to three months to produce antibodies, it's best to practise safe sex until this "window of infection" is passed, and it should only be relaxed if there is

no other potential high risk activity such as intravenous drug use or unprotected intercourse with another person.

WHAT IS THE TREATMENT?

• Following a diagnosis of HIV, treatment is begun to try to slow down the rate of viral replication. Various drugs are prescribed to achieve this aim, and different combinations are being researched and developed all the time.

• These treatments are not without their side-effects but they do seem to decrease the rate of HIV multiplication in the body.

• Treatment of opportunistic infections depends on the specific agent infecting the patient. High dose antibiotics and antiviral drugs are often given routinely to prevent an infection from taking hold.

CAN HIV/AIDS BE CURED?

Although the progression of HIV infection to AIDS may be slowed down, there is still no cure for AIDS, nor is there a vaccine to prevent infection with HIV. The problem is compounded because HIV attacks the immune system – the route by which the body is usually able to fight infections and cancers. HIV-1 and 2 also seem to consist of various sub-types which makes the likelihood of finding a universal vaccine remote.

Death is nearly always due to overwhelming pneumonia or Kaposi's sarcoma. The brain may be affected terminally giving rise to an illness resembling dementia.

TESTING FOR HIV

The usual test for HIV infection involves analyzing a blood sample for signs of HIV antibodies. (Antibodies are substances produced by the body to fight off infection by a particular virus.) The presence of antibodies in your blood, therefore, indicates that there is an infection from the virus present. This is why anyone whose blood tests positive for HIV antibodies is said to be HIV positive. The HIV virus incubates for a period of several months before becoming active, so there is a gap between exposure to the virus and identification that infection has developed. For that reason, if you take an AIDS test too soon after possible exposure it can be negative. It is usually recommended that you take a test about six months after you suspect infection may have taken place.

SEE ALSO:
Contraception
Genital Herpes
Sexually Transmitted Diseases
Thrush

FERTILITY PROBLEMS

Becoming pregnant is usually one of the great joys
of life; failure to become pregnant can therefore
be a huge trauma. In the pages that follow,
both physical and emotional reasons for problems
such as infertility, miscarriage and ectopic pregnancy
are discussed in detail. Possible solutions, such
as surgery, hormone treatment and assisted
conception, are also explored. The accent is
on the positive and practical ways to cope
with the problem and the many effective
solutions now available.

PROBLEMS WITH FERTILITY

Infertility means the inability to conceive or bear a child. Very few women and couples are truly infertile; a much higher number are sub-fertile – in other words, they have difficulty in conceiving. About one in ten couples have some period of sub-fertility in their lives. The fertility of a couple is the sum of their fertilities, and infertility must therefore be investigated with the co-operation of both partners.

WHAT CAUSES INFERTILITY?

In about 40 percent of infertile couples, the problem lies with the man. About 40 per-cent of cases are due to problems in the woman, and the remainder are due to shared problems of one sort or another.

Male problems

Male problems include the complete inability of the testes to produce sperm (fortunately very rare); low sperm count due to an abnormality of the testes; a larger than normal number of abnormal sperm; and impotence, premature ejaculation or inability to sustain an erection.

Female problems

• Failure to ovulate (release an egg) is the most common cause of female infertility, accounting for about a third of all infertile women.
• It may result from imbalances of the hormones that trigger ovulation, or damage to the ovary from infection, surgery or radiation treatment. Hormones

may interfere with conception in other ways, not just by influencing ovulation. For example, progesterone is needed for a fertilized egg to survive – so the egg would be affected if too little is produced, or for too short a time.

• Healthy female reproductive organs are also essential for conception to occur naturally. Problems with the uterus account for at least ten percent of infertility cases. The uterus may be congenitally abnormal, or contain adhesions (bands of scars), polyps or **fibroids**, or it may be affected by **endometriosis**.

• The Fallopian tubes are the pathways that permit the ascending sperm to reach the egg and then allow the developing embryo to reach the uterus for implantation. An **ectopic pregnancy**, **pelvic inflammatory**

Mutual support

It is important to discuss fertility problems, treatments and fears together, and to comfort and help each other, as you try to find out what the future holds.

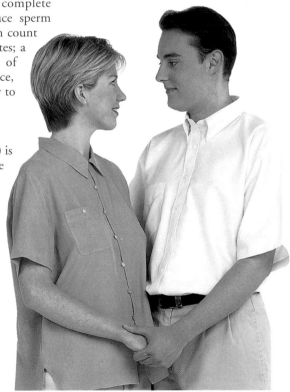

disease, surgical procedures or even an infection of any kind (including sexually transmitted infections) could cause a blockage in the tubes or scarring that would prevent you from conceiving naturally.

• In order to reach an egg to fertilize it, sperm must swim through a large quantity of mucus secreted by the cervix. If the mucus is so thick that the sperm cannot penetrate it, or if it contains antibodies that attack the sperm directly, the sperm will never reach the egg and fertilization cannot therefore occur.

• Age is also a consideration. Around the age of 25, fertility begins to slowly diminish and after the age of 45 only half a woman's cycles are ovulatory. A woman over 45, therefore, has only half as many fertile periods annually as a younger woman.

Shared problems

Between 20 and 30 percent of fertility problems are "shared", usually because of what is called sub-fertility. Sub-fertility occurs when a woman's fertility is marginal, such as when she ovulates infrequently. Usually this only becomes a problem if her partner's fertility is also marginal – if he has a low to average sperm count, for instance - because sub-fertility in one partner can be balanced by strong fertility in the other.

SHOULD I SEE THE DOCTOR?

Whatever your age, if you've been having unprotected sex twice a week for at least a year, and you haven't become pregnant, consult your doctor. However, since some forms of treatment can take several years to complete (see overleaf), you may find that if you are over 35 it is worth consulting your doctor after about six to eight months of unprotected sexual intercourse and failure to conceive.

WHAT WILL THE DOCTOR DO?

• Your doctor will question you closely about your menstrual history, and you may be asked for the dates of your last six periods. You will be asked how long you have been trying to have a baby, when you stopped using contraception and about your family's medical history.

• You'll be asked about your own medical history, including any surgical operations or illnesses that could have a bearing on your fertility, such as anorexia nervosa; and to give details about any specific gynaecological problems you may have experienced, such as **terminations of pregnancy** or sexually transmitted diseases.

• Both you and your partner will also be asked about your frequency of sexual intercourse. Although this may seem too obvious, your doctor will want to rule out the possibility that you are simply not having unprotected intercourse frequently enough to enable conception to occur. There may also be some psycho-sexual difficulties that need to be addressed, and the doctor may therefore refer you to a psycho-sexual counsellor.

• You will then be given a physical examination to check the condition of your reproductive organs and your health in general. The precise examination will depend on your medical history and may involve your doctor looking into your eyes to check the retina or feeling your neck for any differences in your thyroid gland. Your breasts may also be examined to check for normal development.

• Your partner will also be asked about his medical and family history. The doctor will want to know, for example, if his testes did not descend in the normal way. He may also be questioned about his work environment, since environmental factors can sometimes result in a low sperm count. Childhood illnesses, such as mumps, and sexually transmitted diseases are also relevant. The doctor may then examine him to see if there is any obvious physical reason for infertility.

• You and your partner must be honest and thorough in your answers. Investigation of infertility can take a long time and be very

PROBLEMS WITH FERTILITY: CONTINUED

frustrating and sometimes embarrassing. If you are prepared for this, the strain will be easier to bear. While these investigations have been known to cause irreparable damage to a relationship, other couples find that they are brought closer together by the shared experience and their determination to become parents.

• This first examination will help the doctor determine which initial investigations and tests should be carried out. If you are an older woman wanting a first baby, ask for the programme to be speeded up if at all possible as it takes time, and the doctor will optimize the treatment schedule if he can, although different centres have different policies about this.

WHAT TESTS ARE DONE?

• If your doctor suspects some anatomical obstruction is causing the problem, basic tests will be carried out straight away. If, however, there seems to be no immediate and obvious reason for your inability to

conceive, your doctor will first ask your partner to produce a sample of semen for analysis; there wouldn't be much point in carrying on with the various female tests if your partner is found to be infertile. The semen analysis will note the number of sperm, their motility (ability to move) and the number of abnormal sperm.

• The first step in investigating your infertility is to determine whether or not you are ovulating. Your doctor will show you how to put together a basal body temperature (BBT) chart covering a period of three months. This will show whether or not your body temperature rises during the time of ovulation.

• You may also be given a progesterone blood test. If around the middle of your menstrual cycle your blood level contains the normal amount of progesterone, it is assumed you are ovulating.

• Once the semen analysis and preliminary tests have been completed, it should be clear whether it is you or your partner who needs treatment.

WHAT IS THE TREATMENT?

• Actual treatment of course depends on what is thought to be the cause of the infertility, but your doctor is likely to refer you to a specialist fertility clinic for further investigation and help.

• The clinic can employ a whole battery of tests to help discover why you have been unable to conceive, including **ultrasound scanning** of the ovaries to confirm that ovulation is occurring, and **laparoscopy** to determine whether the Fallopian tubes are damaged or blocked, and also to view the uterus for signs of problems that could prevent pregnancy, such as **endometriosis**, **fibroids** or malformations.

• Once the problem has been diagnosed, treatment can usually proceed. This may be by surgery, fertility drugs or assisted conception techniques.

BLOCKED FALLOPIAN TUBES

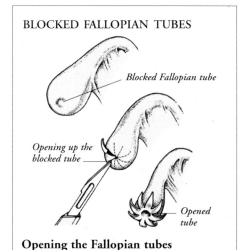

Blocked Fallopian tube

Opening up the blocked tube

Opened tube

Opening the Fallopian tubes
If Fallopian tubes are blocked (top), they can be opened up (centre) with micro-surgery. This enables the opened tube to carry sperm to the egg to fertilize it.

SURGICAL TECHNIQUES

• Blocked Fallopian tubes may be opened with a microsurgical technique known as salpingostomy. **Ovarian cysts** and fibroids can also be removed surgically.

• Other surgical procedures may also have to be considered if you have miscarried recurrently and are unable to carry a baby to term. Abnormalities in the shape of the uterus and an incompetent cervix are two reasons why this happens.

FERTILITY DRUGS

• Fertility drugs are used when a hormone defect has been diagnosed. Specific therapy will be tailored according to your particular needs and often involves more than one drug. The risk of multiple pregnancy is increased and other side-effects of this treatment may include headaches, hot flushes and abdominal pain because the ovaries are enlarged.

• You may be given Clomiphene, which creates a period and then encourages the pituitary gland to secrete oestrogen so that the ovaries produce an egg. Throughout this therapy, during which the drugs are only administered for short periods of time during the cycle, your doctor will check your ovaries with an ultrasound scan to see if ovulation is occurring.

• If this treatment does not succeed in stimulating the ovaries, a daily injection of hMG (human menopausal gonadotrophin) may be given to encourage the ovary to release an egg.

ASSISTED CONCEPTION

• Many childless couples have been helped by techniques to assist conception. These include sperm or egg donation and in vitro fertilization (IVF). However, emotional costs can be high, and it is essential that all the issues involved should be discussed thoroughly before you proceed. Counselling for couples who are considering an assisted conception is provided by fertility clinics and hospitals.

ISSUES TO CONSIDER

There are a number of issues you need to resolve before embarking on what can be an emotional and long-lasting attempt to become pregnant.

• If you were to have a child using donor sperm or eggs, or both, would the fact that the child wasn't "yours" genetically, prevent you from loving him or her as your own?

• Would you feel jealous if a donor's sperm or eggs were used to conceive a child with your partner?

• Would you tell your child how he or she was conceived, or would you try to keep it a secret?

• If you intend to keep it a secret, can you be sure that the truth won't come out, perhaps destructively, during a time of crisis?

• If your child was conceived by the use of donor sperm or eggs, how would you cope if your child wanted to trace his or her genetic parent in later life?

• How long would you persist with infertility treatment?

• What would you do with frozen sperm, eggs or embryos that you do not use?

• Could you cope with a multiple pregnancy? What if one, some, or all of the babies died?

• You should also be aware that in vitro fertilization is a very time-consuming process. If you opt for a non-private IVF clinic, for example, your first appointment may be as much as two years after the date of your first referral. Even when you are eventually accepted for IVF, your treatment may then be delayed by a further year or more. This means that it could be up to four years from the time of referral to receiving treatment, which can be a very long time to wait if you have postponed having a family until your mid- to late thirties.

PROBLEMS WITH FERTILITY: CONTINUED

SPERM DONATION

The most straightforward type of assisted conception is the artificial insemination of a woman with her partner's or a donor's sperm. Donors are often university or medical students, and hospitals and clinics take great care to ensure that potential donors are in good physical and mental health, and have no known inheritable disorders in their family. Donors are always tested for AIDS. They also try to make sure that your donor has similar physical characteristics to those of your partner.

• All information about the donor is strictly confidential. There is no mention of sperm donation in your maternity records, and your joint names can be given on the baby's birth certificate.

• Before you are inseminated, the clinic will have ascertained that you are ovulating using basal body temperature (BBT) charts or a luteinizing hormone (LH) predictor kit. An ultrasound scan just before ovulation can detect follicle growth and, if necessary, you will be given hormones to stimulate ovulation. The donor's sperm is then introduced into your cervical canal or uterus using a syringe.

• Donor insemination can seem to be the ideal solution for many couples, but there are a number of points that should be carefully considered. First and foremost, the feelings of your partner need to be considered. It is not uncommon, for instance, for men to feel inadequate or jealous when a donor's sperm is used to impregnate their partners. In addition, some women are very repelled by the circumstances in which they conceive or by the fact that a different man's sperm can be used at each visit.

EGG DONATION

If a woman is unable to produce an egg of her own, those of a donor may be used instead. The egg is fertilized with your partner's sperm by in vitro fertilization (see below). This has the advantage that both of you are involved in the process: your partner fertilizes the egg and you will carry and give birth to the baby. However, it is a much more complicated procedure than sperm donation.

IN VITRO FERTILIZATION

Since the first test-tube baby was successfully delivered in 1978, tens of thousands of babies have been born by what is called in vitro fertilization (IVF). *In vitro* simply means "in glass", and refers to the glass dish in which sperm and eggs are combined in the laboratory. IVF involves the removal of eggs from the ovaries, fertilization with sperm in the laboratory and transferral of the early embryos into the uterus. The process is as follows:

• First, a test is carried out to ensure that the sperm count is healthy. Then the eggs are collected. Most women only produce one egg per cycle, but because IVF needs several eggs, the ovaries are stimulated to produce more. This involves suppressing the woman's normal cycle, then stimulating the ovaries with special hormone injections so that they produce a number of eggs simultaneously. Over the next week or so, you will make several visits to the clinic so that the development of the eggs can be carefully monitored.

• To collect the eggs, a gynaecologist will use ultrasound to give a clear picture of the reproductive tract. He or she will guide a thin, hollow probe in through the vagina and towards the ovary. Eggs are drawn into the probe by a gentle suction action. The probe is then withdrawn and the eggs are incubated for 24 hours.

• Once the eggs are fully mature, they are carefully placed in a culture medium with 100,000–200,000 sperm from your partner or donor for about 12–15 hours to allow fertilization to take place.

• Alternatively, a single sperm is injected into the centre of the egg through a glass pipette only one-tenth the width of a human hair. This technique is known as ICSI (intracytoplasmic sperm injection).

• After two or three days in an incubator, a maximum of three of the best embryos are then transferred into your uterus. To minimize the risk of having twins, triplets or even more multiple births, many fertility centres suggest implanting no more than two embryos at a time.

OTHER TECHNIQUES

Some fertility specialists use a number of other techniques to try to bring about a successful pregnancy.

• One such is GIFT (gamete intra-Fallopian transfer). Rather than fertilizing the egg in the laboratory, in this method the sperm and egg are transferred together into the open end of a Fallopian tube, which thereby allows fertilization to occur naturally. The resulting embryo can then arrive in the uterus at the correct point in the cycle, allowing implantation to occur. The essential requirement for this is that at least one of your Fallopian tubes must be healthy, and the drawback is that you have no idea if fertilization has occurred, let alone implantation.

• One week after the day of egg retrieval, a blood sample is taken so that your progesterone level can be measured. If you have not had a period by about 16 days after retrieval, a test is then done to detect the pregnancy hormone beta-hCG. Finding the hormone present confirms to your doctor that at least one of the embryos has implanted successfully.

• The actual number of implanted embryos can be ascertained as early as 28 days after implantation, by using ultrasound.

WHAT IS THE OUTLOOK?

Only about ten percent of couples achieve pregnancy on the first attempt at in vitro fertilization and the overall success rate, leading to the birth of a healthy baby, is about 12–14 percent. With repeated IVF cycles, however, the pregnancy rate rises considerably to exceed 50 percent.

SEE ALSO:
Ectopic Pregnancy
Endometriosis
Fibroids
Laparoscopy
Ovarian Cysts
Pelvic Inflammatory Disease
Sexual Problems
Termination of Pregnancy
Ultrasound Scan

MISCARRIAGE

Sometimes called spontaneous abortion, this refers to the loss of a fetus before 24 weeks of pregnancy. The use of the word "abortion" sometimes leads to misunderstanding, but doctors use it to describe any pregnancy that ends suddenly, whether artificially or from natural causes.

Spontaneous abortions are much more common than is generally thought. Many miscarriages go undetected and many are unreported. In fact, up to a third of all first pregnancies miscarry. Excluding unrecognized miscarriages, spontaneous miscarriage occurs in about 15 percent of all conceptions. There is usually a very good reason why a miscarriage occurs during the first trimester of a pregnancy.

SYMPTOMS
- *Bleeding from the vagina, either spotting or heavier*
- *Mucus in blood that has leaked from the vagina*
- *Backache and/or abdominal cramps*
- *Disappearance of the signs of pregnancy*

WHAT CAUSES IT?

A spontaneous abortion can result because of parental, fetal or combined factors. These include:
- Defect in the egg or sperm resulting in an abnormal fetus.
- Abnormally shaped uterus which cannot sustain a pregnancy because of some anatomical problem.
- Uterine **fibroids**.
- Incompetent cervix in which the cervix opens rather than remains closed until labour begins; this is often the result of an unskilled induced abortion or a previous rapid labour.
- Placental insufficiency; the placenta fails or does not develop properly and so cannot nourish the fetus.

- Uncontrolled diabetes or very severe high blood pressure.
- Rhesus incompatibility.
- Maternal infections – bacterial or viral such as **syphilis** or rubella.

SHOULD I SEE THE DOCTOR?

If you know you are pregnant, or think you might be, and experience any vaginal bleeding and/or cramping pain at any time, ring your doctor immediately.

While you are waiting for your doctor, go to bed and keep your feet raised. Wear a sanitary pad if necessary. Do not flush away any of the discharge as your doctor will want to examine it.

WHAT WILL THE DOCTOR DO?

- With a threatened abortion, you will be advised to go to bed for 24 hours to wait and see – bedrest helps by increasing the flow of blood to the uterus.
- Low hormonal levels usually lead to a miscarriage; you will be advised to rest, although unfortunately it probably won't make any difference to the outcome.
- An **ultrasound scan** will determine whether the fetus is still alive or not, or whether there is any tissue left inside your uterus. In some cases of miscarriage there may be a large loss of blood, necessitating a blood transfusion.

WHAT IS THE SURGICAL TREATMENT?

- If some products of conception remain after an incomplete abortion (see panel, right), you will need to be admitted to hospital for an ERPC to remove it. (ERPC stands for "evacuation of the retained products of conception".)
- If there is a "missed abortion", the fetus will have to be removed surgically or by an induced labour. If you miscarry several times recurrently, you will have tests to try to find the specific cause.

• You may be given a **hysterosalpingo-gram** to check out the condition of your uterus and Fallopian tubes.
• Your doctor will examine the aborted fetus and placenta as well in order to treat you accordingly. In some cases, you may be referred to an infertility expert.
• If you have a septic abortion, which means that your internal organs have become infected, you will be given antibiotics in large doses to combat infection, which is the most frequent cause of maternal death following abortion.
• An ERPC will be essential to remove the infected material, as infertility can result from such an infection.

WHAT CAN I DO?

• Whatever the reason for the miscarriage and whatever the treatment your doctor prescribes, the emotional effects can be devastating. As well as the natural feelings of grief, you will probably feel angry that your body has let you down.
• The one emotion you must try to combat is guilt. It is not your fault and, although you may feel like hiding yourself away and perhaps punishing yourself, this is not the way to get back to normal. Try not to isolate yourself and try to be positive about what you can do in the future.
• Anxiety is one of the emotional factors that can result in a failure to conceive. Your doctor should give you an honest answer as soon as possible about whether you can successfully carry a baby to full term without medical treatment. If he says it's possible, keep trying, but try not to become obsessive. If you have a problem that can be treated, don't waste time – seek treatment.
• A miscarriage is a true bereavement and is very difficult to cope with. Counselling might help and is available. If you think you'd benefit from this, ask your doctor to put you in touch with a counsellor.
• You can usually resume sexual intercourse within about three weeks, when the bleeding has stopped and the cervix has

---

TYPES OF MISCARRIAGE

There are several types of first trimester miscarriage (spontaneous abortion):
• *Threatened miscarriage* where there is spotting of blood, sometimes when the period would have been due, but the cervix is closed. This does not invariably lead to the loss of the fetus.
• *Inevitable miscarriage,* which is accompanied by more severe vaginal bleeding and pain because the uterus is contracting. Virtually nothing can prevent the expulsion of the fetus. Inevitable miscarriages are either complete (when both the fetus and placenta are expelled) or incomplete (when the fetus is expelled but parts of the placenta remain).
• *Missed abortion* in which the fetus dies in the uterus but remains there.
• *Recurrent or habitual miscarriage* in which a woman has three or more miscarriages that have occurred at the same time and for the same reason in each pregnancy.
• *Induced abortion* in which the pregnancy is terminated by medical means.

closed. You will probably be advised to wait for at least two complete menstrual periods before trying to conceive again.

SEE ALSO:
D&C/ERPC
Fertility Problems
Fibroids
Hysterosalpingogram
Laparoscopy
Syphilis
Termination of Pregnancy
Ultrasound Scan

ECTOPIC PREGNANCY

When a pregnancy develops in an organ other than the uterus, it is known as an ectopic pregnancy. The most common site is in one of the Fallopian tubes, but the fertilized embryo can very occasionally implant on other organs within the pelvis. The egg is fertilized in the Fallopian tube, and if the tube is damaged in any way, the egg may become stuck there. Ectopic pregnancies occur in about one out of every hundred pregnancies and are more common in first pregnancies, if you have an IUD, are taking the progesterone-only contraceptive pill and with postcoital contraception.

SYMPTOMS
- *Missed period, nausea and tiredness*
- *Colicky type of abdominal pain*
- *Unexpected vaginal bleeding, which could be mistaken for an early miscarriage*
- *Pallor, sweating and faintness if you have internal bleeding*
- *Sharp shoulder pain*
- *Shock; hot and cold flushes and dizziness*

IS IT SERIOUS?

An ectopic pregnancy is always serious because the fetus inevitably outgrows the Fallopian tube through which it bursts, leading to haemorrhage, shock, pelvic infection, peritonitis and, if untreated, collapse and death.

SHOULD I SEE THE DOCTOR?

If there is any chance you could be pregnant and you are suffering pain in either the right or left side of your lower abdomen, consult your doctor immediately. Women with a history of **pelvic inflammatory disease** (PID) are particularly at risk. Home pregnancy tests are not reliable in tubal pregnancies, so don't hesitate even if you had a negative result on the test.

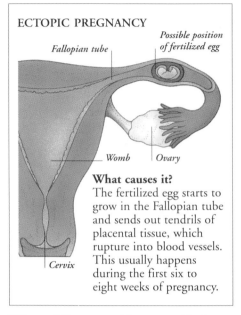

ECTOPIC PREGNANCY

Fallopian tube

Possible position of fertilized egg

Womb | *Ovary*

Cervix

What causes it?
The fertilized egg starts to grow in the Fallopian tube and sends out tendrils of placental tissue, which rupture into blood vessels. This usually happens during the first six to eight weeks of pregnancy.

WHAT WILL THE DOCTOR DO?

- It is possible your doctor will be able to feel the pregnancy by examining your abdomen externally. **Ultrasound scanning** is also used as a diagnostic procedure.
- If a tubal pregnancy is detected, you will need surgery. A specialist will probably perform a **laparoscopy** prior to removal of the pregnancy. If the ectopic pregnancy has burst, the Fallopian tube, possibly even your ovary, will be removed.

ARE THERE ANY COMPLICATIONS?

Even if the surgeon can save the Fallopian tube, it may heal with scar tissue, impeding the passage of the ovum on that side.

SEE ALSO:
Contraception
Fertility Problems
Laparoscopy
Pelvic Inflammatory Disease
Ultrasound Scan

8

INVESTIGATIONS AND OPERATIONS

From time to time, various investigations and operations will be recommended to us, and it is important in making a choice between one form of treatment and another that we understand precisely what is being offered so that we can decide, with our doctors, which is more appropriate for us. Here, the common tests of adult female life and the reasons for them, such as cervical smear and ultrasound, are explained, and surgical operations such as hysterectomy are described and their consequences revealed.

PELVIC EXAMINATION

A pelvic examination is a routine diagnostic check on the health of your pelvic organs and should be done regularly after the age of 35. The first part is an external manual examination of the abdomen, followed by an internal examination, first manual and then by speculum. Although it is uncomfortable, a pelvic examination is not painful.

WHY IS IT DONE?

Pelvic examinations are done as a matter of routine in Well-woman clinics and as an investigation for symptoms such as irregular bleeding, pelvic pain and bladder problems. Other reasons include:

• As a general check before you are prescribed any form of contraception: the contraceptive pill, fitting of an IUD, diaphragm or cervical cap; if a **cervical smear** test is being done; if you have had any bleeding after intercourse.

• To check on any unusual or smelly vaginal discharge so that a sample can be taken for laboratory investigation.

• If you suffer from irregular or unusually heavy menstrual bleeding, any bleeding between periods, or if you have any pain during intercourse (dyspareunia).

• If you suspect that you might have contracted a venereal disease, with any symptoms of pain when passing urine, or sores on the genital area.

• If your mother took the drug DES during her pregnancy.

HOW IS IT DONE?

• An internal examination is done while you lie on your back or your side. Your doctor will do a preliminary manual examination by placing one or two fingers inside the vagina and the other hand on top of the abdomen. In this way, the doctor can feel a cyst, for example, between his or her two hands and get some idea of size, shape and texture.

• The speculum examination is an integral part of an internal pelvic examination. The speculum is a plastic or metal instrument shaped somewhat like a duck's bill, which is inserted into the vagina in order to separate the walls of the vagina so that the cervix can be examined.

• A warm, lubricated speculum is inserted with the blades closed. Once inside your vagina, the blades are gently opened so that the cervix and the walls of the vagina can be checked visually.

PELVIC EXAMINATION

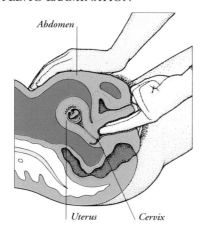

Abdomen

Uterus   Cervix

Manual examination
The size, shape and any abnormalities of the uterus and other organs, are checked by placing the index and middle fingers inside the vagina and pressing down with the other hand on the abdomen.

SEE ALSO:
Cervical Smear
Contraception
Fertility Problems
Genital Problems
Menstrual Problems
Painful Intercourse
Prolapse
Sexually Transmitted Diseases

CERVICAL SMEAR

Also known as the Pap smear after the doctor who originated it, this procedure takes place during a **pelvic examination**. It is used primarily to detect precancerous and cancerous cells on the cervix.

WHY IS IT DONE?

Cervical smears should be performed on all women once they begin having intercourse and then every three years up to the age of 60 – more frequently for women taking the contraceptive pill and those whose mothers were prescribed the drug DES during their pregnancies. The test is also important for those infected with **genital warts**, as this carries a higher risk of cancer. The test also detects urogenital viral infections and sexually transmitted diseases.

HOW IS IT DONE?

• A warmed speculum is passed into the vagina to separate the walls so the doctor can see the condition of your cervix.
• A wooden spatula is wiped across the cervix, and the smear is transferred to a glass slide and sent to a laboratory for analysis.
• The results should be available within six weeks. You should not be menstruating or have had sexual intercourse 24 hours before your test because blood and semen make the results unreliable.

TEST RESULTS

The results of a smear test are classified into four or five categories. Negative gives you the all-clear, some mild dysplasia means that you have some infection and should be screened more regularly, and a positive smear test, though not always indicating cancer, means there is a detectable change in the cells necessitating further investigation. Results and the action needed are as follows:
• Negative: No follow-up needed; next smear in three years' time.
• The mildest inflammation known as mild dysplasia, or CIN I: another smear test in

---

**PERFORMING
A SMEAR TEST**

How is it done?
You lie on your back (right).
A speculum is inserted into your vagina then opened to provide a clear view of the cervix.

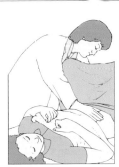

THE PROCEDURE

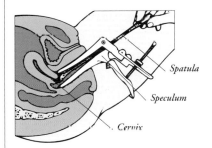

Spatula

Speculum

Cervix

What happens
A spatula is used to scrape cells from the cervix. These are smeared on to a glass slide and sent to a laboratory to be examined. The whole thing takes less than a minute and is not painful.

---

six months' time.
• More severe inflammation called moderate dysplasia or CIN II: **colposcopy**.
• Severe dysplasia with or without non-invasive cancer, or CIN III: colposcopy with or without **cone biopsy**.

SEE ALSO:
**Cervical Cancer
Colposcopy
Cone Biopsy/LETZ
Genital Herpes
Genital Warts
Pelvic Examination**

COLPOSCOPY

Colposcopy is the visual examination of the cervix and vagina, usually recommended after a positive **cervical smear**. It is done by using a colposcope, a magnifying instrument that allows the doctor to get a clear, illuminated view of the area.

Colposcopy is a simple, non-invasive procedure and can be used as a treatment as well as a diagnostic tool. It requires no anaesthetic and can be done in your doctor's surgery.

WHY IS IT DONE?

A colposcopy is recommended to investigate further any abnormalities indicated by a positive smear or, occasionally, by a **pelvic examination**. The colposcope has a series of powerful lenses that pinpoint much more precisely where any abnormal cells occur, and enables the doctor to obtain a biopsy sample for further investigation.

HOW IS IT DONE?

• The doctor will ask you to remove your lower garments and then to lie on your back with your knees raised and apart, supported in stirrups.
• A speculum is inserted into your vagina as for a smear test, the vaginal mucus wiped away and the area washed with either a saline solution or a dilute acetic acid. These solutions are used because they cause abnormal cells to show up either white or patterned on the colposcope instead of the usual pink colour.
• The colposcope is placed at the entrance to the vagina – it never actually enters the vagina itself. The doctor examines the tissue to identify the precise area of abnormal cells. (A smear test only shows that there is some change but does not pinpoint where.) He will then remove the speculum slowly so that he can inspect the vaginal walls too.
• The procedure takes roughly 15 minutes. Sometimes, using special forceps, your doctor will take a biopsy of abnormal tissue

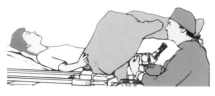

COLPOSCOPY

Telescopic sights
The colposcope is one of the most versatile pieces of equipment in a modern hospital. It is used widely by doctors to monitor pregnancies and pelvic problems, as well as to check on the progress of fertility treatments.

he can see through the lens of the colposcope and this will be sent to a laboratory for further examination.
• If a biopsy is taken, you may have some slight bleeding, but there should be no other side-effects.
• If there are abnormal cells inside the cervical canal, a colposcope will not be able to detect them; if this is suspected, a **cone biopsy** will be recommended, to check on cells from inside the canal.
• If a biopsy sample indicates precancerous change only, the affected tissue can be destroyed by laser treatment or by burning away with a hot loop (**LLETZ**).

SEE ALSO:
Cervical Cancer
Cervical Smear
Cone Biopsy/LLETZ
Pelvic Examination

ENDOMETRIAL BIOPSY

Endometrial biopsy involves removing a small amount of tissue from the lining of the uterus (endometrium) in order to examine it for any abnormality. It is a very common procedure that can be performed under a general anaesthetic, although nowadays it is often done under local anaesthetic during an outpatient visit to the hospital.

As a woman gets older, it becomes more difficult in general to obtain an adequate amount of tissue using this technique, and a **hysteroscopy** and **D&C** may be a more appropriate procedure, especially if the abnormal bleeding persists.

WHY IS IT DONE?

The procedure may be carried out to help determine why a woman is suffering from heavy, irregular or prolonged periods. If an older woman starts to bleed after the menopause, a sample of tissue is also needed to exclude a malignant cause for the bleeding. Occasionally, bleeding after intercourse may lead a doctor to suspect an abnormality in the cells lining the uterus and a biopsy may be performed.

HOW IS IT DONE?

• You will be asked to lie down on a couch in the clinic. A fine plastic "straw-like" instrument is passed into the uterus, via the vagina and cervix, to obtain a piece of tissue that is removed by suction.

• The majority of women tolerate the procedure well; however, some women may find it uncomfortable. Very occasionally the procedure will not be successful, due to a very tight cervix which does not allow the biopsy instrument to pass through it or because the procedure is too uncomfortable for the woman.

• After the biopsy you may find that you have some mild spotting for a day or two. If the investigation was performed with a local anaesthetic, you will normally be able to go home immediately afterwards. However, if you have been given a general anaesthetic, you will need to stay in the hospital for a few hours to recover.

• The tissue biopsy may take a few weeks to be analyzed by the pathology department. You will normally be seen again in the outpatient department in order to go over the result of the biopsy.

• Depending on what is found, the doctor may decide that no further treatment is required, or he can arrange further investigations, which may include an **ultrasound** examination of the uterus as well as a hysteroscopy and D&C. More extensive surgery, such as a **hysterectomy**, may be necessary if the cells that are removed from the uterus are found to be malignant.

WHAT CAN I DO?

Discuss with the doctor the exact reasons why it is thought necessary for you to have an endometrial biopsy; don't be afraid to ask questions about anything you are not clear about.

SEE ALSO:
D&C/ERPC
Hysterectomy
Hysteroscopy
Menstrual Problems
Ultrasound Scan
Uterine Cancer

HYSTEROSCOPY

Hysteroscopy involves examining the inside of the uterus with a small telescopic camera that is passed through the cervix. Hysteroscopy can either be performed under a general anaesthetic, when it is often combined with a **D&C**, or in the outpatient clinic. Various hysteroscopic procedures have been developed to treat specific problems.

WHY IS IT DONE?

Hysteroscopy is used to examine the inside of the uterus to make sure the lining (endometrium) appears normal, and to check for growths. These may be benign, such as polyps, or malignant. It is an integral part of the investigations to find out the cause of heavy or frequent periods or bleeding between periods. It is also performed on older women to investigate postmenopausal bleeding.

Hysteroscopy also has a role in removing misplaced or difficult-to-locate IUDs and, in the investigation of infertility, to check that the uterus is structurally normal.

HOW IS IT DONE?

• The procedure involves passing the hysteroscope into the cavity of the uterus. If the procedure is being performed in the outpatient clinic you may be given pain-killers about 1–2 hours beforehand, and occasionally a local anaesthetic will be injected in and around the cervix to help relieve any discomfort.

• In order to obtain a good view of the cavity, it has to be distended using either a harmless gas such as carbon dioxide, or liquid. The doctor will visually inspect the inside of the uterus, making a note of any abnormal areas.

• If it is carried out under a general anaesthetic, the procedure is often followed by a D&C.

• Other procedures may be carried out using specially adapted hysteroscopes. The lining of the uterus can be burned away to help treat heavy periods. This is useful if there is no evidence of malignancy, if drug treatments for heavy periods have been unsuccessful and to avoid a **hysterectomy**.

• Infertility treatments occasionally use hysteroscopic instruments to divide scar tissue in the uterus and to help correct any congenital structural abnormalities affecting the uterine cavity, including the removal of **fibroids** within the cavity of the uterus.

• For a few days after a hysteroscopy you may notice some spotting. Most women go home the day of the operation. However, some may be required to stay in hospital for a few days if the hysteroscopy has been combined with an operative procedure.

• In experienced hands, complications of hysteroscopy are uncommon but they can, rarely, include uterine infection and perforation if an additional procedure is being performed, such as endometrial resection.

WHAT CAN I DO?

Make sure that you understand why the procedure is being performed and what is going to be achieved. Hysteroscopy is usually not performed if you are pregnant and is best avoided if you are suffering from **pelvic inflammatory disease**.

SEE ALSO:

D&C
Fibroids
Hysterectomy
Menstrual Problems
Pelvic Inflammatory Disease

ULTRASOUND SCAN

This is a way of producing a photographic picture by using sound waves. The picture is formed by the echoes of sound waves bouncing off different parts of the body. The echoes differ in their waves according to the density of the organ. Ultrasound scanning can give pictures of soft tissue in great detail. If it is done during pregnancy, it will show fetal heartbeat and movement. An accurate picture of the fetus *in utero* may be printed out that can be used as a non-invasive means of examining the fetus.

Imaging from sound waves
Ultrasound uses sound waves to look inside the body. The waves are converted into electric signals from the receiver and processed by the computer to form a video image on the linked monitor.

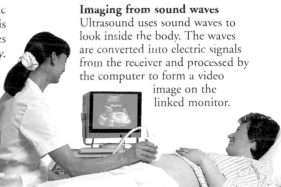

WHY IS IT DONE?

Ultrasound is used in many areas of medicine as a diagnostic tool, particularly to detect breast lumps and the cause of abdominal pains, such as gallstones or hiatus hernia. It can also sometimes be used to treat abnormalities. For example, high levels of ultrasound waves can destroy stones in the bladder. In gynaecological investigations ultrasound is used:

• To detect endometrial thickness.
• To detect **fibroids**.
• To investigate **uterine cancer**.
• To detect polyps.
• To investigate swollen tubes.
• To investigate **ovarian cancer**.
• To detect an **ectopic pregnancy**.

Ultrasound scanning is also used widely in fertility treatment and to tell whether a pregnancy is viable or not.

HOW IS IT DONE?

• The procedure is painless and takes about five to ten minutes. It is done when the bladder is full.
• Warm oil is poured over your stomach and a receiver is passed over it by the technician. The receiver passes back signals that show up on a black and white monitor.
• If you have ultrasound during pregnancy, it is particularly exciting to see your baby in the womb; modern ultrasound monitors can show the baby moving. Ask the technician to point out the head, limbs and organs to you.

WHAT ARE THE RISKS?

• There appear to be no risks to the unborn child or to the mother, but there is no evidence that it is completely safe either. However most centres try to use ultrasound sparingly on pregnant women. Scans are only done during pregnancy if doctors and midwives think it advisable.
• If you are extremely worried about something, such as having twins, then your doctor would probably comply with your request for an ultrasound scan. Older women tend to be scanned more frequently.

HYSTEROSALPINGOGRAM

This is an X-ray picture of the womb and Fallopian tubes. In the simplest form, the outline of the organs is achieved by pumping up the abdominal cavity with air or carbon dioxide, known as tubal insufflation. This gives a sufficiently clear picture to determine whether the cavity of the uterus is clear and that the Fallopian tubes are not blocked. If a more accurate and detailed picture is required, such as precisely where the blockage is, a radio-opaque dye can be injected directly into the uterus and tubes so that their cavities show up on X-ray. If there is no blockage, the dye passes into the cavity and is harmlessly reabsorbed into the body. A blockage of either the uterus or the Fallopian tubes can be easily seen because the dye does not flow beyond it.

WHY IS IT DONE?

An hysterosalpingogram (HSG) is most commonly used as part of investigations for infertility. It may also be performed after an **ectopic pregnancy** to establish the site and extent of scarring or deformity, or a blockage of the Fallopian tubes. The X-ray pictures will show whether there is any distortion in the uterine cavity, such as that caused by a **fibroid** or polyp. It will also show if the Fallopian tubes are blocked and pinpoint where the blockage occurs. What it can't do with any accuracy is show the state of the organs, and if there is any doubt remaining after the hysterosalpingogram, the doctor will probably arrange for you to undergo a **laparoscopy** so that the organs can be viewed directly. Laparoscopy has largely replaced HSG because of this.

HOW IS IT DONE?

• Usually HSG takes 10 minutes and can be done either under a local anaesthetic or without anaesthetic. It is performed on an outpatient basis, which is quite safe and allows you to go home on the same day.

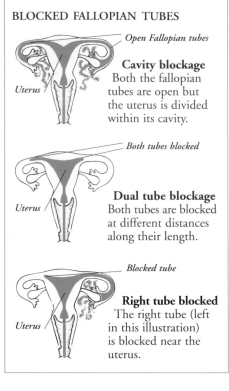

BLOCKED FALLOPIAN TUBES

Open Fallopian tubes

Cavity blockage
Both the fallopian tubes are open but the uterus is divided within its cavity.
Uterus

Both tubes blocked

Dual tube blockage
Both tubes are blocked at different distances along their length.
Uterus

Blocked tube

Right tube blocked
The right tube (left in this illustration) is blocked near the uterus.
Uterus

• Firstly, the cervix is exposed by the insertion of a speculum into the vagina. A hollow metal tube is passed through the cervix, and a radio-opaque dye injected into the uterus and X-rays taken.

WHAT ARE THE RISKS?

This is not a difficult procedure although, as the dye is injected into the uterus, there may be some cramping sensations. It is painful, so take painkillers beforehand.

SEE ALSO:
Ectopic Pregnancy
Fertility Problems
Fibroids
Laparoscopy

LAPAROSCOPY

Certain conditions can be diagnosed accurately only if the organs are directly seen. Laparoscopy is a procedure that enables a doctor to see both the inside of the abdominal cavity and organs such as the gallbladder, liver and uterus through an instrument called a laparoscope.

The most common use of laparoscopy is in gynaecology. The procedure is used to view the pelvis and pelvic organs. The long metal tube with a lens and a light at one end and a telescope at the other allows the abdominal cavity to be seen through the telescopic eyepiece.

WHY IS IT DONE?

The advantages of laparoscopy are that the patient suffers less than with other, more invasive, procedures, and that the surgeon obtains a better view of the internal organs. Laparoscopy is most commonly used for the following:

- Tubal surgery, including **sterilization**.
- Infertility investigations.
- **Ovarian cysts**.
- **Fibroids**.
- **Ectopic pregnancy**.
- Laparoscopic **hysterectomy**.
- Bladder operations for stress incontinence.

HOW IS IT DONE?

- If laparoscopy is for a minor operation such as tubal ligation, you may be offered an epidural anaesthetic, but generally it is done under a general anaesthetic.
- A tiny cut is made in the abdomen, usually just below the navel so that no scar is visible afterwards. A needle is inserted into the abdomen and carbon dioxide gas is pumped into the abdominal cavity so that organs can be visualized.
- The laparoscope is passed in and the doctor can angle it to get a clear view. If other instruments are being used, these are inserted through a second incision above the pubic line.

- The procedure usually takes about 30–40 minutes and you will have one or two stitches in the skin.
- After about two hours, depending on the reason for the laparoscopy, you should be allowed to go home.
- You may have a little discomfort from any gas that remains in your pelvic cavity, and the incision site may be sore. However, laparoscopy is very safe and you should have few problems.

SEE ALSO:
Ectopic Pregnancy
Fertility Problems
Fibroids
Ovarian Cysts
Pelvic Inflammatory Disease
Sterilization

MYOMECTOMY

Myomectomy is the name given to the operation to remove **fibroids**, which are benign growths of muscular tissue in the wall of the uterus. Fibroids, which may be single or multiple, can grow to a large size and may be in the wall of the uterus or within its cavity.

WHY IS IT DONE?

Myomectomy allows for the removal of fibroids without the necessity for a **hysterectomy**, so is generally reserved for those women who have not yet completed their families. Occasionally, if you have large multiple fibroids or if there is a suspicion of malignancy, your doctor may recommend a hysterectomy rather than a myomectomy.

HOW IS IT DONE?

• Myomectomy is performed under a general anaesthetic. The doctor may ask for your agreement in advance for proceeding to a hysterectomy if the myomectomy is too technically difficult.

• Prior to surgery you will probably have an **ultrasound** examination of your uterus to help determine the size and number of fibroids. Some doctors may treat you with special drugs over a period of several months to help shrink the fibroids prior to surgery, especially if they are very bulky. This often helps the surgeon make the smallest possible incision and can minimize blood loss during the operation.

• The operation involves making an incision in the abdomen. This incision is either along the "bikini line" – a Pfannenstiel incision – or occasionally, because of the size of the fibroids, it may be lengthways (a midline incision), along the centre of the abdomen.

• The operation involves making small cuts along the surface of the uterus and then removing each fibroid individually. The operation may take quite a long time to complete, especially if multiple fibroids are found or if they are in particularly difficult-to-reach positions.

• Post-operative management involves an intravenous drip to provide fluid and nutrients, a catheter to help drain away urine and an abdominal drain to help get rid of any blood that may leak from the uterus. After the operation, you will be required to stay in hospital for seven to ten days. You will normally be seen in the outpatient department six weeks after the operation.

ARE THERE ANY SIDE-EFFECTS?

• Myomectomy can be a technically difficult operation. Blood loss can be significant, which may mean that a blood transfusion will have to be given. In addition, it does not remove small "seedling" fibroids, which over the years could grow to cause troublesome symptoms again.

• Women who are experiencing difficulties in conceiving because of fibroids must remember that removing fibroids does not necessarily guarantee that a successful pregnancy will be possible.

WHAT CAN I DO?

• You must make sure that you discuss the possibility of a hysterectomy fully with your doctor before surgery is attempted, and come to a mutual understanding.

• Be prepared for quite a long post-operative recovery period. You will have had a long operation and possibly blood loss, and your body will need time to recover.

SEE ALSO:
Fibroids
Hysterectomy
Menstrual Problems
Ultrasound Scan

HYSTERECTOMY

A hysterectomy is the surgical removal of the uterus. In the United States, 25 percent of all women over 50 have had simple or radical hysterectomies (see below). The operation is often performed for no good reason, such as the removal of small **fibroids**. Some doctors even advocate it once child-bearing is over to forestall the risk of cancer, which is unjustified.

In Britain, until recently there has been a reluctance by doctors to remove the uterus unless the symptoms really warranted it, and not without full discussion and perhaps a second opinion. However, in some cases the American attitude is creeping in. The decision to have a hysterectomy should never be taken lightly and, in young women, the instant menopause that results must be treated with HRT.

WHY IS IT DONE?

The operation is undertaken for the following reasons:
• To remove cancer in the pelvic organs.
• To treat any severe and uncontrollable pelvic infection.
• To stop severe haemorrhage.
• In certain conditions affecting the intestines and bladder which threaten a woman's life, when it is impossible to deal with the primary problem without removal of the uterus.
• To remove multiple fibroids which are causing bleeding and pain.
• The operation is sometimes done to treat **prolapse**, as a method of **sterilization**, to treat severe **endometriosis**, because of injury to the pelvic muscles at childbirth, severe enough to interfere with bowel and bladder function and for uncontrollable uterine bleeding.

WHAT SHOULD I DO?

• Question your doctor very carefully about the reasons for your hysterectomy and be satisfied in your mind that it is absolutely necessary. Explore all the possible alternatives, and involve your partner and family fully.
• Check to see whether your ovaries need to be removed as well as your uterus, and find out about hormone replacement treatments available for premature menopause if your surgeon insists they should be removed. It is no longer medically accepted that ovaries should be removed in case cancer should develop, so don't be persuaded by this argument.

TYPES OF HYSTERECTOMY

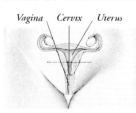

Vagina   Cervix   Uterus

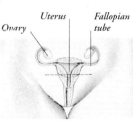

Uterus   Fallopian tube
Ovary

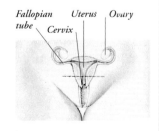

Fallopian tube   Uterus   Ovary
Cervix

Radical hysterectomy
The uterus, cervix, surrounding tissue, lymph glands, part of the vagina, Fallopian tubes and ovaries are all removed.

Subtotal hysterectomy
The uterus only is removed in a subtotal hysterectomy.

Total hysterectomy
The uterus and cervix are removed in a total hysterectomy. The ovaries and Fallopian tubes are left behind.

HYSTERECTOMY: CONTINUED

HOW IS IT DONE?

• For the abdominal route, an incision is made under general anaesthetic in the lower abdomen, and the uterus, and possibly the ovaries and Fallopian tubes, are removed.

• After the operation you will have an intravenous drip for fluids or blood, and perhaps a catheter to drain urine. There will be some discharge from the vagina for a day or two after the operation.

• If your ovaries were removed, hormone replacement treatment will be planned. You will be encouraged to get out of bed after a couple of days.

• Alternatively, you may have a vaginal hysterectomy, in which the abdominal cavity isn't opened but the uterus is removed through the vagina. A woman's recovery is quicker this way and the complications are either minimized or avoided altogether. This is the ideal operation to correct uncomplicated uterine prolapse. Vaginal hysterectomy is only performed if the uterus is not too bulky and if the supporting structures are not too tight.

• An incision is made in the uterus and high in the roof of the vagina, and, if necessary, the ovaries are removed from below.

• The normal hospital stay is five days, and you will be seen in the outpatients department six weeks later. Provided that there are no problems, intercourse can be resumed after this visit.

• A combination approach called LAVH (laparoscopic assisted vaginal hysterectomy) has now become more common. The technique involves using a laparoscope inserted into the abdominal cavity to help perform the operation vaginally.

WHAT CAN I DO?

• When you go home after the operation, maintain a moderate level of activity, but stop the minute you feel pain.

• Gradually build up your strength. Gentle activities can be started by the fourth week after the operation; moderate activity like light shopping or housework can be undertaken by the fifth week. By the sixth week you should start to feel nearly back to normal, though you may still feel tired.

• By the eighth week you can resume sexual intercourse, as the top of the vagina will have healed. There is no reason why sex should be any different for you; many women report increased satisfaction.

ARE THERE PSYCHOLOGICAL CHANGES?

• Nearly half of women who have hysterectomies are satisfied with the operation. The vagina will be the same size as it was before, unless the operation was a radical hysterectomy.

• Dissatisfaction is related to whether the operation was done for a very good reason and after full consideration by the woman of the options available.

• Women who want more children find it difficult, as do those whose ovaries are removed premenopausally.

• The majority of women who suffer depression after hysterectomy are those for whom the operation was undertaken for a non-life-threatening condition. It seems easier to bear if you know that the operation saved your life.

SEE ALSO:
Cervical Cancer
Endometriosis
Fibroids
Laparoscopy
Ovarian Cancer
Pelvic Inflammatory Disease
Prolapse
Sterilization
Uterine Cancer

CONE BIOPSY/LLETZ

A cone biopsy, or conization, is one of the methods used to remove suspect tissue from the cervix for investigation or treatment. It is also known as LLETZ (large loop excision of the transformation zones). **Colposcopy** is the less invasive method of diagnosis and, where available, is preferable for investigating and diagnosing any changes to cervical tissue.

WHY IS IT DONE?

A cone biopsy is performed if one or more **cervical smear** tests indicate dysplasia or the presence of cancerous cells in the cervix. Dysplasia (cell abnormality) occurs if the skin on the outside of the cervix changes. This is symptomless and presents no risk to health, although in some cases cancer develops after a long period of time. It is detected as the result of a routine cervical smear test when some change in the cells is noted. Cone biopsy is performed if a colposcopy has failed to pinpoint the location of the diseased cells. This is most likely to be the case for women over 35, as less of their cervical tissue can be seen on inspection due to retraction caused by age, or when the full extent of suspicious cells cannot be determined accurately.

HOW IS IT DONE?

A cone biopsy is usually performed under a general anaesthetic. The entire area of affected tissue, usually cone-shaped, hence its name, is removed with a scalpel or laser beam. Often a **D&C** will be performed at the same time to check the lining of the uterus for any spread of cancer. The area will be sutured by using diathermy or freezing to reduce bleeding, although it can also sometimes be stitched. The tissue is then sliced and examined microscopically to confirm the diagnosis. Although used as a diagnostic tool for **cervical cancer**, a cone biopsy can result in successful treatment if the entire cancerous area is removed. If this is not so, further surgery or radiotherapy will be required.

WHAT HAPPENS AFTERWARDS?

You will be able to remain in hospital for two or three days. There will probably be some bleeding and this may be staunched by packing your vagina with gauze. If the bleeding recurs, consult your doctor. You will still require regular smear tests.

ARE THERE ANY RISKS?

There is some risk to the cervix with this procedure; the cervical canal may narrow, bringing about some reduction in fertility. Carbon dioxide laser has recently been introduced as another means of removing tissue for analysis. The risk of bleeding and other complications is reduced by using this method and it can also be performed on an outpatient basis.

CONE BIOPSY

Affected area of the cervix

Cone of cervix tissue

Cervical biopsy
After the area of the cervix containing the abnormal cells is removed (above right), the wound is sutured by stitching, diathermy or cryosurgery (freezing).

SEE ALSO:
Cervical Cancer
Cervical Smear
Colposcopy
D&C/ERPC

D&C/ERPC

D&C (dilatation and curettage) is a gynaecological procedure in which the lining of the uterus (endometrium) is scraped away. A form of D&C (in effect a curettage without dilatation) is carried out after an incomplete abortion, when it is called an ERPC (evacuation of the retained products of conception). ERPC is carried out after a **hysteroscopy** has identified what remains in the uterus. A D&C is usually performed under a brief general anaesthetic, on a hospital outpatient basis.

WHY IS IT DONE?

These days, a D&C is usually done to remove the lining of the womb in order to find out the cause of heavy menstrual bleeding (**menorrhagia**), or for other uterine problems such as polyps or misplaced intrauterine coils.

In scraping away the lining, D&C can treat the problems it finds at the same time. It was traditionally used as a means of terminating an early pregnancy, although it is very rarely employed for this purpose these days.

HOW IS IT DONE?

- First, a speculum is inserted into the vagina to separate the vaginal walls so that the cervix can be seen. A series of rods are then inserted to dilate the cervix.
- If the procedure is being performed to check for polyps, the cervix is dilated and a polyps forceps explores the uterine cavity, grasping and removing any polyps that are found. Finally a spoon-shaped instrument, a curette, is inserted into the womb to scrape away the lining.
- The scrapings from the curette are examined for abnormalities under a microscope in a laboratory.
- After the D&C you will need to rest and recover for several hours before going home. You should take it easy for a day or so afterwards, but you shouldn't experience any problems. You can resume sexual relations within a week or so, or whenever you feel comfortable. Your menstrual cycle will recommence within about six weeks.
- To perform an ERPC after an incomplete abortion, the procedure varies a little. There is usually no need to dilate the cervix (it will remain open if any conception material remains), so a sponge forceps is used with a curette to gently clean out the placenta and any fetal material.

DILATATION AND CURETTAGE

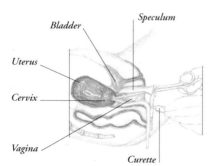

Bladder
Speculum
Uterus
Cervix
Vagina
Curette

A simple procedure
For dilatation, a speculum holds the vaginal walls apart while rods are inserted into the cervix to dilate it. For curettage, a curette is inserted into the womb and the walls are carefully scraped with it.

SEE ALSO:
Endometriosis
Fibroids
Hysteroscopy
Menorrhagia
Menstrual Problems
Miscarriage
Termination of Pregnancy

STERILIZATION

This is a supposedly permanent surgical means of birth control that makes it impossible for an egg to be fertilized and conception to take place.

The simplest sterilization is carried out on men. It involves tying the tubes (*vas deferens*) that connect the testicles to the penis. Ejaculate is still emitted during orgasm, but it contains no sperm and therefore is not capable of fertilizing an ovum. This operation is called a vasectomy and is performed under a local anaesthetic in about 20 minutes. It does not affect virility and sexual performance, nor does it increase susceptibility to illness.

In women, the usual method is tubal ligation, which closes off the Fallopian tubes. This creates an obstruction that stops the ovum moving through to the uterus or sperm from reaching the ovum, thereby preventing conception from taking place.

WHY IS IT DONE?

Sterilization is usually only performed on men or women who have already had children and do not want to have more. As it is a permanent operation that is very difficult to reverse, doctors are generally unwilling to sterilize childless women or women under 30.

For some women the decision is a difficult one. While they may be freed from the fear of having an unwanted pregnancy, they need to come to terms with their feelings about taking this irrevocable step. They may also have to deal with their partner's refusal to have a vasectomy, which is a far less invasive procedure.

HOW IS IT DONE?

• There are several different methods of female sterilization, using either the abdominal or vaginal approach. All are carried out under general anaesthetic or occasionally an epidural.

• Carbon dioxide gas may be introduced into the abdomen to inflate it so that the internal organs can be more clearly seen. While all the procedures involve tying or closing the tubes in some way, a small portion of the tube itself is almost invariably removed.

• Some other forms of surgery, such as **hysterectomy**, result in sterilization, but these operations should never be used solely for this purpose.

• The tubes are either tied or cut, clamped with rings or clips, plugged or frozen. This can be carried out by means of laparotomy, culdoscopy or **laparoscopy**.

STERILIZATION

Male sterilization
In vasectomy, the *vas deferens* (the tube that carries sperm from the testes) is cut in two, the ends bent back and closed to prevent the tube from reforming.

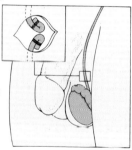

Female sterilization

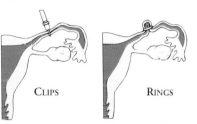

CLIPS   RINGS

Two common ways to carry out female sterilizations are to clip the Fallopian tubes or to close them with a tight elastic ring.

Continued on next page

STERILIZATION: CONTINUED

Mini-laparotomy

First, a slim surgical tool is inserted into the vagina to manipulate the top of the uterus close to the abdominal wall. The surgeon then makes a small incision – about 2.5cm (1in) – into the abdomen, near the uterus, lifts out each Fallopian tube in turn, and clips and ties it.

Laparoscopy

This is the most commonly used technique to perform tubal ligation. A laparoscope, which contains a fibre-optic filament, is inserted into the abdomen, often through a tiny incision in the navel and, under direct vision, the Fallopian tubes are clamped. The stay in hospital should only be one day, but laparoscopy can be done on an outpatient basis at some clinics.

Culdoscopy

In this procedure, an incision is made in the vagina just below the cervix. A clamp on the cervix is used to position the uterus so that the tubes can be seen. The tubes are then brought down one at a time, cut, tied, clipped or blocked.

WHAT ARE THE AFTER-EFFECTS?

• After the sterilization, you won't notice any change in your normal menstrual pattern, and you will have a normal menopause when it occurs because your ovaries have not been affected by the procedure. The ovum produced every month will be absorbed into the body as it would have been normally at any time when fertilization did not occur.

• Some women have a routine **D&C** when they are sterilized; this is a check of the uterus for any growths or problems. Usually there is bleeding from the vagina for a day or two and some local discomfort at the site of any incision. You may also notice pain in your shoulder, caused by irritation from the carbon dioxide gas.

• You may also have a reaction to the general anaesthetic. If you've had a reaction to a general anaesthetic during previous surgery, suggest to your doctor that an epidural might be used.

• If you had a vaginal sterilization, you will not be able to have intercourse for a couple of weeks because of the danger of infection, but you'll have no external scar.

WHAT ARE THE RISKS?

There are few serious risks or complications with any of the methods of sterilization described here, except those normally expected of any surgical procedure. Tubal ligation by the vaginal route has a slightly increased risk of infection.

IS IT EFFECTIVE?

• Sterilization has a higher efficiency rate than any other means of contraception and it is permanent. After the operation no other form of birth control is necessary.

• The operation is considered irreversible, although microsurgery, in a few cases, has succeeded in sewing the tubes back together again. There will be no effect on your libido or sex life.

• Men often feel their potency has been interfered with after vasectomy; but this is only in the mind and has no basis in reality.

SEE ALSO:
Contraception
D&C/ERPC
Hysterectomy
Laparoscopy

TERMINATION OF PREGNANCY

With changes in attitudes to termination of pregnancy, this is now legally performed in the United Kingdom before the 24th week of pregnancy, for both medical and psychological reasons. In some countries, abortion is illegal, and even in those countries where it is allowed, the terms under which it is performed and the time of gestation differ considerably depending on where you live.

Unfortunately there are still many myths about terminating a pregnancy, which may be dangerous. If you are considering terminating a pregnancy, remember that:
• There is nothing you can take by mouth that will safely and efficiently result in a termination of pregnancy.
• Hot baths, bottles of gin and jumping from a great height will not cause abortion if the fetus and placenta are healthy.
• Procuring an illegal abortion may result in heavy bleeding. Any heavy bleeding should be treated immediately. There may be some retained placenta or an infection, which should be treated as an emergency.

WHAT ARE THE RISKS?

On average, five women die each year in England and Wales from an abortion. Medically induced abortion, whether legal or illegal, brings the following risks:
• Infection of the uterus.
• Infection of the Fallopian tubes.
• Blockage of the Fallopian tubes leading to sub-fertility or infertility.
• An increased likelihood of an **ectopic pregnancy** later.
• The cervix becomes so stretched that it becomes incompetent.
• Perforation of the uterus.
• Retained placenta leading to haemorrhage and risk of death.

WHY IS IT DONE?

Women seek abortions for many different reasons, and these can include: personal or financial reasons; failed contraception; medical tests that have shown the fetus to be abnormal; and rape. With sophisticated antenatal tests, more damaged babies are being discovered in early pregnancy. When the results of the tests are known, the parents of the unborn child are usually offered counselling, which will include discussion about termination.

Medical reasons for abortion would be:
• Continuing the pregnancy involves greater risk to your life than the abortion.
• Continuing the pregnancy involves a greater risk of injury to the physical and mental health of your living children.
• There is a substantial risk that the child will be born seriously deformed or suffering from a life-threatening disorder such as haemophilia or cystic fibrosis.
• Trauma and unnecessary misery would result from the birth of a child conceived through rape.

HOW IS IT DONE?

Try to plan far enough ahead so that the abortion can be performed at the best time, before the 14th week of pregnancy, and preferably before 12 weeks. After 14 weeks, the procedure is not only more difficult but also more dangerous.

At this later stage, termination is induced with prostaglandins that result in an abortion within 12–36 hours. It can be very painful, like labour. Unfortunately, even when an abortion has been approved, waiting lists can cause you to wait until you are more than 16 weeks, and only an induced labour is open to you.

Suction termination (4–8 weeks)
• This is a very early termination and may be carried out with a local anaesthetic if it is sufficiently early in the pregnancy. It is certainly the safest and least traumatic form of termination. It takes about five minutes and can be done in a doctor's office, clinic or outpatients department in hospital.

TERMINATION OF PREGNANCY: CONTINUED

• A small tube is inserted through the vagina into the uterus. A syringe or pump gently sucks out the uterine lining and fetal material through the tube.

ERPC (After 4 weeks)
• As above, but an ERPC is carried out under general anaesthetic or epidural. The procedure takes about 30 minutes and recovery will involve some painful cramps.
• You may be given drugs to help the uterus contract afterwards to reduce bleeding and the possibility of infection.

Induced labour termination (16–24 weeks)
• By 16 weeks the walls of the uterus are thinner and can be perforated more easily. The fetus is larger, so an induced labour with its attendant emotional and physical pain is usually necessary.
• A cervagen or mifepristone tablet is given to induce labour. You will have painful contractions and should be offered painkillers. You may be given drugs such as oxytocin to increase contractions. The fetus and placenta are expelled relatively easily. The fetus is recognizable and may live for a few minutes, which is upsetting.
• You may then have an ERPC to check that there is nothing left in your uterus, and drugs to suppress lactation will be given to you. You will probably stay in the hospital for about three days but because of the shortage of hospital beds, you may be in wards with women who have had babies or those who cannot. This is upsetting and you should seek to avoid this if possible.

Hysterotomy (16–24 weeks)
This is rarely performed because it is a major operation requiring a general anaesthetic. It is only used for women who cannot have prostaglandin treatment or for whom the other methods have been unsuccessful.

AFTER A TERMINATION

What happens to you after your termination depends very much on you, and on the stage of pregnancy you were at when you underwent the procedure. The following are sensible guidelines to bear in mind in the days immediately after the procedure.
• Get treatment immediately if you have any heavy bleeding, severe abdominal pain or a smelly vaginal discharge.
• Your period should probably resume within a month to six weeks of the operation. Don't use tampons for the first menstrual period.
• Abstain from sexual intercourse while you still have spot bleeding after the procedure (this should disappear after a few days); thereafter you can resume whenever you feel comfortable doing so.
• An early abortion should mean that you are back to normal physically within a week. For a later termination (after 16 weeks) allow two to three weeks.
• Even if you don't think you need it, you would be wise to seek some counselling after a termination; suppressed guilt, shame and regret can be traumatic and damaging – and can potentially affect current and future relationships if they aren't dealt with.
• Have a check-up six weeks after the termination.
• Start using some form of contraception immediately.

It is rather like a Caesarean section when the fetus is removed through an incision in the abdominal wall and uterus.

SEE ALSO:
Ectopic Pregnancy
D&C/ERPC
Miscarriage

BREAST CARE

A woman's breasts undergo some of the most visible
and radical development of any part of her body. Indeed,
breasts continue to change even after they are fully grown.
A basic knowledge of the elements that make up your
breasts and their working parts will prepare you
to face a lifetime of changes with confidence.
The health of your breasts is in your hands, too.
It's important for your emotional well-being as well as
your physical health that you take on the responsibility of
caring for them, particularly by doing regular breast
self-examination (BSE) and, later, with regular
screening. This way, you'll be doing the best you can
to keep your breasts healthy all through your life.

The breasts sit outside the ribcage and the pectoral muscles, and are cushioned by a layer of fat. This surrounds their working parts – the glandular tissue that contains the lobes and ducts.

The inner surface of the breasts lies closely against the pectoral muscles. The breasts extend vertically from the second to the sixth rib and horizontally from the breastbone across the ribcage, with an extension into the armpits. This extension is called the axillary tail.

The proportion of glandular tissue tends to be higher in young women. Older women have a higher proportion of fat in their breasts.

It's the fat that determines the size and shape of the breasts. The pectoral muscles, when well developed, also marginally influence breast size.

KNOW YOUR BREASTS

With a good understanding of the workings of the breast, a woman can learn to recognize when a problem needs medical attention. Then, if it does, she can get a feel for the treatment options that are open to her, participate fully in discussions with her doctor about the possibilities, and take an active role in deciding on the ultimate line of therapy for any conditions that may arise.

ELEMENTS OF THE BREAST

Breasts have two main components: the glandular elements, comprising the lobes and ducts, and the connective tissue that forms the supporting structure. Both of these elements are literally floating in fat, which at body temperature is liquid and accounts for most of breast volume.

The breast merges imperceptibly with the body fat around it, except for the part that extends into the armpit, the axillary tail, which pierces the upper layers of the muscles of the chest wall.

Lobes and ducts Each breast is divided into lobes of glandular tissue, where milk is produced, and each of these lobes contains 15–25 milk or lactiferous ducts, which lead towards the nipple. Some of them join together on the way, and each duct widens to form a collecting sac (lactiferous ampulla) just behind the nipple.

The nipple and areola While the skin covering the breast is smoother, thinner and more translucent than on most of the rest of the body, the skin of the areola is thinner still and contains complex sweat and sebaceous glands (these secrete an oily lubricating substance called sebum) and hair follicles. The surface of the areola is marked by a number of small bumps, called the tubercles of Montgomery. These bumps are sweat and sebaceous glands. They become more prominent in the second half of the menstrual cycle and grow throughout pregnancy.

The nipple can be flat, round, conical or cylindrical in shape. Its colour comes from the pigmentation and thinness of its skin, and it is either soft or firm according to the tone of the smooth muscle fibres within it. These tiny muscles are quite complex: they are embedded in connective tissue and the fibres run in three different directions – around, across and up – and extend into the connective tissue of the areola. It is these muscle fibres that make the nipple so responsive to cold or sexual arousal and cause it to stand out during breastfeeding so that the baby can take it in his mouth; all the fibres contract at once and the nipple becomes firm, ridged and elongated while the areolar skin puckers markedly. The core of the nipple is pierced by 15–25 milk (or lactiferous) ducts and sinuses that open up at its tip. The nipple itself has many sebaceous glands that keep it lubricated during breastfeeding.

Blood supply The same major arteries that supply the chest wall also supply the breast. The axillary artery comes from the armpit (axilla) and supplies the outer half of the breast; the internal mammary artery passes from the neck down the chest and supplies the inner half of the breast. It is the drainage of blood from the breasts through a network of veins that is more significant, however. Malignant tumours of the breast can spread to the rest of the body by shedding cancer cells into the blood like leaves from a tree; wherever these cells settle, a secondary breast cancer can form. The veins from the breast take blood back to the heart via those of the armpit and rib spaces, and then into veins deeper within the chest.

Nerve supply The large number of sensory nerve-endings that carry signals such as touch, pain and temperature are responsible for the exquisite sensitivity of the areola, particularly the nipple. As well as sensory nerves, the breast enjoys the bonus of extra nerves from the autonomic nervous system, which controls involuntary body functions such as digestion and sweating. Autonomic nerves form the connection whereby stimulation of the nipple can cause arousal and erection of the clitoris. This phenomenon is reported by very many women – indeed, some women can achieve orgasm simply by stimulation of the nipple.

The breast's lymphatic drainage Within the breast there is a network of delicate lymphatic vessels. These vessels communicate with a network in the skin, especially around the nipple under the areola, and there may even be another deep sub-mammary collection of tiny lymph vessels that lie on the surface of the chest muscles.

The lymphatic channels within the breast eventually end in the lymph nodes in the armpit, called the axillary lymph nodes. These nodes receive and filter 75 percent of all the lymph from the breast. Of the rest, about 20 percent passes to the lymph nodes around the breastbone and the other five percent pass deeper into the chest.

LYMPH DRAINAGE OF THE BREAST

Lymphatic fluid flows around the body, bathing cells and organs in the same way as oil lubricates an engine. It drains into regional collecting points – the lymph nodes – which filter it and attack harmful organisms, preventing most infection from passing into the bloodstream. Seventy-five percent of the lymphatics in the breast drain into the lymph nodes in the armpit and from there to those above the collarbone. Lymph nodes around the breastbone receive almost all the rest.

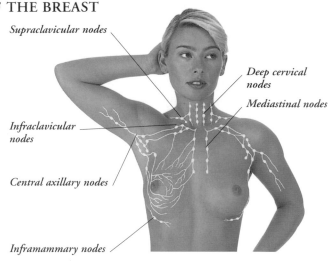

Supraclavicular nodes

Deep cervical nodes

Mediastinal nodes

Infraclavicular nodes

Central axillary nodes

Inframammary nodes

The lymphatic drainage of the breast is of particular importance because of its relevance to the diagnosis and treatment of breast cancer; the axillary lymph nodes can be affected if a cancer spreads through the lymphatic vessels from a primary tumour in the breast. This is why feeling for lumps in the armpit forms an essential part of breast self-examination; you are not checking for tumours in these areas, but for swollen lymph nodes.

BREAST DEVELOPMENT

Although breast growth can't be seen until puberty, breast development begins very early in the embryo and can be discerned within just a few weeks of conception.

Adolescence The first external signs of breast development appear at the age of 10 or 11, although it can be as late as 14. The ovaries start to secrete oestrogen, leading to an accumulation of fat in the connective tissue that causes the breasts to enlarge. The duct system also begins to develop, but only to the point of forming cellular knobs at the end of the ducts. As far as doctors know, the mechanism that secretes milk doesn't develop until pregnancy.

The breasts may appear fully grown within a few years of puberty, but their development is not properly complete until their biological function is fulfilled – that is, until a woman carries a pregnancy to term and breastfeeds her baby, when the breasts will undergo further changes.

The ageing breast As women get older, the breasts tend to sag and flatten; the larger the breasts, the more they sag. With the menopause there is a reduction in stimulation by the hormone oestrogen to all tissues of the body, including breast tissue; this results in a reduction in the glandular tissue of the breasts so that they lose their earlier fullness. In some women, however, the menopause can bring with it an enormous increase in the size of the breasts.

Development and benign breast change As the various components of the breast continue to develop over the years, changes take place in all the tissues, which can give rise to lumps, cysts and sometimes nipple discharge. At one time these changes were thought of as diseases. Doctors no longer see them even as abnormal but simply as aberrations (or variations) of normal that are benign and require no treatment.

WHAT IS NORMAL?

All breasts are normal, regardless of size and shape. Other variations (usually due to quirks of development) are still common enough to be regarded as normal and harmless.

Hairs on the nipple There's hardly a woman who doesn't have at least one hair on her breasts, usually around the areola, and some women have many. Occasional shaving or plucking or using a depilatory cream is enough to remove them. Another option is permanent removal by electrolysis.

Inverted nipples In its usual form, the nipple is everted (turning outwards). Inverted nipples (turning inwards) are quite common, however, and are simply a variation of the norm, although they can be a cause of great concern for women. "Suction" devices such as nipple shells are widely available. A common worry is that breastfeeding will not be possible, but in fact the use of a breast shell can often solve this problem. It is possible to have cosmetic surgery to correct an inverted nipple. A previously everted nipple may become inverted as the result of nipple disease.

Asymmetry It is extremely rare for a woman's breasts to be entirely symmetrical; one is usually larger and consequently may be heavier and sit lower than the other. The difference between the right and left breast is rarely very great, but occasionally it is quite obvious. For some women, having asymmetrical breasts is of no concern but for others it is disconcerting and, if desired, can be corrected with plastic surgery, by enlarging one breast or by reducing the other.

LARGE BREASTS

How the breasts develop at puberty (see far left) depends on the sensitivity of breast tissue to the secretion of the hormone, oestrogen, which can vary among women.

Sometimes breast tissue can be hypersensitive to small amounts of oestrogen and the breasts enlarge and become heavy very rapidly, even making stretch marks in the skin.

The uncontrolled overgrowth of the breasts in pubescent girls is called juvenile or virginal hypertrophy. If unsupported, the suspensory ligaments that hold the breasts will become overstretched and the breasts will sag. Very heavy breasts can become pendulous even with good support.

Teenage girls who have extremely large breasts should be informed of the possibility of surgical breast reduction and offered counselling. The results of the operation are usually very good.

Moving the nipple and areolar skin is a part of such operations and it may affect the ability to breastfeed, although this depends on the surgical technique used. Ask your surgeon about operations that can preserve the milk ducts.

SUN PROTECTION

The breasts of white-skinned women can very easily become sunburned because the chest skin contains few melanocytes. These are the cells that protect the skin from sunburn by producing the tanning pigment, melanin.

• *Until a tan has become well established, you should apply a sun block with a sun protection factor (SPF) greater than 15 every two hours or so and after swimming or being in water.*

• *A gentle run-in period will help the skin accommodate itself to the bright ultraviolet rays. Have no more than five minutes' exposure on the first day, no more than ten minutes on the second, and a further five minutes on each day after that, up to half an hour.*

• *Even after this regime, you may be sunburned if you expose your breasts to sun for longer than two hours before they are given the opportunity to tan slowly.*

EVERYDAY BREAST CARE

The breasts don't need much in the way of beauty routines, but they do need to be treated with care, since their skin is extremely delicate. While many "beauty" treatments for the breasts exist, these are generally entirely worthless.

SKIN CARE

The skin of the breasts, particularly over the areola and the nipple, is thinner and more translucent than elsewhere on the body because the lower layers contain less collagen. This delicate skin needs to be treated gently, and should never be subjected to scrubbing or rough towelling since this can make the nipples sore and tender, particularly in the week prior to menstruation. The nipple and areola may become dry and flake premenstrually, so it's a good idea to moisturize them twice a week by gently massaging in an unperfumed moisturizer. If you are white-skinned and want to expose your breasts to the sun, make sure they are properly protected (see left).

Eczema can occur on the nipples. If you get a persistent patch, consult your doctor for a precise diagnosis and specific treatment, since in rare cases it can be a symptom of a more serious condition – a form of very slow-growing cancer called Paget's disease.

CAN BEAUTY REGIMES HELP THE BREASTS?

When I was a girl, the favourite technique among my friends for keeping your breasts pert was to bathe them first with hot water and then with cold water. This puckered up the areola and made the nipple erect, which was perhaps taken as a sign of uplift. It represented only a change in the slackness of the skin, however, and a transient one at that.

All kinds of beauty products are peddled in the hope of convincing women that potions, lotions and creams rubbed into the skin will help them keep the shape of their breasts or even increase their size. In fact, the only way to maintain the shape of the breasts is to start wearing a bra as soon as there's any weight in them. Nothing applied to the skin can alter their shape or consistency, both of which are determined by your own individual response to oestrogens secreted during puberty and thereafter with each menstrual cycle. Your breasts can be changed only from the inside, by the hormones manufactured inside your body.

BREAST EXERCISES

Exercises won't actually change the shape or size of your breasts. What you can achieve with exercise is to strengthen and tone your pectoral muscle. The suspensory ligaments supporting the breasts are attached to the pectoral muscle, so it's just about conceivable that exercises to tone this muscle could lift the breasts maybe 1 centimetre (½ inch) or thicken the pad of muscle on which the breasts sit, thereby increasing your bust measurement by perhaps 2 centimetres (¾ inch). If you're interested in increments of this order, try these exercises. You will need to do them regularly.

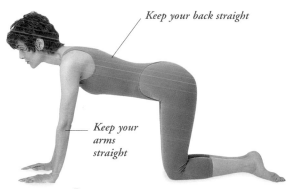

Keep your back straight

Keep your arms straight

PUSH-UPS

1 Kneel comfortably on all fours, with your hands shoulder-width apart and your palms flat on the floor.

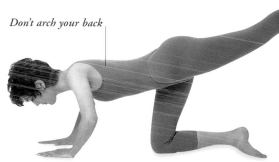

Don't arch your back

Keep your leg straight

2 Stretch your left leg out behind you with your toes pointing back. Bend your elbows to lower your chest nearly to the floor, keeping your shoulders in line with your hands. Repeat this several times, then repeat the whole sequence with your right leg out behind.

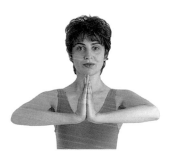

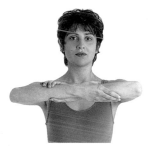

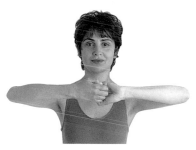

Palm presses
Press the palms and heels of your hands together in front of your breasts. Hold for five seconds. Repeat ten times.

Forearm grip
Grasp your forearms with your hands at shoulder level and pull outwards without letting go. Repeat ten times.

Finger lock
Curl your fingers, lock them together at shoulder level and pull outwards. Hold for five seconds. Repeat ten times.

ABOUT BREAST SELF-EXAMINATION (BSE)

Most women who regularly examine their breasts will never find a lump, let alone a malignant (harmful) one. Breast self-examination (BSE) is simply a way to explore your body and become familiar with it. You don't have to feel that you're looking for anything in particular; you're simply getting to know what your breasts usually feel and look like so that you can recognize something unusual if it appears. Every girl should start doing BSE as soon as she develops breasts and keep on doing it until she dies. There should be no time when you stop or interrupt this routine.

WOMEN WHO DO

Research shows that women who do breast self-examination have a positive attitude to life and to BSE; they think it's a good thing to do, and they're right. They are likely to be better educated, younger and in higher socio-economic groups than women who don't examine their breasts. They also engage in other preventive health measures such as having regular cervical smears and dental checkups.

Women who do BSE feel that breast cancer is the worst imaginable disease to affect women, but they're optimistic about the likelihood of being cured with early treatment and believe it is something they can control by doing BSE regularly. They don't think that doing BSE will inevitably lead to finding a cancerous lump and so they don't feel nervous about doing it. This is the kind of approach and attitude you should try to cultivate.

WOMEN WHO DON'T

Unfortunately, nine out of ten women don't do BSE. There are many reasons for this. Good information on BSE is hard to find and poor information tends to make women anxious. Even many health professionals who can tell you how to examine your breasts are unclear about what you're looking for because they're uncertain themselves. Not every health educator is a good communicator, and you may end up with a confusing message. Many books and pamphlets tell you that you have to look for a change but don't explain what the precise changes are. You have no clear idea, there-fore, of what you're searching for, and that in itself provokes

"I love examining my breasts. I'm proud of them, and I want them to be healthy. It makes me feel I'm in control of my life."

Sue, 25, Musician

anxiety. Normal findings, such as premenstrual lumpiness (see right), can be very frightening if you don't know that they are normal, and can put you off BSE, since whatever is causing the lumps seems to be widespread.

It seems rather surprising in this day and age that women can actually be embarrassed about touching their breasts, yet many women in their fifties and sixties – the age group for which breast cancer is most common – grew up with the view that it was somehow bad, except in the bath, for a woman to touch her own body. A woman who considers that it is somehow improper to touch, let alone examine, her breasts can remain unaware for a long time of dramatic changes, even large, ulcerating tumours.

Sometimes women are put off BSE because they feel that there can't be a positive outcome if they find something needing medical attention. Only very few of the lumps that cause concern turn out to be cancerous. And even when they do, most women with breast cancer don't die from it. Early detection of breast cancer vastly improves the chances of a cure. I feel there's great room for optimism because while you're doing BSE you're in control of your health.

WHEN TO DO BSE

Most authorities advocating BSE suggest that you perform your examination at the same time every month – ideally in the week after your menstrual period – so that you have a consistent basis for comparison. When you're starting, however, I'm in favour of your examining your breasts at different times of the month because they will change in consistency and texture as you go through your monthly menstrual cycle (see right). I feel that all women should be aware of these changes and know how their breasts feel to touch. I also believe that it is better to perform BSE more often – say every two weeks instead of once a month – in a low-key, relaxed way so that it quickly becomes a habit and part of your normal life.

You should never feel tyrannized by BSE; if you don't want to do it, or if you sometimes miss a month or two, no harm will befall you. If you find that the idea of examining your breasts yourself makes you anxious, go along regularly to your doctor, say every three months, so that he or she can perform the examination for you, and if appropriate take advantage of other early detection techniques such as mammograms.

HOW TO DO BSE

There are two elements to breast self-examination: looking and feeling (palpation). You will need a warm place where you can have some privacy and be free from interruptions. Just before going to bed is a good time, or when you are about to have a bath or shower.

LOOKING AT THE BREASTS

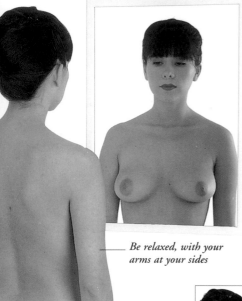

Be relaxed, with your arms at your sides

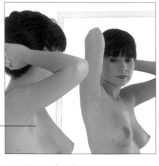

Don't forget to look at the upper part of the breast that leads into the armpit

2 Raise both your arms above your head. Turn to one side so you can see your breasts in profile, and repeat your observations, as in Step 1. Do the same for the other side.

1 Undress to the waist and stand or sit in front of a mirror. Look at each breast carefully for changes in their appearance, size or the colour of the nipples; a difference in level between the nipples; patches of eczema on the nipples; or any dimpling of the skin.

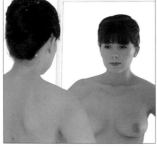

3 Turn to face the mirror. Place your hands firmly on your hips and press in hard. You should feel your chest muscles tense. Repeat your observations.

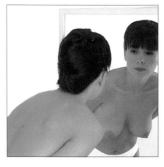

4 Now lean forward from the waist. Look again for dimpling or puckering of the skin, a change in outline of the breast or if the nipple appears to be drawn in.

FEELING THE BREASTS

1 Lie back in a relaxed position and put your right arm behind your head. This shifts the breast tissue towards the centre of your chest, giving you better access to it and making it easier to feel. If your breasts are very large, a pillow under your left shoulder may help.

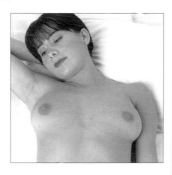

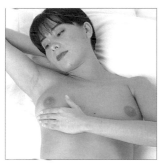
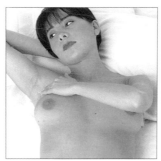

2 Touching firmly, use your left hand to examine your right breast. Use one of the patterns (right) or your own, as long as it's systematic.

3 Check your armpit and along the top of your collarbone for lumps (if the lymph nodes are swollen, you will feel them as lumps).

4 Put your left arm behind your head and, using your right hand, examine your left breast in the same systematic way. Remember to check the armpit and collarbone.

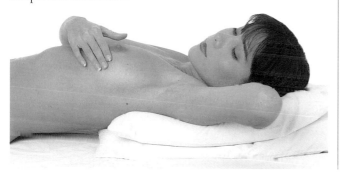

PATTERNS OF FEELING

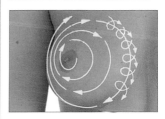

Concentric circles
Start with a big circle around the outside of the breast, making smaller circles with your fingers as you go around the breast. Work inwards until you reach the nipple.

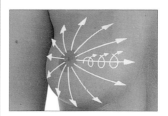

Radial pattern
Mentally divide the breast into a clock. Work out from the nipple towards 12 o'clock, then 1, 2, 3 o'clock and so on to check the whole breast.

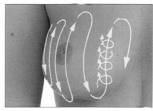

Up and down
Imagine the breast as a series of vertical bands; go up and down each one. Move your fingers in small circles as you work around the breast.

WHAT YOU MIGHT FIND

Above all, you are looking for a change in your breasts. You won't be able to recognize change, however, until you've examined your breasts a few times and established what is normal for you. Here are some of the things you may find in your breasts. They are all quite normal and healthy.

Lumps and pseudo-lumps   You may observe many subtle changes in your breasts. Cancer is not subtle, so don't panic over a very tiny and discrete lump, particularly if its size varies over your monthly cycle. Remember, your breasts may be lumpy naturally or pre-menstrually.

Losing weight often makes natural breast lumpiness more evident. The breastbone (between your breasts) makes joints at either edge with the ribs, which may be prominent. If you're very thin, one of the hard lumps that you feel could simply be breast tissue felt over the end of a rib.

You may feel a swelling of breast tissue between the nipple and the armpit, or directly above the nipple. During the pre-menstrual period, both of these areas are more likely to swell up and become tender. There is also a ridge of tissue in the lower part of the breast that feels thicker and more lumpy than other parts of the breast. Under the nipple is a hollow spot where the milk ducts rise to the surface.

Scar tissue from an infection or surgery (even a biopsy) will always remain as a palpable lump or ridge. (If your doctor examines your breasts, do mention this and the date it occurred, to avoid concern and unnecessary tests.)

Pain   Soreness and discomfort are extremely common in women's breasts. In the vast majority of cases they are connected with menstrual hormones, and they are very rarely symptoms of cancer. If soreness persists or if it is causing you problems, however, your doctor will be able to help, normally by prescribing oil of evening primrose.

SIGNIFICANT CHANGES

Once you have been doing BSE long enough to get used to what is normal in your breasts, you will need to be on the alert for any changes that require a doctor's attention (there are several characteristic ones that might be of concern). First, when looking at your breasts, you might observe:

Normal findings
When examining your breasts, you may find changes that cause you concern. Many of these things, however, are quite normal and healthy and are shown below. If you are at all worried about any changes, consult your doctor at once.

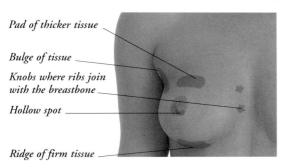

Pad of thicker tissue

Bulge of tissue

Knobs where ribs join with the breastbone

Hollow spot

Ridge of firm tissue

- veins that are visible through the skin more prominently than usual
- change in the size of either breast
- change in the colour or texture of the skin
- new dimpling or puckering of the skin over the breast and nipple, or change in the breast outline
- change in the appearance of the nipple such as redness, scaling, crusting or drawing in
- discharge or bleeding from the nipple.

When feeling, you are really looking for only one thing: a new, discrete lump that is constant in size and doesn't vary with your menstrual cycle. It may be attached to the skin, causing puckering, or fixed to the tissues deeper in the breast. If you feel such a lump, your next step should be to examine the armpit to see whether or not any of your lymph nodes are swollen, and run your finger along the top of your collarbone to see if there are any swollen nodes there too. There are three main criteria for deciding that a lump needs medical investigation:

- the lump is new
- it is very distinct, not just a thickening of breast tissue
- it is unchanged through one or two menstrual cycles.

If you find something but can't decide whether it's serious or not, see your doctor anyway, if only to set your mind at rest. The vast majority of lumps detected by BSE are not cancerous and are quite normal.

WHAT TO DO IF YOU FIND A LUMP

First, check the same part of the other breast. If what you have found is symmetrical, it's just the way your breasts are made and nothing for you to worry about. If the lump is asymmetrical, don't panic. Phone your doctor's surgery to make an appointment for a breast examination at the earliest opportunity. If he or she is at all worried, you will be referred very quickly to see a hospital specialist and further tests will be done. Make a mental note of exactly where the lump is in your breast and try not to keep feeling it to see if it's still there or if it's tender.

Now sit down, phone your best friend and ask her to come round straight away. However rational you think you can be about it, you will be glad of moral support before, during and after your medical appointment. Just keep on reminding yourself that the majority of breast lumps are not cancerous and turn out to be harmless.

DISCHARGE

Some pamphlets and books about BSE tell you to squeeze your nipples and check for discharge. You should not do this as part of your breast self-examination routine.

Squeezing the nipple can create discharge where there was none before, because it increases the hormone, prolactin, in the body, which in turn causes the breasts to produce liquid (although not proper milk).

The way to check for discharge is simply to examine your clothes, and you should do this at least every time you do BSE. Discharge is cause for concern only if it appears without any squeezing of the nipples, if it is persistent or if it's from one nipple only (gently squeeze your other nipple to check this). In all these cases, you should consult your doctor.

MAMMOGRAPHIC SCREENING

To have a mammogram done, you'll be asked to strip to the waist and remove any deodorant or talc from your breasts. The reason for this is that they may show up as microcalcifications.

You will then be asked to stand in front of the machine and the radiologist will compress your breast between two plates. The procedure is described as painless, but it is not without a degree of discomfort, particularly if the plates are cold; the sensation lasts no more than 10 or 15 seconds, however, so it's easily bearable. Two views of each breast will usually be taken.

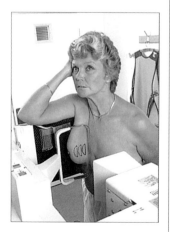

Obtaining the image
The radiologist compresses each breast in turn between two plates so that a good image is obtained.

SCREENING

Breast self-examination is recommended for all women, at all stages of their lives, but additional checks are advisable for older women, who have a higher risk of breast cancer, and for women in other high-risk groups – with breast cancer in the family, for instance. In the UK, there is a screening programme to make sure that women between 50 and 65 years of age attend screening clinics regularly. Screening involves having a physical breast examination – a doctor will examine your breasts in the same way that you do at home for BSE – and a mammogram (see left and below), which can detect smaller abnormalities of the breasts than a physical examination.

There now exists clear evidence that early detection by screening and treatment cuts down the number of women dying from breast cancer. Studies performed in Sweden and the USA have shown that screening can reduce by up to one-third deaths from breast cancer in women between the ages of 50 and 65. Early detection automatically means earlier treatment and therefore increases the chances of a full recovery if a lump is found that turns out to be breast cancer. Early detection also means that you can have greater choice in how your cancer will be treated.

It's understandable to feel anxious about having regular mammograms. However, it is likely that you will be one of the 99 women out of every 100 routinely screened who are found not to have cancer.

MAMMOGRAPHY

A mammogram is a low-dose X-ray of the breast. It is such a refined method of imaging the breast that it can pick up small cancers and other abnormalities that neither you nor your doctor can feel on manual examination.

Mammograms are not done with the same frequency in all age groups. Because breast cancer is comparatively rare in women under the age of 50, it is only after 50 that mammograms are recommended for screening purposes. Women who fall into high-risk groups will be offered annual or biannual mammograms at an earlier age than usual (see above). At present in the UK, mammography is offered to women over 50 every three years, although there is currently some debate about this, and the frequency may be increased to every two years.

Mammography is less effective in women under 50, since their breast tissue is more dense and abnormalities don't show up so well, but it is still more sensitive than BSE. This is why it can be used as a diagnostic tool, to investigate a lump found in physical examination, for example, or to look for further lumps when one has already been found.

GETTING THE RESULTS

The films are developed and examined by a radiologist who specializes in interpreting mammograms. The results usually take only a few days to come through and most women will be told that they're fine and just need regular screening. A small number will be asked to come back for further tests. This can be worrying, but the chances of getting the all-clear are still high. Although mammograms are good for detecting small lumps, they're not much use in determining a lump's precise character, so extra tests may be needed.

Microcalcifications These are tiny deposits of calcium that show up as very fine specks on a mammogram. They may be quite normal and many women have them but, because they have been linked with cancer in a small number of cases, the radiologist will always mention their presence. They are only worrying if they suddenly appear in a cluster in one breast. If it's your first mammogram, your doctor may recommend a further one in about six months' time, which is long enough to see if there is any change. If the pattern of microcalcification is very abnormal, a biopsy will be carried out at once.

Lumps If your mammogram shows any kind of lump, further tests will be necessary. A lump that's large enough to feel easily with your fingers can be aspirated by inserting a fine needle to draw off some of the tissue. This is called fine-needle aspiration cytology, or FNAC.

If the lump is fluid-filled, it's a cyst, which is perfectly harmless; your doctor will draw off the fluid with the needle and send off a specimen for laboratory tests. If it's solid, some of the cells that have been drawn off will be smeared on a slide, stained, and examined in the laboratory.

If the lump isn't easy to feel, you will probably have an ultrasound scan to determine whether it's a solid lump or a cyst. Either way it will be investigated with FNAC or cutting-needle biopsy. When a lump can't be felt, both of these specimens are taken with the guidance of ultrasound so that the tumour can be precisely located.

"After my first screening session, I felt ambivalent really. You know, glad that nothing was found but scared that something will show up next time."

Claire, 53,
Tour Operator

OTHER IMAGING TECHNIQUES

Mammography is the most widely used method of imaging the breast, but there are some other techniques that you may come across, particularly if you are referred for other tests after a routine screening mammogram.

XERO-MAMMOGRAPHY

Xero-mammography requires different equipment from the standard X-ray machine that takes a mammogram. It is not necessarily any more accurate than mammography; it just gives a different end-product: an image on paper rather than on film. Accuracy of interpretation depends on the experience of the radiologist, whatever method is used.

ULTRASOUND

Many of us have come across the painless ultrasonic scans during pregnancy. Ultrasound can produce a picture very similar to an X-ray photograph. The patterns are produced by the echoes of sound waves, which vary in intensity according to the solidity of the tissue that they bounce off. Ultrasound can be particularly useful when examining very dense breasts, so it's good for younger women, and it can detect very small lumps that can't yet be felt, particularly tiny cysts. It's very accurate with larger, palpable lumps, and it can distinguish between solid lumps and those that are filled with fluid. Ultrasound also detects calcification, and can show up the blood supply to a tumour; a rich supply of blood is characteristic of cancerous lumps.

THERMOGRAPHY

Less familiar than X-rays or ultrasound, this is never a first-line investigation. The heat-sensitive photographs usually support manual examination and mammography.

Rapidly growing and dividing tissue such as cancer has a higher temperature than the tissue that surrounds it. Thermography works by mapping out the temperatures in different tissues, so a growing cyst or a tumour will show up on a thermogram as a more intense area of heat than its surroundings. The patient undresses and holds her arms up or stretched out from her body to allow the breast skin to cool. Photographs are then taken with an infrared camera.

10

BENIGN BREAST CHANGES

Many changes in the breast reflect quite normal,
harmless conditions. Such changes do not
necessarily indicate cancer or even disease.
A woman should be helped to maintain a calm and
rational response to benign breast changes, such as cyclical
and non-cyclical pain, cysts, solid lumps and nipple
discharge, and be reassured as to diagnosis and options for
treatment, if it is needed. For her own peace of mind and
well-being, a woman needs to understand that benign
breast changes are simply the normal effects of
her age, menstrual cycle and lifestyle.

CHANGE OR DISEASE?

Cysts, solid lumps and nipple discharge are all normal, harmless conditions that arise in the breast. Since there's no abnormality present, it's misleading to call such conditions "diseases", and well-informed doctors now use the term "benign breast change". This is crucial to a woman for whom the word disease implies something abnormal or dangerous. It's imperative that doctors too stop thinking of these conditions as disease because they have been trained to believe that disease justifies intervention. If your doctor refers to a breast condition in ambiguous terms, always ask for clarification of the terminology. Defer treatment until you have a second opinion if you don't understand.

A NEW APPROACH TO CLASSIFICATION

Until about 18 years ago, breast conditions were not well understood and there was confusion as to what was normal and what was abnormal. In 1980, researchers in Cardiff, Wales, developed a new and logical classification system for breast conditions that has a scientific basis. This system relates the most common breast conditions to normal changes that take place in the breast throughout a woman's lifetime, and has been accepted in most countries where breast research takes place, including the US and the UK. It provides a rational explanation for practically all benign breast conditions. The Cardiff researchers decided to rename benign breast conditions as Aberrations (changes) of Normal Development and Involution (shrinkage), giving the acronym ANDI.

WHY ANDI?

The ANDI classification is based on two facts about benign breast conditions. First, most conditions relate to the normal pattern of breast development with its stages of growth and shrinkage. Second, each condition fits into one of the three main periods of women's fertile lives (puberty to 25 years, 25 to 35 years and 35 to 55 years), so certain symptoms are more common at certain ages.

Take the development of a fibroadenoma for example. Common in teenagers and women in their 20s, this lump is nothing more than a breast lobule of unusual size, shape and consistency. Under a microscope, the cells from a normal lobule and a fibroadenoma look identical.

Your age is therefore of particular importance if you discover a breast lump. Under the age of 35, the chances are overwhelmingly that you've found a fibroadenoma, which is benign and nothing to worry about. If you're between the ages of 35 and 55, the chances are that the lump is an innocent cyst. But if you're over the age of 55, cancer must be a possibility and your doctor will take immediate steps to make a firm diagnosis.

In the light of these observations, doctors can now interpret the majority of benign breast conditions as age-related variations on the normal; they are therefore better thought of as aberrations or "mistakes" rather than diseases. Such aberrations for most women are symptomless, so they rarely prompt you to consult a doctor. Only a few cause symptoms such as pain (see right), and even fewer lead to disease. Most never get beyond the state of being simply a variation on normal development.

ANDI AND DISEASE

There is no evidence that aberrations inevitably progress to disease. On the contrary, it seems that for this to happen some additional factor is needed – often an external one, such as smoking or an excessive alcohol intake. Duct ectasia, for instance, rarely if ever goes on to infection or an abscess except where a woman smokes.

ANDI, therefore, usefully defines the spectrum from normal to minor aberrations that encompasses most benign breast conditions. Disease, on the other hand, is associated with other possibly external triggers.

YOUR CONCERNS

Almost all women fear breast cancer, so any breast symptom can cause alarm. Indeed, most women with breast symptoms seek reassurance even before they consider treatment. The women most at risk, and therefore those who should be most concerned about breast cancer, are those who are under 50 years old with a first-degree relative (that is, mother or sister) who developed breast cancer at a young age. If you know you have a high risk of developing breast cancer or are especially worried about your breasts, ask your family doctor for referral to a special breast clinic; it's your right to do so. Should you develop breast cancer, don't accept treatment from a general surgeon who treats fewer than 30 breast cancers a year.

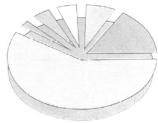

KEY

▷	65%	LUMP, WITH OR WITHOUT PAIN
▷	16%	PAIN (MASTALGIA)
▷	8%	PAINFUL LUMPINESS
▷	5%	NIPPLE DISCHARGE
▷	4%	OTHER
▷	2%	NIPPLE RETRACTION

Breast symptoms
The vast majority of benign breast disorders give rise to three main symptoms: a lump or lumpiness, pain and nipple discharge. Taken singly, breast pain is the most common complaint women report: at one breast clinic it appeared in 170 out of 480 women (35 percent). But not all women who suffer breast pain ever seek help for it; it's thought that seven out of ten women suffer to some degree from breast pain, tenderness and lumpiness.

SEE A BREAST SPECIALIST IF...

Pain is not the only symptom that should make you visit a breast specialist. Any of these symptoms will require further investigation and you should not be put off seeking the necessary help and advice. See a breast specialist if:

• your pain is associated with a breast lump; pain doesn't respond to your doctor's treatment; you are post-menopausal and have persistent pain in one breast.

• you find a new, discrete lump or a new lump in pre-existing general lumpiness; a cyst persistently refills after being drained; you notice asymmetrical lumpiness at the beginning of your menstrual cycle for more than one cycle.

• you have nipple discharge associated with a lump; there is sufficient discharge to stain your clothes; you have bloodstained, persistent or painful discharge.

BREAST PAIN

Is breast pain real? To the 60 percent of women who experience mastalgia, to give breast pain its medical name, the question seems ludicrous. Of course it's real – so real that for some women just having the breasts touched can be excruciating. Less than 20 years ago, however, breast pain, like gynaecological pain such as menstrual cramps, was thought to be all in the mind; for decades it had been labelled neurotic, hysterical and psychosomatic.

The unsympathetic and largely masculine trend of labelling breast pain as "a nervous disorder" was started in the nineteenth century by an eminent British surgeon, Astley Cooper, but was still widespread in the 1950s and 1960s. It was not until 1978 that Professor Robert Mansel of Cardiff, Wales, investigated this notion and reported that mastalgia sufferers were indeed psychologically stable and deserved a sympathetic approach to treatment. Largely due to Mansel's work, breast pain has become recognized as a legitimate complaint.

Breast pain can be classified into two types: cyclical, which is associated with menstrual periods, and non-cyclical. Non-cyclical pain may originate in the breast or in the nearby muscles and joints, in which case it is not true breast pain.

Treating women with breast pain Studies carried out in Manchester, England, indicate that women suffering from breast pain don't always get the understanding and treatment they deserve; and it's clear that too many women seeking help aren't being examined or treated appropriately. Although more than half the women studied had seen their family doctor, they still needed help and treatment. Other women avoided their doctor out of fear or embarrassment. Still others had been met with the attitude that breast pain was a "nervous" or "neurotic" disorder.

It is still common for doctors to prescribe ineffective remedies – diuretics or even antibiotics – to treat mastalgia. Some doctors suggest evening primrose oil, which is widely available in over-the-counter products, although evening primrose oil is effective only in high doses that are expensive unless obtained on prescription.

Effects on lifestyle Although mastalgia can significantly disrupt daily life and even be incapacitating, not all women feel justified in consulting a doctor about it. In one study,

60 percent of women said that they felt they had to cope without medical help. Although women may be reluctant to consult a doctor, the pain often causes them to ring a breast helpline – indeed, mastalgia is the most common reason for women calling such a helpline. Researchers in the UK have demonstrated just how seriously breast pain can interfere with normal daily life. The following figures give the percentages of women who suffered from varying degrees of breast pain:

• sufficient pain to make them particularly aware of the breasts: 42%
• discomfort wearing a bra or light clothing: 26%
• uncomfortable running up or down stairs: 19%
• too uncomfortable for close physical contact: 17%
• cannot bear any physical contact or pressure; pain would interrupt sleep and preclude sex: 9%.

Fear and breast pain Even if breast pain does not interfere radically with normal life, fear of breast pain can be crippling because sufferers fear that cancer is the cause. Studies from Cardiff demonstrate that almost nine out of ten women with mastalgia are much more worried about the possibility of cancer than about the pain itself. This includes the one in six women who suffers from incapacitating pain.

It's reasonable to be fearful of getting breast cancer, but it's not reasonable to be paranoid about it. If you have breast pain and are worried about it, you should visit your doctor. Bear in mind, though, that breast pain is rarely a symptom of breast cancer. And it would be very wrong indeed to think that the worse the pain, the greater the chance that it's caused by malignancy (a cancerous tumour). In fact, the opposite is true. The worse the pain, the less likely it is to be due to a malignant growth. Looked at this way, breast pain is a reassuring symptom since its presence all but excludes breast cancer.

Psychology and breast pain All breast conditions can give rise to anxiety. For many women the symptoms are stressful in their own right, and as such may lead to psychological disorders. On the other hand, psychological disorders may show up as – or be the cause of – breast symptoms, although in saying this I am not suggesting for a moment that the symptoms are imaginary.

Ironically, the highest levels of anxiety are found in women who are subsequently diagnosed as having purely benign disorders. Studies using internationally accepted

Locations of pain
Pain that seems to be in the breast may in fact originate from some other part of the body, typically the bones or muscles. Locating the pain precisely helps a doctor decide whether the pain is true breast pain.

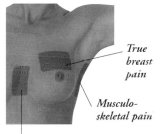

True breast pain

Musculo-skeletal pain

Musculoskeletal pain

113

DIAGNOSING CYCLICAL PAIN

One of the first things your doctor will want to establish is whether the pain is cyclical or not.

A chart known as the standard Cardiff chart allows you to record your pain each day – whether there is no pain, mild pain or severe pain – so that you and your doctor can see whether a pattern emerges.

The first day of each menstrual period is marked with a tick. Put a cross through any dates that don't apply (such as 29 February). After a couple of months, the relationship between the menstrual cycle and breast pain will emerge.

methods for measuring anxiety also came up with the startling finding that the degree of stress felt by women with severe mastalgia is similar to that felt by women with operable breast cancer on the morning of surgery.

Given this degree of pain and anxiety, it is very important for women to realize that they can receive simple and effective treatment for mastalgia.

Lumpiness and breast pain It used to be thought that breast lumpiness, including cyclical lumpiness, could cause breast pain and that, conversely, breast pain would eventually lead to lumpiness. However, neither of these concepts has any medical foundation whatsoever. When mammography was used to measure lumpiness, it was found that women with severe lumpiness had no more breast pain than women with no lumpiness at all. Then again, when women with mastalgia had ultrasound examinations, only half had lumpy breasts. Nor does the degree of lumpiness reflect the degree of pain that a woman experiences. Both lumpiness and pain are common, however, so it is hardly surprising that they often occur together. The association between pain and lumpiness is mainly true of cyclical pain.

As well as lumpiness, breast pain is commonly associated with swelling, hardening and a feeling of tension in the breast. Your doctor may refer to this as engorgement, but it's not the same as the engorgement a breastfeeding mother experiences when her breasts become over-full with milk.

CYCLICAL BREAST PAIN

The commonest kind of breast pain is associated with the menstrual cycle and is nearly always related to fluctuations in hormone levels that every woman experiences as part of the cycle. Pain is probably related to the sensitivity of breast tissue to hormones and this can differ within a breast and between your two breasts. Hormones aren't the whole story, however, because in the majority of women the pain is more severe in one breast than in the other. Most women experience some degree of breast pain when their breasts become sensitive just prior to menstruation. Some women, however, may experience soreness and tenderness starting in the middle of the cycle with ovulation and continuing for about two weeks until menstruation takes place. Others find that this pre-menstrual soreness becomes even worse after the birth of their first child.

The degree of pain varies. Sometimes it's hardly noticeable, but for some women the pain is so great that they wince when hugged, can't stand to wear anything tight around their breasts and can't lie on their stomachs. Sometimes the pain spreads out towards the armpit and occasionally down the arm to the elbow, which can cause women to fear that the pain is due to cancer or heart disease.

Causes of cyclical pain There are many theories as to how hormones may be responsible for causing cyclical breast pain. One possibility is that the pain is due to changes in the production of prolactin, the milk-producing hormone, in response to changes in levels of thyroid hormone. We know that some women are very sensitive to thyroxine and respond to it by producing very high levels of prolactin, which induces breast pain. It's thought that abnormal "pulses" of prolactin may underlie cyclical mastalgia.

Breast pain can be affected by stress, and another theory suggests that it may be related to the many hormones that flood the body during stress. These include adrenaline, noradrenaline, hydrocortisone and thyroid hormone.

French research has shown that mastalgia may occur when there's a lowered production of progesterone, thus changing the normal ratio of progesterone to oestrogen in the second half of the menstrual cycle. Not all doctors agree with this theory, or with the practice of using progesterone to treat mastalgia. At the times in women's lives when hormonal swings are greatest (during puberty, pregnancy or the menopause) breast pain may be intense. During the menopause this may be caused by the ovaries secreting oestrogen without producing progesterone; this changes the normal ratio of progesterone to oestrogen.

Treating cyclical breast pain If a man suffered breast pain 13 times a year, he wouldn't hesitate to demand effective treatment. Neither should you. I believe that every woman with mastalgia has the right to try evening primrose oil, which is effective and safe, on prescription.

Evening primrose oil has to be taken in a large dose (three grams daily) to be effective. It also needs to be taken over a long period of time since its effect builds slowly – in most cases it takes as long as four months to see if there is a good response to the treatment. Notwithstanding the large dose and prolonged usage, evening primrose oil has very few side-effects, which is why it should be the first line treatment of choice.

SEQUENCE OF TREATMENTS

If your doctor establishes that your pain is not cyclical, it will be treated according to cause. If it is cyclical, there are a number of possible treatments.

* *For mild pain, reassurance is often all that is required.*

* *For severe pain, your doctor will first prescribe evening primrose oil.*

* *If pain persists, your doctor may go on to danazol.*

* *If danazol is ineffective, bromocriptine may be tried.*

* *If there is no response and you still have severe pain, your doctor may try hormone treatment with tamoxifen or goserelin.*

SELF-HELP FOR CYCLICAL PAIN

Although I firmly believe that all women with mastalgia should receive medical treatment if they want it, there are self-help remedies that are worth trying. The following remedies are in no way dangerous and are easy to implement.

• *Vitamin E is said to help, although this is unproven.*

• *Water retention doesn't cause cyclical mastalgia, but it can make it seem worse if you're generally retaining fluid pre-menstrually.*

• *If you're bothered by water retention, you might try taking naturally occurring diuretics such as parsley and capsicums (sweet peppers). Coffee is one of the most powerful natural diuretics known and could greatly help to eliminate fluid.*

• *Early research suggests that a diet low in animal fat can reduce cyclical mastalgia. Although this is still unproven, such a diet is healthy anyway.*

Danazol – a drug that blocks ovulation – has a success rate of nearly 80 percent and this makes it the ideal second-line treatment. Despite its success it is not suitable for everyone: some women may experience side-effects such as weight gain and irregular periods. Danazol is given in a dose of 200 milligrams daily for two months; if it has been effective after this time the dose will be gradually reduced.

Bromocriptine works by blocking the hormone prolactin, and may be advised for women who have not responded to evening primrose oil. It has about the same success rate as treatment with evening primrose oil, but it is more likely to have side-effects – nausea, vomiting and headache are among the most common. Giving it in a low dose at first (1.25 milligrams nightly) and gradually increasing the dose to 2.5 milligrams twice daily can help to avoid these. You should always take bromocriptine with food.

NON-CYCLICAL BREAST PAIN

There are two types of non-cyclical breast pain: firstly, true breast pain, which comes from the breast but is unrelated to the menstrual cycle, and secondly, pain that is felt in the region of the breast but is actually coming from somewhere else. This latter kind of pain nearly always involves the muscles, bones or joints and for this reason it is called musculoskeletal pain. Two-thirds of non-cyclical mastalgia is pain of musculoskeletal origin. Sometimes what appears to be breast pain is due to underlying lung or gallbladder disease.

Diagnosing non-cyclical pain Non-cyclical breast pain is relatively uncommon and feels quite unlike cyclical breast pain. It doesn't vary with your menstrual cycle at all and is entirely unrelated to hormones. It's nearly always confined to one spot and you can usually point to exactly where the pain is – it's impossible to do this with cyclical breast pain. Keeping a record of your pain on a daily pain chart over a period of months will show that there is no cyclical pattern and that the pain is therefore unrelated to menstruation.

If your doctor suspects non-cyclical pain while examining you, you may be asked to lean forward so that the breast falls away from the chest. This helps to clarify whether the pain is located in the breast or in the chest wall. As with cyclical pain, a proper diagnosis is important otherwise you may worry needlessly about breast cancer or your heart.

True non-cyclical breast pain There are some benign breast conditions that may be associated with true breast pain. Burning or stabbing pains centred around or under the nipple are nearly always caused by ectasia and tend to run an intermittent, although harmless, course.

A tender spot accompanied by occasional stabbing pain or an ache is common. Its cause is unknown, but it is no reason for anxiety. The pain can be relieved by an injection of local anaesthetic mixed with prednisone, which will help to reduce any inflammation. A cyst occasionally underlies a tender spot.

Pain of non-breast origin Pain that originates in the chest wall or spine may be felt in the breast area. The most usual cause is a form of arthritis, called costochondritis, which affects the ends of the ribs where they join the breastbone; this condition is called Tietze's syndrome. If your pain is worse when you take a deep breath or press on your breastbone and ribs, it's likely to be this kind of arthritis. Taking an analgesic (painkiller) such as paracetamol or a non-steroidal anti-inflammatory drug such as ibuprofen is often effective, so confirming the diagnosis.

Very occasionally pain felt close to the breast originates from a pinched nerve in the neck. An X-ray of the cervical spine will reveal a condition called spondylosis, the natural erosion of the joints between the vertebrae due to ageing. Another possibility is spondylitis, which means that there's some inflammation of the inter-vertebral joints.

In both of these conditions, spurs of new bone are laid down on the sides of the vertebrae and press on the nerves. The resulting pain may be felt in the neck, shoulder, chest, arm or hand. Treatment includes analgesics to relieve the pain, manipulation and physiotherapy, and exercises that are specifically designed to strengthen the muscles of the neck and shoulders.

Although rare, inflammation in the veins of the breast, called Mondor's syndrome, causes pain very like that of an infection or an abscess (you may also hear your doctor use the word phlebitis, which means inflammation of a vein). Careful examination may reveal the inflamed vein, which feels a bit like a string under your fingertips. This condition is not harmful – a blood clot hardly ever escapes from an inflamed vein. Treated with hot and cold compresses and analgesics, it will settle down in about a week.

SELF-HELP FOR ANY BREAST PAIN

For any breast pain, whether it's cyclical or non-cyclical in origin, the following ideas are well worth trying.

- *Invest in a good support bra that is comfortable enough to wear at night.*

- *Consider learning mental techniques such as deep relaxation, meditation and visualization. Some women find them helpful.*

- *Hypnosis is still controversial, but with an expert practitioner results can be as good as with oil of evening primrose.*

ASSESSMENT OF BREAST LUMPS

If you consult your family doctor with a breast lump, you will be referred to a breast specialist who will first try to establish whether the lump is benign or malignant.

To do this, doctors use a "triple assessment" approach to check out the lump: that is, manual examination, mammography or ultrasound, and fine-needle aspiration cytology (see column, right).

Physical examination alone won't reveal whether the lump is filled with fluid or solid. An ultrasound scan will make this distinction, however, and may pick up other lumps that are too small to feel.

If microscopic examination reveals malignant cells, your doctor will move on to a biopsy. Surgeons will remove any lump in the breast of a post-menopausal woman regardless of whether the cells are benign or malignant.

Physical examination
Your doctor will note the location of the lump in one of four quadrants (see below) and examine your armpits for swollen lymph nodes.

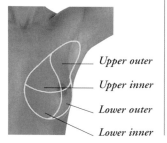

Upper outer

Upper inner

Lower outer

Lower inner

BREAST LUMPS

The commonest breast lumps belong to a group of harmless conditions that have no sinister implications whatsoever, but can cause anxiety if you don't understand how they arise and develop. Every woman has a lump (or general lumpiness) of one sort or another, although it may often be too small to feel. Practically all lumps are merely a variation of normal; they do not develop into cancers and they won't kill you. There is no actual disease. This is very important information for all women because on discovering a lump in their breasts they can be reassured that it probably belongs in the harmless category.

There are only two kinds of common benign breast lump: fibroadenomas and cysts. These lumps are not diseases – they are part of the normal changing growth pattern of the breasts throughout women's lives. There is a third type of lump called a pseudo-lump which, as its name implies, isn't really a breast lump at all. A pseudo-lump can occur at any age and is nearly always extreme normal lumpiness, but it should be checked to make certain that all is well. (Other pseudo-lumps, such as the end of a rib or scar tissue, are discussed on page 104.)

Doctors have no idea why these non-cancerous lumps appear, although they're probably related in some way to natural fluctucations in hormone production. Cysts and fibroadenomas grow only during a woman's fertile years, although they may be detected years later. They occur at opposite ends of the hormonal spectrum, fibroadenomas being most common in the early part of a woman's fertile life and cysts during mid-fertile life.

Lumpiness A special word needs to be said about lumpy breasts. Lumpiness in both breasts is never sinister and needs no treatment, especially if it's worse pre-menstrually. Some doctors still dub it fibrocystic disease, which all experts agree is an alarmist misnomer. The danger is that some doctors still believe fibrocystic disease to be generally precancerous, whereas this is very rarely so. Once a doctor is thinking this way, however, preventive measures may be recommended to you – even bilateral mastectomy (complete removal of both breasts). If your doctor suggests this, get a second opinion from a breast specialist. Bilateral mastectomy is hardly ever justified for lumpy breasts.

Triple assessment of breast lumps To check out a lump, breast specialists take a "triple assessment" approach, using manual examination and mammography or ultrasound (see far left) and a procedure called fine-needle aspiration cytology (FNAC, see right). Since this approach is so thorough, false positives and false negatives are exceedingly rare.

Ruling out cancer Breast cancer is rare in women under 35 years of age, whatever the symptoms. If you're under 35, the odds are that your lump is a fibroadenoma. If you find a new – and the emphasis is on *new* – discrete lump, your doctor will always refer you to a hospital for assessment. The presence of a lump overrides any other symptom and you should expect your doctor to act accordingly, whether he or she believes the lump to be cancer or not. All doctors have the same priority – to exclude cancer.

The picture may be unclear if you already have some lumpiness in your breasts since this occasionally obscures a very small cancer. If you're under 35 and your other breast is also lumpy, however, cancer is unlikely – in fact, even if the lump is new, large, discrete and mobile, cancer is most improbable. If you're between 35 and 55, the lump is probably a cyst – this can be confirmed immediately with FNAC (see right). Cysts are uncommon in women over 55, when the risks of developing cancer increase.

Keeping the lump Excellent research has been done in Edinburgh, Scotland and Oxford, England, showing that most women with benign breast disorders are happy to forego surgery once they have been reassured that the condition is indeed benign. This is sensible and humane, especially since there is no connection between malignant change and most benign breast conditions. Because it's now possible to identify the vast majority of benign lumps without surgical removal, you have the right to keep your lump undisturbed. The only exception is a cyst where the simple procedure of FNAC will collapse and cure it. Most doctors will be happy to leave your lump untouched if:

- on examination, the lump feels smooth and is mobile;
- mammography or an ultrasound scan shows that the lump looks harmless;
- FNAC shows nothing untoward;
- follow-up examinations after three and six months show no change in the size or appearance of the lump. Although some doctors do not require follow-up examinations, you should always return if you notice any changes.

WHAT IS FNAC?

One of the three procedures in assessing a breast lump (see far left) is FNAC; the letters stand for Fine-Needle Aspiration Cytology. It is used to sample cells from the lump.

Under mammographic guidance, or ultrasound if the lump can't be felt, a fine needle is inserted into the lump.

If fluid is withdrawn, the lump is a cyst; the fluid can be aspirated (drawn off) and the cyst will disappear.

If the lump is solid, a sample of cells is removed and spread on a glass slide for staining (a smear) and microscopic examination.

FIBROADENOMAS AND CANCER

Fibroadenomas that are extremely large (that is, larger than a lemon) may undergo cancerous change at their centres. This kind of cancer grows slowly, does not spread to other parts of the body and does not kill.

The fact that some large fibroadenomas may become cancerous is therefore not a justification for removing all fibroadenomas, especially since this kind of change is rare. Having a fibroadenoma does not in itself increase your risk of developing cancer.

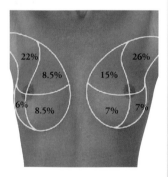

Locations of fibroadenomas
Although fibroadenomas can occur anywhere in the breast, they are often found near the nipple and are slightly more common in the left breast than in the right. No matter which breast they appear in, however, they are far more likely to occur in the upper outer quadrant and are seldom found in the lower ones. The picture shows the percentages found in each quadrant of either breast.

FIBROADENOMAS

These breast lumps are common in teenagers and women in their 20s (although they can occur at any age up to the menopause, or later if you're on HRT). They're simply over-developed lobules and are completely benign. You don't always need to have one removed, as long as you agree to further ultrasound and examination after six months. Most women opt for observation rather than removal.

Fibroadenomas can be very large – they vary from pea size to larger than a lemon. While they can grow anywhere in the breast, quite often they're found near the nipple. They feel smooth, firm and quite distinct, and move freely in your breast. Most doctors can recognize one simply by feeling it, but mammography or ultrasound and fine-needle aspiration cytology will clinch the diagnosis.

Most women who get a fibroadenoma will never get another one, but a few women will have several over their lifetime. It is also possible to have more than one at a time or a single large fibroadenoma involving more than one lobule. In extremely rare cases there may be a tendency for fibroadenomas to run in families.

Treatment options Once the diagnosis is confirmed, you can decide whether or not to have the lump removed. Most fibroadenomas come to nothing and shrink, so it's not unreasonable for your doctor to take a flexible attitude according to your age. If you're not worried, there's no need to have it removed. If you're under 25, cancer is so rare that a typical fibroadenoma can be left without risk, but you can have it removed if you wish. Fibroadenomas usually remain static, but if yours enlarges you can have it removed. Young women are often advised to watch and wait rather than undergo surgery and the resulting scarring. Where the picture is not clear, however, removal is wise.

Surgery is very simple and is done under local or general anaesthetic. To remove the lump, a small incision is made along the natural tension lines of the skin over it. The scars should be virtually invisible when they heal. Removal of a very large fibroadenoma can leave the breast misshapen, so discuss with your specialist the possibility of having your breast surgically refashioned, either in the same operation or later. This option will be available in most breast units. If not, the lump can be removed through an incision in the skin fold under the breast to give the best cosmetic result.

CYSTS

The blockage of glands as they change through a woman's life causes cysts, so cysts are a variation of normal breast anatomy, not a disease. A cyst is a fluid-filled sac similar to a large blister buried in breast tissue. When you feel it you can usually detect its smooth outline and you may even be able to bounce it between two fingers as you push the fluid from side to side. This is particularly so when the cyst is near the surface; when it's buried deep in breast tissue, however, it will simply feel like a hard lump.

Quite often a cyst will seem to appear suddenly – even overnight. This is a very reassuring sign because anything that appears so suddenly is almost certainly harmless. Cysts are most commonly found in women in their 30s, 40s and 50s with the peak just prior to the menopause. It's possible, although rare, for cysts to occur in young women or in post-menopausal women.

Your doctor may be able to identify a lump as a cyst simply on physical examination, but most breast specialists will wish to confirm the diagnosis by following up with an ultrasound examination or a mammogram (mammography will detect a cyst but cannot distinguish between it and other breast lumps, however). Your doctor will then probably suggest fine-needle aspiration cytology (FNAC) as the next step to confirm the diagnosis.

Treatment With cysts, FNAC serves as both diagnosis and treatment in one. Aspiration can be done quickly, simply and painlessly as a routine procedure in the breast clinic. No local anaesthetic is necessary since all you will feel is a needle prick. The needle is pushed through the skin into the cyst and the fluid is aspirated into a syringe, causing the cyst to collapse and disappear. The whole procedure may be carried out under ultrasonic guidance, allowing you to watch as your doctor inserts the needle and aspirates the cyst and it disappears. Large cysts that are easily felt can be aspirated without the help of ultrasound.

The fluid from the cyst can be any colour – brown, yellow, greenish or milky white. (In breastfeeding women, a milk-filled cyst can form, and this is called a galactocele.) Studies have shown that there is no point in the aspirated fluid from the cyst being examined since the risk of cancer is so minute. If the fluid is bloodstained, however, it is sent to the laboratory for analysis of the sediment.

CYSTS AND CANCER

Cysts are rarely malignant, or not harmfully so. In a very few cases, a small cancer may grow inside the cyst, but it usually doesn't spread beyond the cyst into the surrounding breast tissue, and it cannot kill you.

If any evidence of cell growth is found in the cyst, your surgeon will operate on it.

If you have a simple cyst, you will not have any increased cancer risk.

Occasionally cysts reform. If this happens, you should return to your doctor to have the cyst aspirated (drained); although the cyst is harmless in itself, it could obscure other changes in the breasts.

A cyst that persistently refills after being drained carries a slightly increased risk of cancer.

PERIDUCTAL MASTITIS

Infection is the usual cause of periductal mastitis, which means inflammation around the milk ducts. Inflammation can also occur without infection; this form is thought to be due to irritation by stagnant secretions leaking from a dilated duct.

A bacterial infection may result in chronic inflammation of the milk ducts, and may cause the tissue behind the nipple to stand proud and be manifested as a lump – this is known as a granuloma.

Such an infection can be difficult to root out, even with antibiotics, so an abscess or a fistula (a seeping abscess with a permanent opening to the skin) may form. Whatever the cause of the mastitis, the end result is the same: gradual retraction of the nipple.

NIPPLE CONDITIONS

Benign disorders affecting the nipple are less common than lumpiness and pain, but can be equally worrying; like all breast complaints they warrant prompt diagnosis to eliminate a rare cancer and decide appropriate treatment.

DILATATION OF THE MILK DUCTS

The underlying change in the normal anatomy of the milk ducts as a woman grows older is called ectasia, or dilatation. Frequently this leads to blockage of the ducts with pooling of fluid behind the blockage. Infection may lead to chronic inflammation and sometimes an abscess forms.

Ectasia of the milk ducts occurs in the last part of the breast's development cycle. This condition is normal and may thus affect both breasts, but it should not usually cause change in the nipple. If an infection develops and affects the dilated ducts, surrounding inflammation (periductal mastitis, see left) can lead to the formation of scar tissue, which contracts and draws in the nipple. An infection that arises from ectasia is not normal, however. Fortunately, this complication hardly ever occurs except in women who smoke, and it won't heal if a woman continues to smoke.

The normal dilatation of the milk ducts with ageing, and inflammation or infection of the ducts, account for most nipple problems in women over 50, including recurrent subareolar abscesses (infected lumps) and nipple retraction. Occasionally ectasia causes breast pain.

NIPPLE DISCHARGE

Nipple discharge is far less common than pain and lumps, and is of no consequence when it appears only if the breast and nipple are squeezed. It's also normal for premenopausal women who have had children and for women who smoke to produce nipple secretions. The risk of cancer in a woman with nipple discharge is very low, especially if both breasts are involved. To establish the cause it's important to find out if the discharge is coming from one duct or several.

Diagnosis To evaluate nipple discharge, your doctor will perform a biopsy of the duct, also removing tissue under the nipple. Mammography often reveals the characteristic little needle-shaped deposits of calcium around and pointing towards the nipple. Surgical removal of the involved ducts may be suggested if the discharge is embarrassing.

If a lump is found in conjunction with nipple discharge, investigating it takes priority. A lump beneath the areola in a breastfeeding woman is nearly always due to lactational mastitis (see below) complicated by an abscess.

Multiple duct discharge This is due to simple changes like ectasia and is nearly always benign. It is best left alone unless it's profuse and sufficient to stain clothes and cause embarrassment, but this is rare. Discharge caused by ectasia can be whitish, brown, grey or green, and watery or very thick. Surgical removal of the dilated or infected ducts won't be undertaken lightly; it can leave a woman unable to breastfeed and affect the sensation in the nipple and areola.

Occasionally, nipple discharge as a result of ectasia is accompanied by inflammation around the ducts, leaving the areolar skin red, hot and hard. If left untreated, this can lead to fistulae, although mostly in heavy smokers.

Single-duct discharge To doctors, discharge coming from a single duct is more significant than that from several ducts, but provided mammography shows no abnormality, surgery won't be required. Bloodstained discharge is usually due to a small benign papilloma (a wart-like growth) inside a duct, or to an ulcerated duct. The affected duct can be surgically removed. Rarely, a bloody discharge will be due to a ductal cancer; this doesn't have serious implications since this type of cancer is usually non-invasive.

NIPPLE INFECTIONS

The milk ducts are vulnerable to infection because bacteria can enter from the outside. Although such infections are unpleasant and often quite painful, they can be treated and are almost never a sign of something more sinister.

Lactational mastitis Nipple infections in a breastfeeding mother are the most common type. They nearly always arise from cracked, sore nipples; bacteria from the baby's mouth enters the lactiferous ducts through cracked skin and multiply rapidly in the milk. Occasionally, infection can result from a blocked duct. In both cases, the breast becomes tense, hot, reddened and painful.

Treatment Antibiotics combat the infection and analgesics deal with pain; neither should affect the baby. The breast should be rested for as short a time as possible because the baby's sucking keeps the milk flowing and this helps to overcome the infection; milk should be expressed in the meantime to keep the supply going. About one infection in

SUBAREOLAR INFECTIONS

Chronic infections of the breast around the areola usually affect women in their early thirties and are due to inflammation around the ducts. Smoking has been implicated as the most important cause, but how it damages the ducts isn't clear.

If the area is left untreated, it will become inflamed and an abscess may form. A mammary duct fistula is then a possibility if the abscess breaks down at the edge of the areola, and this can give rise to a permanent opening through the skin.

Antibiotics are the treatment of choice, but these infections are notoriously difficult to treat, especially if the patient goes on smoking. If the abscess fails to heal, an ultrasound scan will determine its extent and FNAC will exclude an underlying cancer. The abscess can be drained but it may recur. A fistula must be surgically removed.

If the abscess is very large, or the nipple has become badly inverted, or infections recur even after removal of the fistula, larger-scale surgery may be recommended.

Surgery may be disfiguring, so seek a second opinion, especially if mastectomy is recommended. Most women are happy with major duct excision if they're forewarned of the consequences such as lopsided breasts and loss of nipple sensation.

PAGET'S DISEASE

Although it looks like eczema, Paget's disease is actually a form of very slow-growing cancer, and tends to be associated with its in situ *form. It's therefore not a benign condition but is mentioned here because it is important to consider Paget's disease whenever eczema of the nipple occurs (see right).*

Paget's disease can sometimes be distinguished from eczema just by looking: it invariably starts on the nipple as a non-scaly, moist and erosive patch with a florid, raw, red surface, a definite outline and profuse discharge. Generally only one nipple is affected; it is rare for it to affect both nipples.

Another distinguishing characteristic of Paget's disease is that it develops slowly and is persistent – it won't clear up spontaneously and then recur like eczema. If Paget's disease is suspected, your doctor will recommend a biopsy and perhaps a mammogram.

ten goes on to form an abscess, which must be drained in hospital, under general anaesthetic if necessary. Once this has been done and the pain has subsided, you can breastfeed again. Sometimes ultrasound will show a small abscess, which can be treated by drawing out the pus with a needle.

Non-lactational mastitis Nipple infections are very rare if you are not breastfeeding. Women with lowered immunity, diabetes or who have had breast surgery are most at risk.

SKIN CONDITIONS

The skin of the breasts is thin and sensitive but need not be more prone to problems than skin elsewhere on the body provided proper care is taken.

Cracked nipples During breastfeeding, the skin around the nipples is exposed to milk and vigorous sucking, both of which can damage the skin. Prevention is the best approach: the nipples should be gently dabbed clean after each feed and a baby who is properly latched on will not need to suck hard to feed well. Applying a drop of baby lotion to your breast pad can also help. If the nipples do become cracked, it's important to get advice on positioning the baby correctly on the breast and taking her off. This is best done by pushing down gently on the baby's chin to break the airtight seal between her mouth and the nipple. Treatment for cracked nipples must be prompt, since they are vulnerable to infections.

Eczema Classically, eczema starts on the areolar skin and later spreads to the nipple; it usually appears on both nipples and can be localized or associated with generalized eczema elsewhere on the body. It develops quite quickly and may clear up but then recur. The involved skin is usually scaly, red, itchy and moist and the patch of eczema is likely to have an irregular outline. Eczema will normally respond to one percent hydrocortisone cream.

Areolar gland disorders There are three kinds of gland in the areolar skin and all of them can lead to problems. The apocrine sweat glands can become infected and form cysts; the sebaceous glands can also form cysts; and the accessory mammary glands can discharge or become infected.

Treatment Infection of the sweat glands can usually be cleared with an antibiotic cream, but the glands very often have to be removed if the infection persists. Cysts can be removed under local anaesthetic if they are troublesome. Discharge and infection usually respond to antibiotics.

BREAST CANCER

Understanding the causes and effects of a disease such as breast cancer can greatly improve your chances of avoiding and defeating it. Knowledge of risk and preventive factors can help you to reduce your own risk of getting breast cancer. This includes making both life choices – such as having your first baby before 30 years of age and breastfeeding – and lifestyle changes, such as keeping your weight down and your consumption of alcohol low. Early detection and diagnosis play an important role in the successful treatment of breast cancer, and in the prognosis and long-term outlook. Modern techniques of grading and staging mean that doctors can tailor treatment to the particular needs of each patient.

UNDERSTANDING BREAST CANCER

Cancer of the breast need not be fatal. Only one breast lump in ten ever turns out to be cancerous and, of those that do, a considerable number are of the non-invasive type – that is, they do not spread beyond their place of origin and therefore cannot kill. A cancer that is less than 1 centimetre (½ inch) in diameter is still at a very early stage; there is therefore only a small chance that it has spread and less risk of its being fatal. One of the main aims of this chapter, therefore, is to curb the panic that may grip you when you discover a lump, so that you seek advice immediately and give yourself the best chance, rather than succumb to the paralysing fear that the prospect of cancer may bring.

The psychological reactions to finding a lump and being given a diagnosis of cancer are complex. Breast cancer has social, emotional and sexual consequences that will affect not only a woman's health but her relationships, her lifestyle and her body image. A knowledgeable and well-informed woman is best placed to take an active role in her treatment, and to cultivate the positive state of mind that can contribute to the defeat of the disease.

It's important for you to know that, even when a diagnosis of breast cancer is made, there are different types. Not all cancers have the same degree of invasiveness or potential for spread, so not all have a poor outlook. A positive attitude is a real asset, possibly as vital as some medical treatments.

THE NATURE OF BREAST CANCER

Breast cancer is a family of conditions, not a single entity. The common feature of every type, however, is that certain cells start to grow out of control. Cell growth is normally restricted to simple repair so that an organ is kept up to scratch; it is held in check by chemicals that ensure growth is orderly and never gets out of hand. Cancer starts when the brakes on growth are taken off, or when they are no longer effective, or when cells become insensitive to them. Cell growth then becomes uncontrolled and disorderly and the cells themselves may start to look abnormal. Because cell growth is rapid in a cancer, it absorbs a great deal of body energy. This is why cancer is often accompanied by weight loss, although this is rare in breast cancer.

Tumours and spread The word tumour simply means a lump. Most tumours are not cancerous. They are usually benign; the growth of cells is confined to the area where the tumour starts. Tumours whose cells don't spread to other parts of the body are not fatal. In contrast, the cells that make up cancerous tumours are invasive. They spread beyond their original location, not just into adjacent tissues, but to other distant parts of the body, and as they invade tissue they destroy it.

The original tumour is known as the primary. Tumours that arise from these cancerous cells that have spread elsewhere are called secondaries or metastases. To determine how aggressive cancer cells are and how far they have spread, if at all, grading and staging tests are done. These tests also serve as a basis for deciding on treatment.

Spread through the lymphatic system Cancers of the breast often spread first into the lymph nodes in the armpits (the axillary lymph nodes), causing swelling. They may also spread to lymph nodes under the breastbone and above the collarbone. (This is why you should always check your armpits and collarbone for swollen lymph nodes whenever you do your regular breast self-examination.)

Cancer in the bloodstream While the first sign of spread may be enlarged lymph nodes, spread via the bloodstream is probably more important in determining the final outcome of the disease. The most recent research suggests that breast-cancer cells, or particles of them ("seeds"), enter the bloodstream relatively early in the course of the disease. This is why modern treatments, like chemotherapy, are aimed at eradicating cancer cells from the body *as a whole* rather than just dealing with the tumour locally.

PUTTING BREAST CANCER IN PERSPECTIVE

- Breast cancer, over a lifetime, affects 1 in 12 women and causes around 15,000 deaths a year in the UK.
- Five times more women suffer from the disease than die from it. In a given year, of 100,000 women who live with breast cancer, 80,000 do not die.
- More than 70 percent of women who have operable disease will be alive and well five years after the diagnosis.
- By the age of 50, your chances of dying from breast cancer will have dropped dramatically from 12 in 70 to 1 in 70, and the odds get better with every year you live after that without developing it.

FIBROBLASTS

Some research has centred on whether there may be a link between the character of a woman's breast tissue and her risk of getting breast cancer.

Researchers now suggest that it may not be the glandular elements of the breast that determine whether cells change from normal to cancerous, but cells called fibroblasts.

Fibroblasts lie among the fat and connective tissue of the breast and produce a number of chemical messengers called growth factors. These seem to communicate with breast cancer cells, stimulating their growth and ability to spread.

Cancer cells need a rich blood supply to support their rapid growth, and fibroblasts appear to encourage the formation of new blood vessels in tissues surrounding the cancer that provide the necessary blood.

It's probable that fibroblasts in some women are more likely to support the growth of cancer cells than fibroblasts in other women. This finding may help in part to explain why some breast cancers are hereditary.

Fatal diseases

This chart shows that stroke and heart disease cause many more deaths than breast cancer among women of all ages in the developed world.

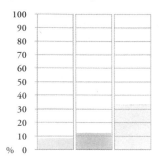

KEY

☐ DEATHS FROM BREAST CANCER

▨ DEATHS FROM STROKE

☐ DEATHS FROM HEART DISEASE

Your chances of dying from something else

Breast cancer (represented on the graph by the green area) is the most common cause of death in women between 35 and 55. While it is more common in women over 55, it is less likely to be the cause of death in this age group.

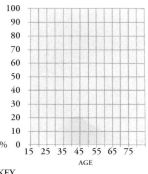

AGE

KEY

☐ DEATHS FROM OTHER CAUSES

☐ DEATHS FROM BREAST CANCER

- In statistical terms, breast cancer accounts for almost one in five of all new cancer cases among women.
- In women between 35 and 55, it ranks as the commonest cause of death overall, *but*
  - for every breast lump found to be cancerous, ten others will prove to be benign and therefore harmless;
  - even with cancerous lumps, six or seven out of ten will be treated without removing the breast. For three or four the cause of death will be something other than cancer;
  - if the lump is diagnosed and treated early, you'll be one of the 85 percent of women who survive at least five years;
  - in post-menopausal women, deaths from breast cancer pale into insignificance when compared with the number of deaths caused by heart disease;
  - by the time you are in your mid-60s, your chances of dying from breast cancer are probably less than half what they were when you were 50.
- So, although the chances of getting breast cancer increase as women age, the chances of dying from it become less with each successive year that they live.

THE GENETICS OF CANCER

A healthy cell has a well-defined shape. It is a responsible "team player", multiplying only when the balance of signals is favourable. Built into cell growth, however, is the hazard of genetic mutations, or random changes. Then, the cell becomes damaged; it may appear normal, but it is slightly less responsive to external signals. As genetic damage accumulates, a cell can become deaf to external messages that inhibit growth and start to show signs of malignancy. In particular, it loses its regular shape and outline and multiplies uncontrollably. Cancer probably develops because cells suffer irreversible damage to their genes. Events that cause damage to genes are called trigger factors and those that facilitate cell growth are called promoters.

The development of a cancer cell takes time, even several lifetimes. On the other hand, it can take as little as ten years depending on how damaged the genes were when they passed from parent to child. Severely damaged genes may respond quickly to an environmental trigger, such as prolonged exposure to menstrual cycling (see right) in the case of breast cancer. Two breast cancer genes have been identified: BRCA1 and BRCA2, but there are likely to be many more.

RISK AND PROTECTIVE FACTORS

Some women are more likely to get cancer of the breast than others: the risk can be connected with geographic location, particular cultures, specific personal traits and lifestyle features. Some women inherit a susceptibility to the disease, which then requires one or more environmental risk factors in order that breast cancer should develop. Genetic factors therefore interact with environmental factors, but unfortunately doctors don't know how.

Doctors do know enough, however, to help them to identify women who are at high risk. This in turn promotes early detection of breast cancer and enables some women to change their lifestyles and make life choices to reduce their risk. Try to take a positive attitude and remember that some risk factors can be turned upside-down to become protective factors: if having your first baby late increases the risk, you might consider having an early first child to lower your risk.

Hormones The patterns of a woman's hormones and their fluctuations during menstruation, pregnancy and lactation all play an important part in determining her risk of developing breast cancer. Hormones from other sources, such as the contraceptive pill and hormone replacement therapy, may have an effect, although this is much less.

Menstruation The risk of breast cancer appears to be increased both by an early onset of menstruation, medically termed menarche, and by a late cessation of menstruation, which is called menopause. In the developed world, the average age at which a woman starts to menstruate seems to be getting earlier, and the average age at menopause getting later, and this lengthening of "menstrual life" could be a contributory factor in the apparent increase in breast-cancer rates.

Researchers are coming to believe that the *total number of menstrual cycles* in a woman's lifetime determines her cancer risk. The number of menstrual cycles before the first pregnancy may be even more important, however. It is possible that the breasts are more sensitive to the action of hormones before they have fully developed – that is, before they have produced milk – and this would explain why age at first pregnancy is so important.

TYPES OF RISK

There are two different ways of describing risk: relative risk and absolute risk.

Relative risk describes how a single factor may increase risk. Take the risk factor of having a family history of breast cancer. The relative risk of a woman whose mother had breast cancer is 2, meaning that she is twice as likely to get the disease as a woman with no family history of breast cancer.

Absolute risk is more precise, and denotes the number of likely cases of breast cancer in a specific number of women over a given time. The absolute risk of breast cancer, however, is 1 woman per 1,000 per year; this means that one woman in one thousand will get breast cancer in a year. For women with a family history of breast cancer, therefore, the absolute risk is 2 per 1,000 per year.

MENSTRUAL LIFE AND RISK

Your "menstrual life" links three important risk factors for breast cancer – age at first period, age at menopause and number of pregnancies – that determine your total exposure to oestrogen. The longer the exposure, the greater the risk. Even quite small differences between women can add up to significant differences in overall risk, as the following two examples show.

Liz

Age at menopause	*48*
Less age at first period	*–14*
Less time spent pregnant (years)	*–3*
Total years' exposure to oestrogen	**31**

Joan

Age at menopause	*52*
Less age at first period	*–12*
Less time spent pregnant (years)	*–1½*
Total years' exposure to oestrogen	**38½**

It is also possible that a fertile lifetime of menstruation is, in biological terms, an abnormal state for the human female and so predisposes women to develop breast cancer. It's only relatively recently that women stopped spending a great proportion of their reproductive life either pregnant or breastfeeding, and it's only in the twentieth century that women in any numbers have lived long enough to reach the menopause at all. The average girl in the developed world now starts to menstruate before the age of 12, but will then wait until she is 25 or 26 years old to have her first baby, exposing her to almost 14 years of continuous menstrual cycling before her first pregnancy. This doesn't happen in many other cultures. An African girl may not start menstruating until she's 17 or 18 because she's under-nourished, and may then become pregnant almost at once, saving her from years of exposure to cyclical oestrogens.

Protection in pregnancy Having babies undoubtedly protects women against breast cancer; this may be because it saves a woman from being exposed to cyclical oestrogens for nine months. The major protection seems to be conferred by the first pregnancy, which must be carried to term to be protective; a first pregnancy that ends in abortion or miscarriage does not have any protective effect.

Not having children and having a first baby late in life both seem to increase the chances of developing breast cancer. For women who have their first child after the age of 30, the risk of breast cancer is about twice that of women who have their first child before the age of 20. Women who remain childless are at increased risk, and this may partly explain why infertility in older women is linked to breast cancer. Surprisingly, women who have their first child after the age of 35 appear to be at an even higher risk than women who have no children.

The contraceptive pill The oral contraceptive pill was introduced 30 years ago and has been used by about 150 million women. Huge long-term research studies have not uncovered any *substantial* increased risk of breast cancer in women who take the pill. Breast cancer is fairly common, as is the practice of taking the pill, so if breast cancer develops in a woman who is on the pill, it can't be assumed that the two are related; it might have happened anyway.

Against these very small increases in risk, doctors have to weigh the fact that the pill has a protective effect against ovarian cancer. For a woman at risk of ovarian cancer, this protective effect would outweigh the breast cancer risk. Some studies have shown a reduction in benign breast disease among contraceptive pill users, which could reduce the risk of breast cancer.

Hormone replacement therapy Menopausal symptoms have been successfully treated with hormone replacement therapy (HRT) for more than 50 years. There has been no dramatic increase in breast cancer, however, since the use of HRT became fairly widespread some two decades ago, suggesting that any risk is very small. Most researchers in this field agree that in the first ten years of use there is no increased risk associated with HRT. After that time there may be a very small increased risk, but for the average healthy woman, it would appear that the use of HRT does not increase breast-cancer risk any more than having a first baby after the age of 30.

As with the contraceptive pill, there are also benefits to be weighed against any possible risk. HRT has a protective effect against cancers of the lung, colon, ovary and cervix. It also protects against heart disease, the major killer of women, and osteoporosis. Women on HRT who develop breast cancer usually have a less invasive form of cancer and are more likely to respond to hormone treatment. Women who develop breast cancer after having taken HRT for eight years have an improved survival rate. Finally, women who have used HRT seem to have a lower mortality rate at any age from any cause than those who have not.

Even for women who have had breast cancer, HRT needn't be ruled out as long as there is careful follow-up from a doctor who is expert in this field. If you fall into this category, you should talk it over with a gynaecologist as well as a cancer specialist.

Family history A family history of breast cancer is a strong risk factor in itself and makes all other risk factors potentially more significant. The increase in risk depends on how close the relative is and on how many relatives have had breast cancer. The risk is greater if the affected relative developed breast cancer under the age of 50, and increases still further if *two* female relatives are affected. The risk is greatest if your mother developed breast cancer under the age of 35.

A woman whose mother developed cancer in both breasts before the age of 35, for instance, has a 50 percent chance of developing breast cancer herself. This familial susceptibility to breast cancer is now known to be related

Family history and risk
The more relatives a woman has with breast cancer, and the younger they are when they develop the disease, the higher her own risk becomes.

25 TIMES NORMAL RISK

MOTHER WITH BILATERAL BREAST CANCER UNDER 35

MOTHER AND SISTER WITH BREAST CANCER

SISTER WITH BILATERAL BREAST CANCER UNDER 40

SISTER WITH BILATERAL BREAST CANCER UNDER 50

FIRST-DEGREE RELATIVE (MOTHER OR SISTER) WITH BREAST CANCER

SECOND-DEGREE RELATIVE (AUNT OR GRANDMOTHER) WITH BREAST CANCER

NORMAL RISK

BREAST CANCER "LEAGUE TABLE"

The following list shows the relative positions of 24 countries in a "league table" of breast cancer rates, with countries in Western Europe at the top of the league.

1 England and Wales
2 Denmark
3 Scotland
4 Northern Ireland
5 Netherlands
6 Belgium
7 Switzerland
8 New Zealand
9 Canada
10 Germany
11 United States
12 Hungary
13 Czech Republic and Slovakia
14 Australia
15 Argentina
16 France
17 Norway
18 Sweden
19 Portugal
20 Poland
21 Bulgaria
22 Greece
23 Hong Kong
24 Japan

to two genes, labelled BRCA1 and BRCA2. Being born into a "breast-cancer family" carries the greatest risk, and it's important to identify these women who are at high risk of developing breast cancer.

Age Given that environmental factors can react with a genetic predisposition to trigger the growth of breast cancer, it stands to reason that the longer a woman lives the more likely she is to be exposed to these environmental triggers and the higher her risk is of developing breast cancer. This supposition is borne out by the statistics: about half of all breast cancers occur in women aged 50–64, with a further 30 percent in women aged over 70. This means that 80 percent of breast cancers occur over the age of 50.

Geography Although the frequency of breast cancer varies widely throughout the world (see left) the disease seems to single out white women living in colder climates in highly industrialized societies, and it's the lifestyle of the developed world that is largely to blame. Women from low-risk areas (for instance Japan, which has one of the lowest rates of breast cancer in the entire world) who move to and settle permanently in higher-risk countries, such as the US, climb into a higher risk group for breast cancer. Environmental factors therefore seem to be stronger than racial or inherited ones. There is even evidence that shows rates of breast cancer increasing as countries become more industrialized.

Radiation Doctors have known for some time that high doses of radiation can promote the development of breast cancer. In the past, women who received high-dose chest X-rays to check on treatment for tuberculosis ran an increased risk of developing cancer. Japanese women who were exposed to enormously high doses of radiation from the atomic bombs at Hiroshima and Nagasaki are still developing breast cancer at higher rates than other Japanese women of the same age living in other parts of Japan.

Protection in breastfeeding Breastfeeding does seem to protect against breast cancer, although pregnancy is even more important; an early pregnancy is protective regardless of whether a woman breastfeeds or bottlefeeds. Some evidence from UK studies suggests that breastfeeding even for a very short time is protective. Since breastfeeding has so substantial a protective effect, and since it is available to all women who give birth, it's astonishing that more women don't do it. I would urge all women to consider breastfeeding, even for as short a time as a couple of weeks.

Diet The Western diet is constantly cited as a risk factor for breast cancer, but the evidence is pretty thin. The original connection came from an observation that dietary fat can cause breast tumours in rats. Such evidence can't be directly applied to human beings, but it was an interesting lead. Studies of total fat intake, however, have not found that women with breast cancer consume a significantly higher amount of fat than women without; the relationship may reflect total intake of calories rather than fat intake alone. Breast-cancer risk seems more influenced by obesity than by fat consumption.

People who eat a diet high in fat tend to eat less fruit and vegetables, so it could be that the risk is due to a deficiency of fibre rather than an excess of fat. Quite recent evidence suggests that a diet rich in cereals and vegetables may protect against breast cancer. Fibre is thought to influence oestrogen metabolism and some vitamin derivatives may have a protective effect, particularly vitamin E and beta-carotene, which is a form of vitamin A.

A study from Cambridge, England, has shown that a soya-rich diet will lengthen the menstrual cycle by two or three days. Over a lifetime this would mean significantly fewer cycles, having a beneficial effect with regard to breast cancer. The active components of soya are isoflavones, which have a strong oestrogenic effect.

Obesity Women who are overweight have a higher risk of dying from breast cancer than their leaner sisters. The pattern of obesity seems to be important in defining cancer risk. When fat is concentrated around the trunk, giving a ratio between waist and hip measurements of greater than one (an "apple shape"), cancer risk is higher than in women who retain a well-defined waist with bigger hips ("pear shapes"). This pattern of obesity is linked with a number of diseases, such as heart disease in men. It's a common fat distribution among post-menopausal and infertile women, in whom breast cancer rates are higher than average.

Alcohol Excessive alcohol intake increases a woman's risk of developing breast cancer in the long term, since alcohol can interfere with the body's metabolism of oestrogen. Both alcohol and oestrogen are broken down in the liver and, after many years of exposure to alcohol, the liver loses its ability to metabolize oestrogen. This results in increased levels of oestrogen in the blood, a factor known to increase the risk of breast cancer.

SMOKING

Rates of breast cancer are lower in smokers than in non-smokers. This can never be advocated as a reason for smoking, however, since the risk of dying from a smoking-related disease such as lung cancer far outweighs that of dying from breast cancer.

It is thought that smoking exerts an anti-oestrogenic effect, accelerating the onset of the menopause; smokers typically reach the menopause three to four years earlier than women who do not smoke.

Smokers tend to be thinner than those who don't smoke; it is known that oestrogens are manufactured in the fatty tissues and that obesity is a risk factor for breast cancer (see left). Smokers also have less benign breast disease than non-smokers and this could partly explain the reduced risk.

The protective effect that smoking confers is greater among post-menopausal than pre-menopausal women, and seems to operate only as long as you go on smoking. When you stop, the protection is lost.

As yet, doctors don't fully understand why smoking has an anti-oestrogenic effect. One study has found that women who smoke have higher levels of male sex hormones, such as testosterone, which has anti-oestrogenic properties.

This link with alcohol is not a great risk and must be kept in perspective. If one thousand women over the age of 30 drank moderately for two years, there would be one extra case of breast cancer among them.

WHAT YOU CAN DO

Although you can't control factors like your family history or age at menopause, you can change some aspects of your lifestyle to make a difference to your risk of breast cancer.

- Restrict the amount of red meat and fat in your diet and increase your fibre intake by eating plenty of wholegrain cereals, fruit and vegetables every day.
- Enjoy alcohol only in moderation.
- Keep your body fat down by eating a balanced diet and taking regular exercise.
- Plan to have your first baby by the age of 30.
- If you have babies, breastfeed – the longer the better.

Comparison of risk
The chart below looks at the different factors that can affect your risk of developing breast cancer and helps you to compare them. Remember that the lowest possible risk has a score of 1.0.

FACTORS THAT CAN AFFECT THE RISK OF DEVELOPING BREAST CANCER

RISK FACTOR	LOWEST RISK		SLIGHT INCREASE		MODERATE INCREASE	
AGE AT FIRST MENSTRUAL PERIOD	16 years (late)	1.0	15 years (late) 11–14 years	1.1 1.3		
AGE AT MENOPAUSE	Before 45	1.0	45–54	1.4	Over 55	2.1
AGE AT BIRTH OF FIRST CHILD	Before 20	1.0	20–29	1.45	Over 30 years or no children	1.9
FAMILY HISTORY	None	1.0	Mother affected before age 60 Mother affected after age 60	2.0 1.4	Two first-degree relatives affected (i.e., mother and sister)	4.0–6.0
BENIGN BREAST DISEASE	None	1.0	Increase in number of cells	2.0	Atypical hyperplasia (see p. 53)	4.5
ALCOHOL INTAKE	None	1.0	1 drink a day 2 drinks a day	1.4 1.7	3 drinks a day	2.0
RADIATION EXPOSURE	No special exposure	1.0	Repeated X-rays	1.5–2.0	Atomic bomb	3.0
ORAL CONTRACEPTIVES	Never used or no longer used	1.0	Currently used	1.5	Prolonged use before pregnancy	2.0
HRT	Never used or no longer used	1.0	Currently used all ages	1.4	Used longer than ten years or currently used over 60	2.1

BREAST-CANCER FAMILIES

A single first-degree relative (that is, mother or sister) with breast cancer doubles anyone's risk of cancer, but in breast-cancer families the risks are even greater. A breast-cancer family is one in which the risk of a woman developing breast cancer is determined almost totally by family history, and appears to be independent of other risk factors, except atypical hyperplasia.

Breast-cancer families, although quite rare, have been studied for more than two millennia and were first reported in Roman medical literature of AD 100. In the 1860s, an American doctor, Paul Broca, described many instances of breast cancer in combination with bowel cancer in several generations of his wife's family. He was describing what we now call hereditary breast cancer (HBC). The word hereditary means that the cancer runs through a family affecting successive generations of women. The pattern of inheritance nearly always suggests that the hereditary factor is extremely strong. The factor responsible has been narrowed down to one or two genes, and since it's so strong, it is known as a dominant gene. Although hereditary breast cancer puts women at very high risk, it accounts for only a small proportion of all cases of breast cancer – between five and ten percent.

A rigorous approach There are several important features of HBC that profoundly affect treatment. The first is the early age of onset. Breast cancer is more common in older women as a rule, with an average age of 62 years among women affected, but in breast-cancer families the average age is 44. Second, there is often more than one tumour in the breast. Finally, the cancer may affect both breasts.

These three characteristics have an enormous bearing on how doctors view familial breast cancer. Women in these families need to be identified, and made aware that they are in danger of developing breast cancer early, and in both breasts. Any woman who is aware of her risk should seek advice from a breast unit while still in her teens or early 20s. Because of the aggressive nature of this cancer, doctors are more likely to be receptive to the idea of prophylactic (preventive) mastectomy together with breast reconstruction, although medically such a radical course is hard to justify when inheritance of the gene cannot yet be conclusively proved.

The shadow cast by the hereditary aspect of HBC falls on all aspects of managing it. Monitoring of the health of the breasts must be rigorous and scrupulous. It must include regular check-ups, mammograms, ultrasound scans where appropriate and biopsies of any suspicious changes.

Identifying women at risk At present, the most important tool for doctor and patient is a thorough family history. There's unfortunately no way of testing for the precise genes and chromosomes associated with HBC and identifying vulnerable women before the cancer appears, although there is hope that such tests will become possible in the next few years. Until then, a careful family pedigree and close surveillance, together with frequent physical examinations and mammograms, are the best defence. Much controversy surrounds the age for starting mammographic screening. The problem with mammograms in younger women is that their breasts are more dense than those of older women and cancers are difficult to pick up. Several studies have shown, however, that early detection is possible, and it is certainly worthwhile in breast-cancer families.

Careful surveillance of cancer families is essential. This is best done by gathering the female members of the family together to explain how cancers can run through each generation in a family, offering counselling and ensuring that each woman is vigorously screened and tested in order to detect any cancers as early as possible.

Breast cancer genes Two of the genes that are responsible for inherited breast cancer were finally identified in 1994, and it is likely that there are more to be found. These two, called BRCA1 and BRCA2, are probably responsible for more than half the cases of hereditary breast cancer. A woman carrying either of them has about an 80 percent risk of contracting breast cancer during her lifetime, and a 70 percent risk after the age of 50. The genes can be passed on by either parent (not just the mother), and there is a 50–50 chance that children will inherit them.

At the moment, no gene test is available (there are many possible gene mutations, presenting complex problems for testing), but it is probable that within the next three years, women from breast-cancer families could be offered a test. Women found to carry the genes would then have the options of increased monitoring to detect cancer early on, including annual mammography from age 35, tamoxifen therapy, or prophylactic (preventive) mastectomy.

PREVENTIVE MEASURES

An overview of breast-cancer risk factors shows there are some that can be controlled to reduce risk, notably diet, alcohol intake, an early first child and – for women who have children – breastfeeding. For women at very high risk, however, some kind of prevention in the form of hormone treatment or surgery may be advisable.

Tamoxifen A complex drug with both oestrogenic and anti-oestrogenic properties, tamoxifen was first used in the treatment of breast cancer and is now being studied as a way of preventing it among high-risk women, particularly those with a strong family history where breast cancer may appear at an early age. Tamoxifen is used to treat women who already have breast cancer; not only does it reduce the risk of recurrence and improve mortality rates, but in the long term it also reduces by half the risk of getting cancer in the other breast, a cause for great concern for women with a family history of breast cancer.

Just as fibroblast growth factors promote breast cancer, other growth factors suppress it. The production of suppressor growth factors is stimulated by tamoxifen, and this is one of the reasons why it could be effective in the prevention of breast cancer.

Because of its action on the production of the hormone, oestrogen, tamoxifen has side effects when taken for long periods, causing menopausal symptoms and an early onset of the menopause. One study has raised the possibility of a slightly increased risk of uterine cancer; others do not. This is being studied to see if any risk actually exists. Tamoxifen has life-saving properties other than reducing the risk of breast cancer, however. It seems to protect against heart attacks – in a recent study in Scotland it led to a significant reduction in deaths from heart disease – and osteoporosis (brittle bones caused by loss of bone protein).

Prophylactic (preventive) mastectomy If you are at high risk of developing breast cancer, you may have seen your mother or sister die from the disease, and may consider mastectomy as an effective way to prevent it in yourself. Prophylactic mastectomy aims to reduce the risk of breast cancer by removing as much breast tissue as possible. Reconstruction may be carried out to rebuild the breast. In such a case, you do not have the option of a subcutaneous mastectomy, which is an operation where the breast tissue

MAKING THE DECISION: PROS

You should consider both the pros and the cons if you are thinking about prophylactic mastectomy.

- *There is no definite evidence to prove that prophylactic mastectomy reduces a woman's chance of getting cancer, but it probably does, as long as the operation is a total mastectomy.*

- *The operation certainly reduces painful symptoms and tender lumpiness in the breast as part of the menstrual cycle, although mastalgia (breast pain) alone would never be a reason for mastectomy.*

- *For women who cannot live normal lives for fear of breast cancer, it can provide a new lease of life.*

- *Modern surgical procedures mean that the breasts can be reconstructed.*

MAKING THE DECISION: CONS

Reconstruction may be done to rebuild the breasts after prophylactic mastectomy. You should consider the risks of this operation as well.

- *General anaesthesia is a risk in its own right.*

- *There may be complications including bleeding, infection, skin loss, nipple loss and damage to the implant.*

- *Capsular contraction may occur, where the capsule of scar tissue that forms around the implant contracts and becomes as hard as wood. Massaging the breasts may reduce the firmness, but if they are very hard, treatment can be quite complicated and may involve further surgery.*

- *Complications can occur if an abdominal flap is used for reconstruction.*

- *The reconstructed breast is rarely as attractive as the original breast, and there may be permanent scarring and loss of sensation.*

- *More than one operation may be needed to achieve the best results or manage complications.*

- *There's no guarantee that cancer will be prevented: not all breast tissue is removed and any that is left behind is still a potential site for breast cancer.*

is removed from beneath the skin and an implant inserted, leaving the nipple and areola intact. The operation *must* be a total mastectomy; anything else is not justifiable. If your doctor should suggest a subcutaneous mastectomy, question its reliability and usefulness and get a second opinion.

Prophylactic mastectomy, in which one or both breasts are removed, is a controversial operation. Many doctors are loath to remove healthy breast tissue when cancer may never develop. Also crucial is whether the operation is effective enough in preventing breast cancer when powerful, non-surgical treatments, such as tamoxifen therapy, could accomplish the same goal. When contemplating prophylactic mastectomy, you must remember that there is no guarantee that breast cancer will be prevented. For these reasons, you will be considered eligible to have both breasts removed only if you fulfil the following strict criteria:

- an unarguable family history and an estimated 50 percent chance of getting breast cancer;
- your clear understanding that you have a 50–50 chance of inheriting the high-risk gene, so that you have an equal chance of carrying and not carrying the gene (the latter would mean you are at normal risk for breast cancer);
- the presence of additional factors that would raise the risk above 50 percent, such as two sisters being affected or atypical hyperplasia.

Other factors that would also be taken into consideration are breasts that are difficult to examine both clinically and radiographically, and severe cancer phobia. You should decide to have prophylactic mastectomy only after careful discussion of your precise risk, details of the operation and the likely outcome with a specialist breast surgeon and the other members of the breast management team. Even better would be counselling by two surgeons who can evaluate your particular risk factors and their implications. Finally, you should also consult close family and friends. Most women, when advised that they have a chance of not carrying the high-risk gene, opt for intensive follow-up screening and testing rather than surgery.

The majority of women at high risk are monitored most effectively by breast self-examination and regular physical examinations and mammograms. In addition, fine-needle aspiration cytology is decreasing the need for open biopsy if a breast lump should occur, and biopsy is available for any suspicious breast areas that may arise.

NON-INVASIVE CANCER

The glands and ducts that make up the breast lobules are in a state of growth, development and shrinkage during a woman's fertile life. Overgrowth of cells or hyperplasia, as it is called, may occur in any part of the lobes or ducts. The word hyperplasia without qualification always implies a benign condition, although it carries a small increase in the risk of cancer. In some hyperplasias, however, the cells become somewhat unusual or atypical. This is referred to as atypical hyperplasia, and has a moderate chance of turning into a localized cancer. (A woman with a family history of breast cancer who develops atypical hyperplasia moves into a very high-risk group indeed.)

Actual cancer comes at the far end of the hyperplasia spectrum, but, at first at least, it is the non-invasive "cancer in situ" (in situ means that the cancer is confined to its place of origin). This term is used for patterns of cell growth that are confined to the duct or lobule where they originated, but carry a high risk of becoming invasive (see right).

PRE-INVASIVE DISEASE

As cell growth proceeds from hyperplasia, which is benign, towards malignancy, it reaches an in-between stage – cancer "in situ". This is a crucial distinction to make, since these cancers by definition are not invasive and they are seldom fatal. There are two kinds: ductal carcinoma in situ (DCIS) and lobular carcinoma in situ (LCIS).

In situ carcinomas are confined to the duct or lobule in which they start growing, and rarely invade the surrounding breast. A true lump is often difficult to detect and, unless there is some other symptom such as nipple discharge, the majority of these lumps are picked up only through screening mammograms, when the characteristic tiny Y-shaped calcifications of DCIS are seen.

In situ cancers sometimes pose a problem for treatment because it is not known how many may progress to invasive cancer, nor how long they may take to do so. Nor has one approach to the treatment of DCIS and LCIS been proved to be substantially better than any other.

Because of the risk that an invasive cancer may develop, preventive mastectomy may be an option. Most doctors, however, would probably adopt the compromise of a wide excision to remove the cancerous tissue and a watch-policy,

UNDERSTANDING HYPERPLASIA

Hyperplasia (cell overgrowth) has four stages. The stage that most concerns doctors is the second: atypical hyperplasia (see below). When assessing hyperplasia, there are several features that doctors look at to decide whether the condition is benign or whether there is a risk of cancer.

- *Deciding features include the rate at which the cells are dividing; the way the cells are organized, and the features of the cells themselves.*

- *In normal circumstances, the cells lining the breast ducts and lobes multiply only under strictly regulated conditions and in response to specific signals.*

- *Overgrowth of cells may occur in any part of the lobes or ducts, and may progress through four stages.*

- *One: Hyperplasia The cells multiply more than necessary, creating a harmless excess that builds up inside the duct.*

- *Two: Atypical hyperplasia The cells lose their normal appearance and are called "atypical". This is still a benign condition.*

- *Three: Carcinoma in situ The atypical cells fill up the duct, forming a carcinoma, but the cells are not invasive.*

- *Four: Invasive carcinoma The atypical cells break out of the duct and spread to the surrounding tissues. This is a true invasive cancer.*

with mastectomy at a later date, if necessary. Ultimately, the choice of treatment depends on a woman's individual risk, whether she has a family history of breast cancer, whether there is calcification in her breast lesion, and her age when it is found.

Lobular carcinoma in situ (LCIS) LCIS in itself does not develop into cancer, but it is useful as a marker, showing that a woman is at risk of developing DCIS. This explains why breast cancer in women who have been diagnosed with LCIS doesn't always develop in the same spot as the LCIS, or even in the same breast. Because of this, removing the affected lobe will not reduce the risk, so the woman with LCIS is in the same position as other women at high risk. She must either have both breasts removed or have close follow-up, with regular breast self-examination, medical checks and mammograms. Most women opt for the latter.

Ductal carcinoma in situ (DCIS) DCIS represents the far end of the spectrum of hyperplasia; a woman with DCIS has 11 times the normal risk of developing invasive cancer. It is most common in breast ducts adjacent to an established cancer (it is often found when a cancerous lump is removed), and so is nearly always treated by some form of breast surgery. DCIS tends to fall into two distinct types: focal (occurring in only one spot in the breast) and multicentric (in several parts of the breast). There is little tendency for the first to proceed to the second.

Total mastectomy will be recommended for multicentric DCIS. If mammograms do not show clearly which type is present, however, a wide excision of the lump, plus a margin of healthy tissue, will be performed; alternatively, the whole quadrant of the affected breast will be removed. The tissue that has been removed is microscopically examined and, if the DCIS is found to have more than one focus, total mastectomy will be done after discussion with the patient.

If the original area of DCIS is the only focus in all the breast tissue removed, a further surgical procedure may not be recommended. Follow-up is crucial, however, because of the increased risk of invasive cancer. It should take the form of monthly self-examination, yearly clinical examination by a doctor and two-yearly mammography. It is unclear if any additional treatment, such as radiotherapy or tamoxifen, is needed, although one US trial suggests that radiotherapy can reduce local recurrence rates. This topic is the subject of a UK trial; your doctor may ask you to take part in it.

TRUE CANCER

As a rule, breast cancers arise from the cells that line the ducts or lobules. The most frequent form is known as ductal carcinoma because it was originally thought to arise from the milk ducts. It is now recognized, however, that both this type and the less common lobular carcinoma usually arise in the breast lobule. All other forms of breast cancer are rare. Both ductal and lobular carcinomas can be pre-invasive or invasive.

Invasive ductal carcinoma Ductal carcinomas comprise over 80 percent of all detected breast cancers. The first symptom is generally a new, hard, ill-defined lump within the breast. As the tumour spreads along the strands of connective tissue between the breast lobes, it pulls on the overlying skin, creating a characteristic dimpling effect. Extreme skin pitting, known as *peau d'orange* because the skin resembles orange peel, is a serious sign. If the tumour spreads along the ducts, it will pull on and eventually invert the nipple; this is why a new inversion of the nipple should always prompt you to visit your doctor, although it can also be caused by duct ectasia, a benign condition. The lymph nodes under the armpits may be involved, and as the tumour spreads it may also involve the underlying muscles. The smaller and less advanced the cancer is at the time of diagnosis, the better the outlook.

Invasive lobular carcinoma Lobular carcinomas account for about 10 percent of breast cancers and behave in a very similar way to ductal cancers, except that they may spread diffusely rather than forming a discrete tumour.

SITES OF CANCER

Breast cancer can arise in the lobes or, more rarely, the milk ducts. If it is non-invasive and remains confined to the lobe or duct, it is termed "carcinoma in situ". Once it spreads to the surrounding tissue, it is a true invasive cancer.

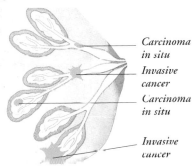

Carcinoma
in situ

Invasive
cancer

Carcinoma
in situ

Invasive
cancer

DIAGNOSIS AND BREAST LUMPS

If you report a lump to your doctor, or something shows up on a mammogram, you will be referred to a breast unit. The initial tests that are done depend on whether there is a high probability of cancer.

If cancer is unlikely, fine-needle aspiration cytology (FNAC) is used to take a sample of cells from the lump. Laboratory analysis of the aspirated cells will distinguish between a benign lump and a malignant one.

If cancer is suspected from your mammogram or because of your age or family history, or if FNAC reveals cancer or is inconclusive, a biopsy is needed to provide a sample of tissue from the lump.

A cutting-needle biopsy or open biopsy is carried out to provide a sample of tissue from the lump. If it can't be felt, wire localization will be used.

Following biopsy, histology (analysis of slices of tissue) will diagnose the cancer type and grade the tumour.

Further tests are carried out to see if the cancer has spread (see Diagnosis of secondary spread), to determine the outlook for the cancer and to help plan treatment.

DETECTION AND DIAGNOSIS

Mammography is your lifeline. Routine mammographic screening can cut the death rate from breast cancer by 20–30 percent. For example, DCIS becomes invasive in 50–75 percent of cases within five years, so early detection is crucial. Mammography can detect cancers less than 5 millimetres (¼ inch) across, whereas a lump cannot be felt by either you or your doctor until it has grown to about 1 centimetre (½ inch). In the UK, screening has brought about a marked lowering of the number of women with aggressive tumours and spread to the axilla. Between 30 and 50 percent of detected tumours now measure less than 2 centimetres (¾ inch) when they are first diagnosed; 20 years ago, the proportion was only 5–10 percent.

There are drawbacks to this routine screening, however. Some doctors are concerned about the number of marginal abnormalities detected by mammography, which may then be treated when they should probably be left alone. If surgeons operate on women who have in situ cancers as if they had invasive breast cancer (perhaps even performing mastectomy), there is the possibility that such women will undergo unnecessary surgery. Despite these questions, you need to remember that mammography is the best screening tool available for the detection of breast cancer and the only screening method for malignancy, the value of which has been proved by rigorous clinical trials.

Special cases for screening Currently, evidence supports the value of two-yearly screening only in women between the ages of 50 and 70, since the incidence of breast cancer is lower in younger women and mammography is less efficient when breast tissue is more dense (as it is in younger women). In some special cases, however, screening should be carried out at an earlier age and more frequently than every three years, which is the recommended interval in the UK.

US guidelines for a woman with a first-degree relative (that is, mother or sister) who develops pre-menopausal breast cancer are that she be routinely screened every two years, starting when she is ten years younger than the age at which her relative developed breast cancer. Women who are diagnosed with atypical hyperplasia are also advised to have mammography every two years.

Identifying cancer Mammography does not reveal only cancer. It also detects benign lumps, which have rounded, smooth edges and a halo of healthy fat around them. Cancerous lumps, on the other hand, are more dense at the centre than they are at the edges, which are often irregular. Mammography may also be able to show other changes, for instance skin thickening, or tethering and distortion of breast tissue around a lump. A deposit of calcium particles may show up as white dots; this is called calcification. In a benign lump, calcification appears as relatively large blobs; with cancer it has a characteristic fine, speckled appearance. To a radiologist experienced in interpreting mammograms, this almost certainly confirms that the lump is malignant.

DIAGNOSIS

When a woman finds a lump in her breast, doctors use many investigative techniques and skills in order to arrive at as specific a diagnosis as possible. The initial sequence of tests varies, depending on whether the lump has been found by the woman herself or has been detected during routine screening on a mammogram, in which case it may be too small to feel. In all cases, however, a sample of cells or tissue will have to be examined under a microscope to determine whether the lump is malignant; if it is, further tests will be carried out to assess the precise origin of the tumour, its grade and its stage.

Clinical diagnosis The doctor will start his examination by looking at your breasts while you sit with your hands by your sides and then with your arms raised above your head, so that he or she can observe any asymmetry between the breasts, nipple retraction (the nipple will appear drawn in), difference in level between the nipples or dimpling of the skin. If you've been doing regular breast self examination, you'll be able to confirm which of these features are new and which you have observed in the past.

You will then be asked to lie back with your arms above your head while the doctor examines your breasts carefully, feeling each quadrant of both breasts with the flat of the hand. The aim is to decide whether there is an obvious, discrete lump or if the breasts are just generally lumpy. The doctor will then check the underarm region on both sides for any lumps caused by swollen lymph nodes, the area above the collarbone (this also checks for swollen lymph nodes) and the abdomen and chest.

CUTTING-NEEDLE BIOPSY

FNAC yields only a tiny sample of cells from breast tissue, so it's impossible to tell whether they originate from an in situ cancer or an invasive cancer. A cutting-needle biopsy provides a core of cells that can be analysed to make this distinction.

• *Under local anaesthetic, a special fine-notched needle with a sheath is inserted into the lump in order to withdraw a fine core of tissue from it.*

• *The sheath is drawn back and some tissue from the lump falls into the notch.*

• *The sheath is closed, trapping a tiny core of tissue from the lump inside the notch, and the needle is withdrawn.*

• *The skin is left virtually intact. Although there may be a little bruising afterwards, there is hardly any discomfort.*

If your symptoms are lumpiness of the breasts or pain or both, but no obvious new discrete lump is found when the doctor examines you, further management will depend on your age. If you are under the age of 40, cancer is unlikely, and you may be asked to return in six weeks. If you still have pain from a lumpy breast, treatment may be advised. If you are over 40, a mammogram may be advised to ensure that no hidden cancer is present. If this shows no evidence of malignancy, you can be reassured and offered treatment for your symptoms if necessary. If there is any suspicion of cancerous pattern on the mammogram, FNAC will be advised and perhaps further tests, depending on the result of the FNAC.

If you have discharge from the nipple, it will be tested to see if it contains blood (this is not always obvious to the naked eye) and the doctor will note whether the discharge comes from a single duct or many. Nipple discharge is usually associated with benign conditions, but in rare cases a bloodless discharge from either single or multiple ducts may require further investigation to rule out cancer. Laboratory tests of the discharge are too inaccurate to rely on, so your doctor will need to perform a biopsy.

If there is an obvious lump that the doctor can feel, the next step is to biopsy it, usually by aspirating the lump. The sample of breast tissue will be sent to the laboratory for microscopic examination.

Open biopsy This kind of biopsy is an alternative to a cutting-needle biopsy (see left). As the name implies, the skin is cut open to reveal the lump and remove it with a margin of healthy breast tissue. Any woman over 30 with an obvious breast lump should have it removed for further analysis, unless she's had a firm diagnosis of cancer from a needle biopsy, in which case she can proceed straight to definitive surgical treatment. In practical terms, therefore, open biopsy nearly always means removing the whole lump (lumpectomy), and this procedure will be carried out in hospital under a general anaesthetic.

Complications of this kind of biopsy are rare (fewer than one in ten cases) but, as with any surgical procedure, they do occur. The two most likely are a haematoma (bruise) and, less often, infection. A haematoma forms due to blood oozing into the tissue surrounding the site of the biopsy, and may show up as a bruise with a vague lump beneath within a day or two of a biopsy having been done. As with any other bruise, the body simply absorbs the blood and recycles it, and the bruise will disappear after a week or so. Infection, if it occurs, will probably show up within a week of the biopsy as pain and a raised temperature; it is usually successfully treated with a course of antibiotics. Very rarely, a haematoma may become infected and an abscess may form. Antibiotics will be prescribed and the abscess can be surgically drained.

Analysing the biopsy The biopsy or lump is sent to the pathology laboratory where it is very finely sliced, stained to show up cancer cells and examined under a microscope; this process is known as histology. If the tissue is found to be cancerous, a very precise diagnosis of cancer, and the type of cancer it is, can be made. The tumour is also graded, providing information about how malignant it is. At some hospitals, specialized tests may be performed on a slice of tumour tissue to reveal features that help to decide treatment and give the patient an idea of what the future outlook may be.

An open biopsy is performed purely to remove the lump and send it for analysis. If cancer is found, the surgeon will wait to discuss the treatment options with the woman and her family before any further surgery is carried out. In the past, a biopsy was analysed instantly while the woman was still under general anaesthetic. If the lump proved to be cancerous, mastectomy was performed immediately. This was extremely traumatic and is no longer done.

Diagnosis of secondary spread In addition to lymph node involvement, spread of the disease to the rest of the body is checked by a series of simple tests, which are generally performed during the initial assessment. They include chest X-rays to detect secondary tumours in the lungs or involvement of the membranes around them, and a blood test to look for anaemia or abnormalities of the blood cells, which may indicate that the bone marrow has been invaded. Any abnormalities of blood chemistry that might indicate spread to the bones or liver are picked up at the same time. If a woman has no clinical evidence of metastases (secondary tumours) and her blood tests are normal, the chances are that the cancer has not spread. In more advanced cases, specialized tests are used to check for secondaries, including X-rays or bone scans of likely sites of bone spread (the skull, spine, pelvis and hips) and an ultrasound examination to assess the state of the liver.

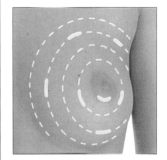

Biopsy incisions
When a biopsy is carried out, the cut is usually made along natural tension lines in the skin of the breast, to help keep scarring to a minimum.

The size of the tumour, the involvement of axillary lymph nodes and the presence of secondary tumours are vital factors in assessing how far the disease has progressed and determining the outlook.

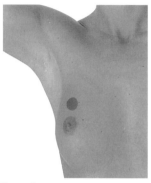

Stage I
The disease is confined to the breast. Dimpling of the skin may or may not be present.

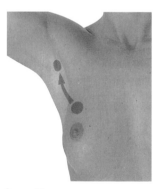

Stage II
The axillary lymph nodes are affected. Stages I and II may be curable by surgery but some adjuvant systemic treatment, such as tamoxifen therapy, is usually advised.

ASSESSMENT

One of the major aims of your doctors will be to get a feel for the "virulence" of your cancer. To do this, they use a series of tests to decide your treatment and assess your long-term outlook. The tests are intended to determine the grade of the tumour, which means the aggressiveness of its cells, and the stage of the disease, which is a measure of how far advanced it is and how far it has spread (if at all) beyond its original site in the breast.

GRADING

When cancer cells are microscopically examined, they can be graded according to their appearance or type. How they look indicates how malignant the cancer is. Generally, the more primitive the cells, the more malignant the cancer.

The degree of cell specialization is known as the grade of the tumour and can give a fairly reliable guide to the long-term outlook for the patient. Tumours of recognizable cells, which look quite similar to their normal cells of origin (that is, breast tissue), are called "well-differentiated" or Grade 1 and carry an excellent outlook. Tumours containing cells that become increasingly unrecognizable as breast tissue are known as "poorly differentiated" or "undifferentiated" and descend through Grades 2 and 3 with a worsening prognosis.

STAGING

Once a breast cancer has been diagnosed and graded, the patient as a whole is staged (see columns left and right). In order to stage every patient individually, three factors are taken into account: the size of the tumour; whether the axillary lymph nodes are involved; and whether there are metastases (secondary tumours) elsewhere in the body.

Although size is a fairly crude predictor of the invasive potential of the tumour, generally speaking the larger the tumour, the more likely it is to have had time to spread to the axillary lymph nodes. Even a small tumour may have spread, however. Most women whose tumours measure less than 1 centimetre (½ inch) and whose axillary lymph nodes are free of disease have an excellent prognosis.

In assessing a patient's outlook, the crucial factor against which all others should be weighed is spread to the axillary lymph nodes; the more nodes that are involved, the worse the prognosis. With a node-negative cancer, seven women out of ten will be alive ten years later; with a node-positive cancer, only five or fewer out of ten. Adjuvant chemotherapy is now routinely given to pre-menopausal women with involved nodes. Most other women, whether their nodes are free of cancer or not, would benefit from adjuvant systemic therapy, usually tamoxifen.

The presence of metastases elsewhere in the body can be detected by tests (see Diagnosis of secondary spread). If the lymph nodes above the collarbone are involved, these are regarded as metastases. Distant metastases in the lungs, liver or bones automatically put the cancer at Stage IV, so their presence is a very serious sign.

Planning treatment Once you have been staged, decisions about treatment can be made. You have the right to discuss all of the possible alternatives so that you and your family participate in all decisions. You can also be helped to come to terms with the diagnosis by being given a tape-recording of the "bad news consultation" to take home, so ask for one, and by having a friend or relative with you for moral support when the news is broken.

Survival Doctors prefer to talk about survival rather than "cure". It is usual to measure five-year and ten-year survival rates and then express them as a percentage. If you are told by your doctor that your cancer has a five-year survival rate of 80 percent, it means this: out of ten women with your disease, with a tumour of the same grade and stage, and of the same degree of aggressiveness, eight could expect to be alive in five years' time.

PROGNOSIS AND OUTLOOK

The stage of the tumour (see right and far left) is crucial in assessing five-year survival rate for breast cancer: the five-year survival rate of 85 percent for women suffering from Stage I tumours falls to less than ten percent for those with Stage IV tumours.

About one in every three women treated vigorously for early breast cancer will go on to have a normal life expectancy. Of the rest, those who get local recurrence can often be treated adequately with radiotherapy. Only about half of the women who see breast-cancer surgeons see them early enough, when the disease is eminently treatable and curable, the other half leave it too long before seeking help.

ADVANCED STAGES

The stage of the tumour is crucial in assessing five-year survival rate. The prognosis worsens when the disease has invaded the lungs, liver or bones, although breast cancer can defy all predictions.

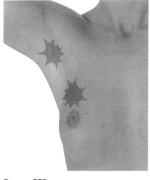

Stage III
The disease has spread and invaded the muscles of the chest wall, the overlying skin, or possibly the lymph nodes above the collarbone.

Stage IV
The cancer has spread to other parts of the body, typically the bones, liver or lungs.

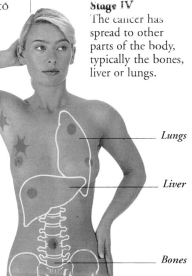

Lungs

Liver

Bones

Most women with breast cancer still have a reasonable expectation of life by comparison with cancers of the lung, stomach or ovary. Many women can expect to live in comfort for many years after treatment, even if their disease cannot be classed as cured. Since breast cancer is mainly a disease of older women, many will die from other causes or simply from old age rather than from their breast tumour.

SPECIAL RESEARCH TESTS

Over the years, researchers have attempted to develop special tests that will provide doctors with an even better idea of the aggressiveness of breast tumours, future outlook and survival. The tests require very advanced technology and are by no means performed at all centres, but it is hoped that their future use will help to identify groups of patients who would do better with one kind of treatment or another.

Oestrogen receptors (ERs)   Approximately 60 percent of cancers contain detectable ERs. A tumour that has ERs is sensitive to oestrogen and has a slightly better prognosis than one that doesn't.

Epidermal growth-factor receptor (EGFr)   All cells have receptors that are "switched on" by growth factors telling the cell to multiply. In altered cells, the receptors don't wait for signals, but cause the cells to multiply uncontrollably. About half of all breast-cancer cases have altered receptors. Tumours that are EGFr-negative generally have a better outlook for recovery than those that are positive.

Ki-67   Put simply, this measures the speed of cell growth and division; in general, the faster the cells are dividing, the more aggressive the tumour. The consequence of this is that the spread of the cancer throughout the body is likely to occur earlier and be faster. The chance of metastases is high and the outlook poorer than with slower cell changes.

erbB-2   Research has shown that women who relapse have extra copies of the altered form of this gene, and higher levels of the protein it produces. The more erbB-2 present, the poorer the prognosis seems to be.

Cathepsin D   Patients with low levels of this enzyme and positive axillary nodes invariably outlive those with high levels of cathepsin D and negative nodes. It is therefore quite a powerful predictor of outcome.

p53   This gene mutation is known to be present in about half of all breast cancers. An abnormality of p53 also gives an increased risk of ovarian and bowel cancers.

ON FINDING A LUMP

So much attention is given to breast cancer nowadays in all the popular media that it would be difficult for any woman to ignore the potential significance of a breast lump. The sad fact is that on finding a lump, practically all women underestimate the chances of survival and overestimate the chances of dying. Finding a breast lump is therefore a shocking experience for everyone.

THE IMPLICATIONS OF DELAY

Finding a lump in the breast will always be scary, but don't become so frightened that you don't seek help immediately. It's been estimated that approximately one in five women with symptoms of breast cancer delay seeking advice for three months or more, and some research has suggested that this delay could well be contributing to the high mortality rates from breast cancer in Great Britain.

The interval between finding a breast lump and having a diagnosis confirmed is the most stressful part of finding a lump in your breast. A group of women who were studied before and after having their lump diagnosed as benign were found to suffer severe impairment of critical thinking and concentration, together with profound anxiety before the diagnosis. Fewer than one in eight women gives breast loss as her primary concern; nearly six out of ten are more distressed at the prospect of having cancer.

ON HEARING THE DIAGNOSIS

Individual strategies for coping and personality factors will affect your response to the news that you have breast cancer. Social support can help you, and the communications skills of your medical carers – especially the surgeon who breaks the news – are extremely important. Your reaction may have several stages; denial, fighting back, brave acceptance, depressed acceptance and a mixture of helplessness and hopelessness are all possible.

Most women are likely at some time to go through stages of depressed acceptance, where they acknowledge that they have a potentially fatal disease but are overwhelmed with fears for themselves and their families. At worst, they may feel that there is no hope for them; whatever they have to live for, they may not be able to muster the energy to fight for it by overcoming the disease.

DENIAL

One of the most common coping strategies is denial, a natural protective mechanism that helps you go on with life in times of stress or shock.

- *You may try to convince yourself that a lump is nothing to worry about until it can no longer be ignored. Such delay in reporting symptoms will worsen the outlook.*

- *By the time you seek help, the tumour is difficult to treat and the chances of survival are therefore much lower.*

- *Individuals most likely to delay reporting a breast lump include older women; women of lower social class or little education; women who are fearful of cancer and surgery and don't feel they can be helped or cured; women who are inhibited about their bodies; depressed or anxious personalities or those who habitually resort to denial when faced with a crisis.*

- *Paradoxically, knowledge as opposed to ignorance about breast cancer may inhibit some women from seeking advice at the proper time; one study showed that female healthcare professionals, especially nurses, tended to report their lumps later and generally had larger tumours than other women.*

SUPPORT

Women who have supportive family and friends are more able to cope with this kind of life crisis. Hearing the bad news in the presence of a close relative or friend reduces anxiety and depression for a long time afterwards, and he or she will probably remember more clearly than you what the doctor said. The presence of a trusted ally, be it spouse, partner, friend or relative, is useful in the long term to help you accept that you have cancer.

THE FAMILY

The needs of your family are sometimes overlooked. It's easy to assume that they will be able to keep their feelings in check and be ready to offer you support. Families do, however, suffer along with you and very often reflect your mood. One study showed that if a patient with cancer is depressed or anxious there is a very high probability that the next of kin will be also.

Partners   Your spouse or partner is likely to feel responsible for helping you to adjust successfully to your disease and to your new body after any necessary surgery. He may suffer considerable emotional distress but pretend to hide this behind a confident pose, assuming that this will help you. Unfortunately this attitude may lead to misunderstandings. You may feel that your partner is not being sensitive to your feelings and doesn't realize the seriousness of the situation or can't share your fears. It is natural when a loved one is in distress to try to offer advice, be cheery, or somehow "sort things out", but this may not be what you need; more often you just want someone to listen and understand.

Close relationships are always affected in some way by a diagnosis of breast cancer; with fragile relationships, this burden may prove to be the final straw. For the majority of women, however, this is a time when the commitment, love and affection of her family and friends are re-affirmed.

At the time the diagnosis is made, good information and counselling should be provided to the person closest to you, since this "significant other" will be a crucial factor in your long-term adjustment. In the end, most couples feel their relationships to be at least the same as before diagnosis, and sometimes even better.

"Waiting for the diagnosis was pure hell. I lay awake at night imagining the cancer was spreading through my body. Nothing could distract me for more than a few minutes – not work, not my family or my friends. I'd been decorating the spare bedroom because my parents were coming to stay, and I just didn't have the heart to go on with it. I kept thinking about what I might have to tell them."

Jill, 36, Potter

12

TREATING BREAST CANCER

The detection and diagnosis of breast cancer is only the first step in combating the disease. You have the right to expect the best possible care. All women should know what their treatment options are – including a clear and detailed explanation of the aims of the proposed treatments, their benefits and any possible side-effects – and have the opportunity to discuss treatment plans with interested and sympathetic breast-care specialists. They should also know what techniques are involved, the impact of treatment and the support they are entitled to receive, especially when coming to terms with life after treatment.

YOUR BILL
OF RIGHTS

*When you find a lump in
your breast, you are entitled
to the best possible treatment.
Your care should include:*

• *A prompt referral by your
family doctor to a team
specializing in the diagnosis
and treatment of breast cancer,
including a consultant.*

• *A firm diagnosis within one
week of being examined.*

• *The opportunity of a
confirmed diagnosis before
consenting to any form of
treatment, including surgery.*

• *Full information about
types of surgery (including
breast reconstruction where
appropriate) and the role of
adjuvant treatments such as
radiotherapy, chemotherapy,
hormone therapy including
tamoxifen, and so on.*

• *A clear and detailed
explanation of the aims of the
proposed treatments and their
benefits and any possible side-
effects (including long term).*

TREATMENT OPTIONS

If you are diagnosed as having breast cancer, it's crucial that you are fully aware of the various treatment options that are open to you. Twenty years ago, radical mastectomies were the rule; today, surgery aims to conserve the breast if at all possible. At the same time, very sophisticated reconstructive surgery has been developed so that a woman who loses her breast has the option of replacing it. Advanced techniques for calculating future risks mean that doctors can place a woman in a very clearly defined group and choose a tailor-made treatment programme especially for her, giving her the best possible chance of a cure.

BREAST UNITS

Women with breast cancer are increasingly treated at specialist units, such as those at Guy's Hospital in London and the Sloan-Kettering Institute in New York. These units offer the best possible care and ensure close co-operation between an interested and sympathetic oncologist, surgeon, pathologist, radiologist and radiotherapist, which allows rapid and accurate diagnosis and appropriate treatment. The team will also include special breast-care nurses or counsellors who deal with the emotional and psychological aspects of breast cancer. Specialist breast cancer units also supervise adjuvant therapy (additional forms of treatment) such as radiotherapy, chemotherapy and hormone therapy, and can arrange for breast reconstruction if desired, so that all your treatments are kept under one roof with a minimum of travel and disturbance during follow-up.

CONSERVING THE BREAST

Women who develop breast cancer today are in a much more fortunate position than in the past; many more treatment options are open to you and preserving the breast need pose no hazard to life. Not so long ago it was thought that mastectomy, including the removal of all the axillary lymph nodes, was necessary in every case to give a woman the best chance of survival. This is no longer true. Doctors have abandoned the idea that this kind of extensive surgery should be routine and – without sacrificing results – have greatly improved recovery after surgery. With conservative treatment, the once worst complication of breast surgery, swelling of the arm, is now rare.

Surgeons today believe in conserving the breast whenever possible or choosing the least extensive operation that is appropriate. With early breast cancer, lumpectomy is nearly always an option. This means that very small tumours can be dealt with, leaving the breast virtually intact.

Because the many different approaches to treatment all offer about the same success rate, there's nothing to prevent your preferences about the choice of operation from carrying weight. The outlook for the disease is affected more by the grade and stage of the tumour when it is diagnosed than by the type of surgery performed.

Any choice should be made in consultation with you and with your family. Not all patients are suitable for breast conservation, however, and you would be well advised to listen to your doctors if they advocate a more radical approach. If lumpectomy is attempted in inappropriate cases (on a large tumour, for example), the cosmetic results and control of the disease can be poor.

THE LOSS OF A BREAST

Whenever the subject of mastectomy is discussed, be sure that you and your family understand precisely the extent of the operation. Ask to see some photographs of women after mastectomy, to give you an idea of how your body will look after surgery. You'll almost certainly need time, space and counselling to get used to the idea of a different-looking body, which at first may seem alien to you.

You'll have much greater difficulty coming to terms with your new appearance than your partner, family and friends will. They are far more concerned about your well-being and long-term health than about your body's appearance. It's understandable, however, that you are not. A woman's self-image is often indistinguishable from her self-esteem. Fortunately, doctors and surgeons now understand this and should be willing to give you all the help you need.

You are entitled to have a cosmetically acceptable result after surgery and to be pleased with your appearance when dressed, even in low necklines. This can be achieved with prostheses. Reconstructive surgery is also widely available to restore both breast contour and a nipple if you so wish. Don't be afraid to ask your surgeon about these things or worry that you will be thought vain or frivolous. You have the right to expect your surgeon to be sympathetic to these concerns, and most surgeons are.

CONSIDERING TREATMENT

Whatever your doctors advise, your have the right to time, space and counselling when considering treatment. Your care should include:

• *Access to a specialist breast-care nurse trained to give you information and emotional and psychological support.*

• *As much time as you need to consider your treatment options and gather information.*

• *A sensitive and complete breast prosthesis service, where appropriate.*

• *The opportunity to meet a former breast-cancer patient who has been trained to offer practical, psychological and emotional support.*

• *Information on all support services (including local and national groups) available to breast-cancer patients and their families.*

BREAST CANCER IN PREGNANCY

It seems that breast cancer is no more likely to arise in pregnancy and behaves no differently during pregnancy than at any other time. Be assured that the hormonal changes of pregnancy, when levels of oestrogen are high, do not seem to make the situation worse.

There is no good reason why breast cancer in pregnant women should routinely lead to termination.

The toxic anti-cancer drugs used in chemotherapy do affect the developing fetus and it therefore seems best to avoid this kind of medication in the first three months of pregnancy. After three months, selected and well-tried drugs may be given with safety.

Generally, radiotherapy is not considered an option in the first six months of pregnancy; even in the last three months, its use is controversial.

An alternative approach would be to perform a mastectomy rather than just a lumpectomy, since this would avoid the need for radiotherapy to the breast.

CONSIDERING CANCER TREATMENT

When your doctors consider the treatment of your breast cancer, they are taking into consideration several different factors that will influence the treatment you have and your long-term outlook. Doctors have to tread a narrow line between establishing the most effective treatment for your condition and needing to cause you the least trauma, both physical and mental. This fine balance is not always easy to achieve and requires your full and frank input as well as your co-operation. In addition, the better informed you are about the issues involved, the more active a part you can take in deciding your own treatment. This will not only help your doctor and surgeon in their task but may also give you added strength in fighting and overcoming your cancer. The first thing you need to understand is that treatment of breast cancer falls into three distinct areas:
- treatment of the lump, usually with surgery
- treatment of the lymph nodes in the axilla if they are involved in the cancer, with surgical clearance as a rule
- adjuvant (additional) therapy where appropriate, which could be radiotherapy to clear any remaining cancer cells from the breast after surgery, or chemotherapy or hormone therapy (with a drug such as tamoxifen) to catch any spread of the cancer to the rest of the body.

Surgery and radiotherapy are both referred to as local treatments, since they treat only the area where the tumour has occurred. Chemotherapy and hormone therapy are both called systemic treatments, since they treat the whole of the body, not just the diseased part.

The state-of-the-art treatment for breast cancer appears to be the one pioneered by Guy's Hospital in London and centres in Paris, Milan, and Boston in the US. The first step is exact diagnosis with cutting-needle biopsy, done under local anaesthetic; a short while later (three to seven days), after you have been fully consulted, a single operation under general anaesthetic will remove the lump and clear the axillary lymph nodes. Precise radiotherapy to the tumour site is given, which avoids excessive irradiation of the skin and deeper organs. This gives results at least as good as mastectomy and with much less heartache. Nearly every woman is considered for some form of systemic adjuvant treatment. If you have a tumour less than 1 centimetre (½ inch) in diameter and are node-negative (that is, the cancer has not spread to the axillary lymph nodes), you belong to the only group of women for whom systemic therapy is not considered necessary.

PLANNING TREATMENT

Breast cancer is usually referred to as early or advanced; this reflects whether the tumour is operable or not. "Early" usually encompasses Stages I and II and "advanced", Stages III and IV. These terms are also used to reflect the aggressiveness of the tumour – some patients do quite well with large, ulcerated cancers that have been present for some time but which are clearly not rapidly growing because they have not spread. A small primary tumour, on the other hand, can spread quickly to other organs if it is very aggressive. With early breast cancer (see right), local control is of prime importance and, as proven at Guy's Hospital, can be achieved largely by removal of the lump with a margin of healthy breast tissue, followed by a course of radiotherapy in some form. If you have a large or aggressive tumour, you'll be asked to consider mastectomy. All patients except those with very early cancer will be given adjuvant therapy in some form; for nearly all older women, this is the drug tamoxifen.

If a tumour is allowed to reach an advanced state, then the likelihood of metastases (secondary tumours) is much greater. For this reason, local treatment alone is deemed inadequate and systemic treatment is the rule. The most common systemic treatment for pre-menopausal women is chemotherapy. This works on cancer throughout the whole body and may shrink your tumour to an operable size.

PRIMARY MEDICAL THERAPY

Research at the excellent breast unit in Milan, Italy, showed that chemotherapy given *before* the operation can reduce four out of five large tumours to less than 3 centimetres (1½ inches) in diameter, allowing them to be treated with more conservative surgery and therefore reducing physical and emotional trauma. Tumours have been clearly seen to shrink and disappear on successive mammograms, although microcalcification may remain. Primary medical treatment, where practised, is always followed by additional surgical treatment to avoid the chance of local relapse.

TREATING EARLY BREAST CANCER

The treatment of early breast cancer – that is, a cancer that has not yet spread beyond the axillary lymph nodes – has three main aims:

- *to control the disease locally (this means at the site of the tumour) and prevent local recurrence.*

- *to treat any micrometastatic disease (tiny, undetectable secondary spread) so as to increase the chances of survival.*

- *to conserve as much of the breast as possible and be minimally disfiguring.*

IMPALPABLE LESIONS

Lesions that can't be felt by physical examination, but show up on mammography as shadows with tiny white dots of calcification, can be accurately located with mammographic guidance.

- *Small solid tumours can also be localized with the use of ultrasound and a small wire (see photograph below).*

- *The surgeon dissects down onto the wire so that the whole of the tumour can be cut out, and removes 1–2 centimetres (½–1 inch) of tissue around it. This is then X-rayed while the patient is still anaesthetized to confirm that the abnormality has been completely removed. With this technique, complete excision (removal) in almost 100 percent of impalpable cancers can be achieved.*

Locating the lesion
Using an ultrasound image for guidance, the radiologist inserts a fine wire into the centre of the tumour. The wire is left in place to guide the surgeon to the tumour.

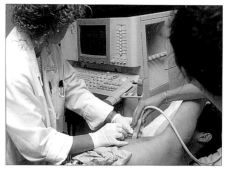

SURGERY

In most cases, local conservative therapy is achieved with surgery. Although it is possible to treat even small tumours with chemotherapy and radiotherapy, these treatments are time-consuming and tend to be reserved for tumours that are greater than 4 centimetres (2 inches) in diameter. In addition, large doses of radiotherapy can produce distortion and disfigurement of the breast tissue.

Lumpectomy is the most common primary treatment for smaller breast cancers and can generally be relied on to give a good cosmetic result (see right). If yours is a large tumour in the centre of the breast or one with several different areas of focus, a mastectomy may be better. A lumpectomy in such instances may not be cosmetically attractive and it may be impossible to provide a satisfactory prosthesis for a very distorted breast. Reconstruction is always an option either during the initial surgery or later. Chemotherapy or hormone therapy prior to surgery may be offered if you have a large tumour, to reduce its size and allow a smaller area of breast tissue to be removed.

Mastectomy is major surgery and you deserve to have an expert, rather than general, surgeon. A British study in 1995 recommended that women with breast cancer be treated only by doctors who see more than 30 new cancers a year, who can offer a full range of treatment options and who work within a team of specialists.

CONSERVATIVE THERAPY

Breast conservation is most suitable if your lump is less than 4 centimetres (2 inches) in diameter, felt on clinical examination or shown on a mammogram. Minimal nodal involvement with no distant metastases (to the liver, lungs or bones) is a requirement. If you have large breasts and a tumour greater than 4 centimetres (2 inches), you might also be suitable. There is no age limit. If you are elderly, provided you are fit, you should be treated in exactly the same way as younger patients.

Breast conservation will not be offered if it would result in an unacceptable cosmetic result. This would normally include the majority of cancers in the centre of the breast and those that are over 4 centimetres (2 inches) in diameter.

Women with more than one focus of cancer have a high local recurrence rate with breast conservation and are better treated with mastectomy, ideally with immediate breast reconstruction (this means during the initial surgery rather than at a later date). Cancer in both breasts can be treated by a bilateral conservation, but you may prefer bilateral mastectomy, again with immediate reconstruction.

LUMPECTOMY

Wherever possible, lumpectomy is now the treatment of choice for breast cancer, because of its cosmetic qualities and because it is less emotionally traumatic. As long as the post-operative dose of radiotherapy is sufficiently high, only the lump itself need be removed, but most surgeons still go for the safety margin of 1 centimetre (½ inch) of normal breast tissue around it. The minimum amount of skin is removed to give the best cosmetic result.

When a large amount of skin needs to be removed (if the lump is very near the surface, for example), the cosmetic results are likely to be rather poor and your doctor should make you aware of this. Most surgeons remove the lymph nodes from the armpit at the same time. The operation itself is a fairly minor procedure carried out under general anaesthetic, and you'll probably have to stay in hospital for four or five days to make sure the scar is healing and there are no complications.

MASTECTOMY

In the past, mastectomy was the treatment of choice for breast cancer, since it was thought that the tumour spread by growing outwards from the primary growth in the centre. It therefore seemed logical to perform ever more extensive surgery in an attempt to get beyond the growing edge of the tumour. Radical surgery is no longer the norm for breast cancer and there are currently several possible variations of mastectomy.

• A partial mastectomy, as its name implies, involves removing part of the breast (other versions of this type of operation remove varying amounts of tissue). A sample of the axillary nodes will be taken at the same time or the nodes may be cleared. The operation can leave a misshapen breast, depending on how much tissue is removed. Knowing this, women frequently opt for a total mastectomy.

BREAST SURGERY

There are several possible operations but in all cases, surgeons will aim to remove the minimum amount of tissue that is necessary to get rid of the cancer. The extent of the surgery is determined by the size and position of the tumour, whether the lump has a well-defined outline, how aggressive it appears to be and whether the cancer has spread.

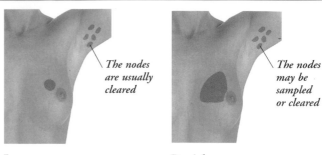

The nodes are usually cleared

The nodes may be sampled or cleared

Lumpectomy
The lump is removed with a 1 centimetre (½ inch) margin of healthy tissue to give the best cosmetic result. The axillary nodes are usually cleared too.

Partial mastectomy
Where the cancer doesn't have a well-defined outline, the lump is removed with a larger amount of surrounding tissue than for a lumpectomy. The axillary nodes are also sampled or cleared.

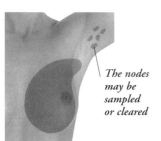

The nodes may be sampled or cleared

Simple or total mastectomy
All of the breast tissue is removed, including the nipple and areola and the axillary tail; the pectoralis minor muscle is not removed. The axillary lymph nodes may be sampled or cleared.

Pectoralis minor muscle removed from behind breast and pectoralis major muscle

The nodes are cleared

Modified radical mastectomy
All of the breast tissue is removed (as with simple mastectomy) and the pectoralis minor muscle. The axillary lymph nodes are cleared.

• A simple or total mastectomy (see above) removes all of the breast tissue including the nipple and areola and the axillary tail. Some or all of the axillary lymph nodes will be cleared (removed) at the same time.

• A modified radical mastectomy (see above) is a total mastectomy. In addition, the pectoralis minor muscle is removed to facilitate complete axillary clearance (removal). This is the favoured operation of many breast units where lumpectomy is not feasible.

• In a radical mastectomy, the pectoralis major muscle is also removed. This extensive operation should probably never be carried out nowadays, however, so don't agree to it without first asking for a second opinion.

Mastectomy is a major operation and you'll have to stay in hospital for four to eight days depending on the type of surgery performed. If your shoulder is stiff afterwards you can do exercises to get it back to normal.

TIMING THE OPERATION

The team at Guy's Hospital, London, first came up with research findings suggesting that pre-menopausal women who had breast surgery during the second half of the menstrual cycle – the so-called luteal phase – had improved survival rates. Their initial findings have now been corroborated by teams in Milan, and at the Sloan-Kettering Institute in New York. The crucial factor seems to be the higher progesterone levels that occur in the luteal phase, and these are linked to a significantly better life expectancy in women with lymph nodes affected by cancer.

A WORD ABOUT MASTECTOMY

More than 80 percent of breast cancers are caught early enough to be suitable for lumpectomy, yet the American College of Surgeons says that only 35 percent are treated in this way. In New York, hospitals just miles apart have widely varying rates for lumpectomy. Why? In Colorado, where three-quarters of women have mastectomies, studies show that it is doctors who are responsible for such low lumpectomy rates, advocating mastectomies even though the profession has had scientific evidence since 1989 to show that lumpectomy plus radiation is just as good as mastectomy. According to some professors in the US, this is because surgeons have not been keeping up to date with medical literature. This is sad because a study has revealed that, when asked, half of mastectomy patients said they'd choose lumpectomy if they could make the decision again.

In 1992, a report in the *New England Journal of Medicine* showed that teaching hospitals, where surgeons tend to keep more up to date, have a higher lumpectomy rate. And women who have lumpectomies return to everyday life more quickly and report better sex lives. You always have the right to a lumpectomy if you're eligible, but you may have to change surgeons to get one.

TREATING THE AXILLA

A lymph node infiltrated by cancer has ceased to perform any useful service to your body. Furthermore, cancer can only spread further. Affected axillary lymph nodes must therefore be removed or treated vigorously. The treatment of axillary lymph nodes is still debated by surgeons and radiotherapists. The surgical options range from sampling, that is, the removal of a limited number of nodes (with or without subsequent radiotherapy) to complete surgical clearance of the axillary nodes. Some radiotherapists would advocate radiotherapy as the first and only treatment. The consensus among specialists in the UK, however, is that complete axillary node clearance should be the first step in treating the axilla, wherever possible.

All doctors treating breast cancer are concerned to know the status of the axillary nodes because it remains the single best predictor of long-term survival. Added to this, some of the most important treatment choices and decisions are based on axillary node status. In order to get a true idea of the axillary node status, some form of surgical sampling is needed, since as yet there are no good imaging techniques for the axilla. The role of axillary surgery is therefore twofold: to stage the tumour and to treat axillary disease. Radiotherapy may treat the axilla effectively enough, but it precludes staging of the tumour – information that most oncologists consider crucial.

STAGING THE AXILLA

The most accurate way to stage the axilla is to examine the lymph nodes, starting with the shallowest – Level I – and working through to progressively deeper levels; III is the deepest. On average, there are 14 lymph nodes at Level I, five at Level II, and two at Level III. When lymph nodes at Level I are not affected by cancer, the chance of disease at Levels II and III is very slight. However, when five nodes are positive at Level I, there is an 85 percent chance of positive nodes at Levels II and III.

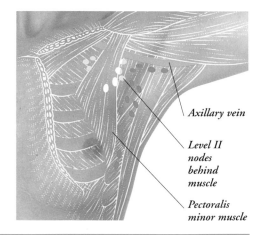

Axillary vein

Level II nodes behind muscle

Pectoralis minor muscle

KEY

LEVEL I   LEVEL II   LEVEL III

Logically, then, surgery is superior to radiotherapy, and many surgeons feel that if they are going to operate on the axilla, complete clearance of the lymph nodes gives a better outlook and chance of survival than just sampling.

DETERMINING SPREAD

Sampling of lymph nodes at Level I (see left) can be a good indication of how far the tumour has spread. Surgical options include single-node biopsy, removing a sample of four nodes, Level I clearance, Level II clearance and Level III clearance. Where surgery is the preferred treatment to radiotherapy, then it's obvious that complete clearance rather than sampling is necessary.

Even a single positive lymph node at Level I may be an indication of involvement at Levels II and III. To be sure that there is no involvement at the deeper levels, however, a large sample of clear nodes is required. Research from Edinburgh, Scotland and Denmark has shown that at least ten lymph nodes at Level I have to be sampled in order to give 90 percent confidence in predicting that there is no lymphatic spread of the breast tumour.

There is a direct relationship between the size of your tumour and whether it has already spread to the axillary lymph nodes. If your tumour was detected by screening, however, it's less likely to have axillary spread than if you'd found it yourself, regardless of its size. For this reason, it has become standard practice in many breast units for patients with breast cancer that cannot be felt to have an axillary node sample taken at Level I as a first step. Patients with obvious lumps are treated with Level III clearance.

TREATMENT OF AXILLARY DISEASE

If disease is found in the axillary lymph nodes, there are two main options for treatment: radical radiotherapy and full Level III axillary clearance. Both give good results, but studies have shown that complete axillary clearance gives lower recurrence rates. It provides more information about ultimate outlook and the need for adjuvant therapy, and it avoids the skin irritation and scarring of radiotherapy. The differences, however, are not dramatic and a 95 percent control rate up to ten years is possible using radiotherapy.

Although surgeons may feel zealous about clearing every scrap of cancerous tissue from a woman's body, there is no doubt that those women who have radiotherapy *and*

RECURRENCE IN THE AXILLA

Do discuss how your doctors intend to treat your axilla so that you are aware of what the treatments mean.

• *With no cancer in the lymph nodes, there is only a small difference in rates of recurrence between surgical clearance and radiotherapy.*

• *With involved nodes, surgical clearance will give you a lower chance of recurrence than radiotherapy.*

• *Bear in mind how mobile you want to be and ask about post-treatment complications.*

• *Also consider whether or not you would like to have breast reconstruction.*

axillary surgery suffer as a result. Complications from the treatment include swelling of the arm, damage to the nerves in the axilla and a reduction in the range of movement in the shoulder. The aim of treating the axilla must therefore be to control disease with the minimum number of post-operative complications.

SURGERY

If you appear to be node-negative, then it's best that your status is determined by the most limited surgery possible, that is, an axillary lymph-node sample. A Level I sample alone can never be considered a safe procedure in a woman who has a single positive axillary node, because the positive node may imply the presence of disease at Levels II and III. This is why complete surgical clearance is preferred to both stage and treat the axilla.

If you're having a lumpectomy, partial mastectomy or total mastectomy for invasive breast cancer, you should have an axillary clearance, thus avoiding the need for radiotherapy after surgery. This is particularly important when you've opted for immediate breast reconstruction, since radiotherapy will significantly affect the cosmetic result.

It may seem like a contradiction that doctors remove the lymph nodes when their purpose is to fight disease, but in medical terms it makes sense. If they have been infiltrated by cancer, they are no longer useful in any case.

THE PLACE OF RADIOTHERAPY

The medical world is somewhat divided as to whether the axilla should be treated surgically or with radiotherapy. If radiotherapy is done without surgery having determined whether the cancer has spread to the axilla, there is a danger that women without axillary disease will be unnecessarily exposed to radiation and any side-effects; four out of ten women do not have axillary spread.

A sensible approach to treatment, therefore, would be radical radiotherapy to the axilla where surgery determines cancer spread, and a "watch policy" for women who are node-negative. Treatment can thus be limited to patients who have axillary disease or develop it later. The watch policy has been justified by clinical trials that showed no difference in overall survival at ten years between women having radiotherapy initially and women who were given radiotherapy only when monitoring revealed cancer spread.

ADJUVANT THERAPY

Most women with breast cancer will have some form of surgery to remove the tumour, either by taking out the lump alone or by removing the whole breast. By the time the breast cancer is diagnosed, however, some of the cells may have spread beyond the lump itself so there is a risk that some cancer cells may be left behind after surgery.

In about 40 percent of cases where a cancer appears to involve only a single site within one breast, there may be other areas of change in the same breast that are either pre-malignant or already cancerous. Doctors know that, even when the spread of the tumour is not detectable, in many cases cancer has already spread to distant parts of the body, since secondaries appear later on. It may be that, by the time a cancer can be felt, in up to 70 percent of cases small deposits of cancer cells have spread through the body by way of the bloodstream and lymphatic system.

If these cells are allowed to grow, cancer could come back at the same site (local recurrence) or could spread to form secondary tumours (metastases) elsewhere in the body. For this reason, additional forms of treatment are often given as an insurance policy to destroy any remaining cancer cells, wherever they are. This is called *adjuvant* treatment, and it has three main forms.

- radiotherapy given to the breast area to reduce the risk of local recurrence
- hormone treatment
- chemotherapy (cytotoxic drugs).

Hormone treatment and chemotherapy are both *systemic* treatments, aimed at reducing the risk of secondary growth elsewhere in the body. Some form of systemic treatment is probably advisable for most patients, even after surgery and radiotherapy combined, because they can reduce the odds of dying in any year by 25 percent. After ten years, one in ten deaths could be avoided. In the UK, 2,000 lives every year could be saved by using systemic adjuvant therapy.

Ideally, an anti-cancer therapy should be able to kill off only cells affected by the disease without harming healthy cells in the body. Unfortunately no anti-cancer treatment is that discriminating, so some healthy cells are bound to be affected, sometimes leading to side-effects. Discuss these with your doctor before deciding to proceed with any treatment.

A BOOSTER DOSE OF RADIATION

When a lumpectomy is performed, your surgeon is faced with the dilemma of trying to take as little healthy tissue as is possible to retain the shape of the breast, yet removing enough tissue to ensure maximum safety.

• *Some surgeons feel they can strike the optimum compromise if a booster dose of radiation is given to completely smash any remaining cancer cells.*

• *The booster dose is given in addition to the standard course of radiotherapy.*

• *The boost can be given in several ways, but common to all methods is the delivery of a large dose of extra radiation in a short time.*

• *In Europe, 60 percent of centres use electron therapy. It is very precise and leaves the lungs unharmed (radiation can scar tissue at the top of the lungs).*

• *Other centres have tried implanting tubes at the site of surgery, which can be loaded with radioactive material after the operation. This procedure has proved to be very labour-intensive, involving specially designated treatment areas, and is therefore not practised widely.*

RADIOTHERAPY

Adjuvant radiotherapy is given to catch any cancer cells that may have been left behind after surgery. Doctors now know that simple mastectomy plus local radiotherapy is just as effective a treatment as radical mastectomy, both in terms of controlling local spread and survival rates. A UK study involving nearly 3,000 women showed that there was no difference in survival rates between the two treatments, but showed a marked improvement in controlling local recurrence in women who received radiotherapy.

At one time, radiotherapy was standard treatment after all mastectomies, but now doctors are more selective. If you fulfil any of the following criteria, you'll be a candidate for post-operative radiotherapy:

• a tumour more than 4 centimetres (2 inches) in diameter
• a Grade 3 tumour
• a node-positive tumour, especially if the disease has spread beyond the axillary lymph nodes.

Even so, deciding who is to be given radiotherapy is not a cut-and-dried procedure, because only about one-third of women with breast cancer are at risk of recurrence. This means that many women would receive unnecessary doses of radiation if all patients were treated.

There's no doubt that radiotherapy should be given to high-risk women with aggressive tumours. For women at lower risk – those with a small, node-negative tumour, for example – it's probably safe to monitor them closely and use radiotherapy only if the cancer returns. Although your hopes may be dashed by local recurrence, try not to get too depressed. It doesn't seem to affect long-term survival rates, provided you get radiotherapy at the time of recurrence.

HOW RADIOTHERAPY IS GIVEN

The aim of adjuvant radiation treatment is to ensure that all the cancer cells in the area of the affected breast are destroyed. Doses of high-energy X-rays are accurately beamed at the breast area of the chest wall and occasionally the axilla and the area above the collarbone. An average course of radiotherapy involves five out-patient treatments each week over about six weeks. Each dose of radiation is meticulously calculated and is then precisely delivered to the area of your skin, which will have been marked with a tiny tattoo of blue dye. Each session can take several minutes, depending on your individual treatment, during which time you will have to lie very still. Otherwise, the experience is not different from that of having an ordinary X-ray. You will be asked not to wash the area during the treatment to avoid irritating the skin. Radiation treatment will not make you radioactive, and there is no danger to adults or children from coming into contact with you.

SYSTEMIC ADJUVANT TREATMENT

The word systemic means affecting the whole. Systemic adjuvant treatment aims to kill off cancer cells throughout your body, thereby preventing any cells that have migrated from the original tumour from causing secondary tumours (metastases) in the bones and organs such as the lungs or liver. The type of systemic treatment that you're eligible for is largely determined by your age. If you are under 50 and pre-menopausal, chemotherapy has been shown to have the most dramatic effect in reducing your odds of dying from the cancer. If you are post-menopausal, hormone treatment in the form of tamoxifen has the same life-saving effect when used for at least two years, especially in tumours that are hormone-sensitive.

HORMONE TREATMENT

Breast cancers may sometimes be influenced by the levels and fluctuations of a woman's hormones, and so lowering oestrogen levels in a woman's body may help in combatting some forms of breast cancer. A few breast cancers are very sensitive to oestrogen levels, and various forms of treatment are aimed at reducing or abolishing a woman's oestrogen production. These include:

- anti-oestrogen drugs such as tamoxifen (the first option)
- surgical removal of the ovaries
- destruction of the ovaries by radiotherapy
- treatment with drugs to stop oestrogen production.

Tamoxifen This drug blocks the stimulatory effect of oestrogen on breast-cancer cells, and it may also have other actions – stimulating the body's own anti-cancer defences, for example. During the last twelve years, tamoxifen has produced a modest but extremely exciting breakthrough in breast cancer treatment. A single 20-milligram tablet taken daily for between two and five years offers a 20–30 percent reduction in the risk of dying from breast cancer. This appears to continue for at least ten years.

SIDE-EFFECTS OF RADIATION

Radiotherapy to the breast area does not cause infertility, nor will your hair fall out. You could find the treatments very tiring, so it's a good idea to put aside rest time on your return from hospital and to be relaxed about chores.

- *Occasionally, sickness or nausea follows treatment and meals have to be planned carefully around each session. Anti-nausea tablets will help.*

- *Skin exposed to radiotherapy may become darker, slightly itchy and sore, as though it had been sunburned. Women with fair skin, particularly those with red hair, are more likely to have skin problems than darker-skinned women.*

- *Small blood vessels in the skin may dilate and burst, forming tiny red marks.*

- *The top of the lungs can be affected because radiation can cause scarring while treatment is in progress, leaving behind a dry cough or breathlessness. This may take a few months to clear up.*

- *Radiotherapy has the potential to interfere with the body's immune system, but this side-effect is now very rare.*

- *Any side-effects will usually subside within a few weeks of your stopping radiotherapy, and by no means everyone experiences them.*

- *After finishing radiotherapy, don't expose the treated skin to the sun for about 18 months.*

Tamoxifen produces few side-effects, although some pre-menopausal women may experience menopausal symptoms such as irregular periods and hot flushes. It acts similarly to natural oestrogen and thus reduces the risk of heart disease and prevents post-menopausal bone loss (osteoporosis).

The benefits of tamoxifen apply to all women regardless of age or the stage of their cancer, but women over the age of 50 seem to gain most. The majority of post-menopausal women are therefore given tamoxifen for at least two years after breast-cancer surgery, irrespective of tumour grade, stage or lymph-node involvement. The role of tamoxifen in pre-menopausal women is less certain. However, tamoxifen is now being studied as a way of preventing breast cancer in high-risk groups.

Destruction of the ovaries (ablation) Abolishing the secretion of oestrogen by the ovaries with either surgery or radiotherapy has been shown to increase the overall survival rate for pre-menopausal women with breast cancer by about 10 percent. It also reduces the number of women who get a recurrence by about 25 percent. Most specialists prefer not to use this treatment in younger women unless they are at very high risk because it causes an immediate menopause and loss of fertility.

Goserelin Injecting the drug, goserelin, inhibits the brain hormones that control the ovaries' production of oestrogen. The reduction in oestrogen levels may cause menopausal symptoms in pre-menopausal women. However, the effects are reversible when treatment is stopped. Treatment will continue depending on its efficacy and side-effects.

CHEMOTHERAPY

This treatment, mainly for younger women, uses cytotoxic drugs that find and kill cancer cells anywhere in the body. They are often given after breast-cancer surgery, especially to pre-menopausal women whose axillary lymph nodes are involved or who have particularly aggressive tumours. Chemotherapy will delay relapse by 30 percent and lower the risk of dying by up to 25 percent.

If you do not want surgery or your tumour is unsuitable for surgery, chemotherapy may be the first or only treatment. Since there are many anti-cancer drugs, which are used in different combinations, success rates and side-effects vary. Prolonged multiple drug treatment (cyclical combination chemotherapy), with a combination of cyclophosphamide, methotrexate and 5-fluorouracil (known as CMF), is the most commonly used regimen. The drugs used should be discussed in some detail with your doctor and all possible side-effects carefully considered.

Treatment Adjuvant chemotherapy is usually given by injection or through a drip inserted into a vein in your arm. Treatment tends to be given in cycles at monthly intervals for six months. Although out-patient treatment is possible, an overnight hospital stay after each treatment is not a bad idea so that any side-effects can be dealt with quickly.

Side-effects of chemotherapy The most worrying effect of chemotherapy is possible damage to the bone marrow that replenishes blood cells; white cells are the most vulnerable. To check that levels of white blood cells remain normal and the body's immune system is intact, a blood sample will be taken before each treatment. If the white-cell count is too low, your next course of treatment will be put off or the dose reduced until the white-cell count returns to a safe level. Antibiotics or a blood transfusion during a course of chemotherapy may be needed to ameliorate this side-effect.

Other side-effects include tiredness, nausea, some hair loss, mouth ulcers, loss of appetite and diarrhoea. Any or all of these can make you feel miserable and ill. Simple remedies such as mouthwashes can help to combat mouth soreness, and powerful drugs have been specially developed to stop the nausea associated with the treatment. If your appetite is affected, whether it is suppressed or increased, your doctor or special-care nurse will be able to advise you about your diet. Some foods have been found to react with the drugs used in chemotherapy, but this is rare.

Given correctly, anti-cancer drugs need not necessarily cause complete hair loss, although you may find that your hair thins a little during the treatment. For some women, this is the most distressing side-effect, especially coming on top of the trauma of disfiguring breast surgery. Your hair will grow back after treatment or even before the treatment is completely finished, but it may be a little more curly and may have changed slightly in colour.

Anti-cancer drugs can often disrupt menstruation, and it may stop altogether. About 40 percent of women who are treated with chemotherapy will become infertile, and you should discuss this possibility with your doctor before treatment begins. The younger you are, the more likely your periods are to resume when chemotherapy ends.

STEM-CELL TREATMENT

About 17 years ago, it appeared that women with advanced breast cancer who received very high doses of chemotherapy were likely to live longer. However, doses of the cytotoxic drugs used are constrained by the poisonous effect on bone marrow.

- *To combat this, researchers developed a procedure that is called autologous stem-cell transfusion. This uses the woman's own bone marrow to rescue her from otherwise toxic high doses of chemotherapy.*

- *Stem cells, the cells that produce all other blood cells, are removed from the patient's blood or bone marrow and frozen. Then a course of high-dose chemotherapy is given over a period of four to five days in doses that would usually be sufficient to kill the stem cells (leading ultimately to the patient's death).*

- *Doctors can reinfuse the previously harvested stem cells after chemotherapy is complete. Because these cells have not been affected by chemotherapy, they can once again begin to form healthy blood cells.*

- *Stem-cell treatment remains controversial, traumatic and very expensive. It is not generally available in Europe, although it is in some centres in the US. In addition, the procedure is unfortunately not as successful as was first hoped.*

BREAST RECONSTRUCTION

If you have lost part or all of your breast, you can have reconstructive surgery. This involves the creation of a natural-looking artificial breast through plastic surgery. Although a reconstructed breast may look very real, there will be little or no feeling in the transferred skin. The psychological benefits and increased confidence you will experience in the way you look tend to outweigh the disadvantage of reduced sensation of the nipple and areola.

Every woman has the right to consult a specialist about reconstruction. If your doctor is reluctant to consider the option, seek a second opinion. Even the most well-adjusted woman flinches at the thought of mastectomy. It's reasonable to see the changes you have to make to the way you dress and to your lifestyle as a threat to your femininity and body-image. Above all the mastectomy scar may serve as a reminder of the cancer you once had. Reconstruction can go a long way to making you feel whole again. You'll no longer need prostheses (false breasts) or special bras, or feel so restricted in the kind of clothes you wear. Reconstruction can contribute a great deal to your self-esteem and your optimism about the future. About half of all mastectomy patients choose to have breast reconstruction, finding that it helps them to put their cancer behind them.

Reconstruction in no way restricts the treatments open to you. It doesn't interfere with radiotherapy, chemotherapy or hormone therapy. Post-operative follow-up is made no harder and recurrence can still be easily detected.

TIMING

Some consideration should be given to the timing of reconstruction. It may be possible for you to have it immediately after your mastectomy and under the same anaesthetic, or at any time afterwards. This means that a woman who had a mastectomy many years ago when breast reconstruction was not available can opt to have it now.

With immediate reconstruction you will wake from your operation with your breast still present even though it will have altered. The psychological stress associated with breast removal is greatly reduced and, in addition, you don't have to cope with the prospect of more surgery later.

Despite these advantages, immediate reconstruction isn't carried out very frequently because it involves two specialist surgeons (a cancer surgeon and a plastic surgeon) working together at the same time. This makes it a lengthy, difficult and complicated operation. There's also evidence that some women are less happy with the reconstructed breast if the reconstruction is done as part of the mastectomy operation, and some surgeons prefer waiting several months to make sure that the breast has healed completely.

You may not be able to take advantage of immediate reconstruction in the clinic that you attend but, if this is what you want, it may be possible for you to be transferred to a specialist breast unit that does offer it.

SUITABILITY FOR RECONSTRUCTION

Don't worry if you are slightly unfit; reconstructive surgery can be performed on any woman except the very frail. Even if you have widespread disease, your life expectancy may still be several years and the quality of your life during this time can be greatly improved by reconstruction.

Although half of all breast cancer patients will not need a mastectomy, even women who have conservative surgery may lose quite a lot of breast tissue. They too can take advantage of reconstructive surgery.

METHODS OF RECONSTRUCTION

Reconstructive surgery remoulds your breast mound, areola and nipple. The mound can be reconstructed using your own tissue or an artificial implant. Two kinds of implant are available: fixed-volume implants and tissue expanders. Both types have a textured silicone shell filled with either saline (salt in solution) or silicone gel.

It's important to realize that the link between silicone implants and cancer is entirely unproven. Bear in mind, too, that implants have been around for more than 30 years and have been used in nearly two million women, not to mention the large number of people who use other silicone products, for instance contact lenses. In 1989, the FDA (Food and Drug Administration) in the US concluded that "a carcinogenic [cancer-producing] effect in humans could not be completely ruled out, but if such an effect did exist, the risk would be very low". Breast surgeons in the rest of the world have found this statement sufficiently reassuring to go on using silicone implants.

ARTIFICIAL IMPLANTS

A fixed-volume implant is placed behind the muscles of the chest wall. Although this is the simplest operation, it's not suitable for all women since there may not be enough skin in the breast area to accommodate the implant.

If too little skin remains after your mastectomy to cover a fixed-volume implant, your doctor may recommend an expander implant (see right) – an empty sac with a hollow tube and small valve attached that is placed behind the muscles of the chest wall in the same way as a fixed-volume implant. Over a period of several months, your doctor will gradually fill the implant (through its attached valve) with saline solution, allowing the skin to stretch so that a fixed-volume implant may eventually be inserted.

YOUR OWN TISSUE

The simplest kind of breast reconstruction is carried out with an implant but there are several methods that use your own tissue. These reconstruction procedures (see right) all involve "flaps" and produce a better result than implants.

Skin, muscle and fat are taken as a flap from either your back or your abdomen. The flap from your back is called the latissimus dorsi flap; the flap from your abdomen is known as the rectus abdominis or TRAM (transverse rectus abdominis myocutaneous) flap. In this procedure, tissues with their arteries and veins intact are swivelled up to your breast area so that they can "take" in a similar way to a skin graft. The flap is tunnelled underneath your skin to the breast area and is fashioned into a breast mound resembling your other breast as closely as possible. Many women find implants of their own tissue preferable to the artificial kinds. However, these breast reconstructions require quite complex surgery, and occasionally there are side-effects such as a weakening of the abdominal muscles if a large amount of tissue has to be moved.

The final kind of reconstruction takes tissue from your buttocks as a free flap – the gluteus maximus flap. In this procedure, blood vessels supplying the tissue that is moved are cut and rejoined to blood vessels in the chest wall where the implant is placed. This is the most complex kind of reconstruction and for some patients it may be the most satisfactory. There is a small risk that the blood vessels will fail to join, in which case the implant may not take.

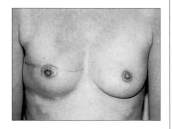

Reconstructed breast
In this example of a reconstruction, both the right breast and nipple have been reconstructed after a total mastectomy.

RECONSTRUCTION PROCEDURES

Tissue expander implant

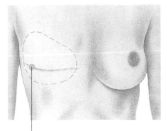

Valve under the skin allows saline to be injected later

Latissimus dorsi flap (own tissue implant)

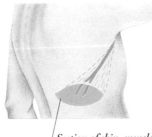

Section of skin, muscle and fat to be moved

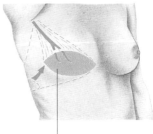

Flap brought under skin to front of chest

Artificial implant
A hollow sac with a valve is put in place. Over a period of months, saline fluid is injected into the valve, allowing the skin to stretch gradually and naturally. The expander implant can then be replaced with a fixed-volume implant.

1 A flap of skin, muscle and fat is taken from the latissimus dorsi muscle on the back. The section of tissue to be moved keeps its feeding artery and blood vessels intact even after it has been moved to the new site.

2 The flap is tunnelled under the skin to the site of the mastectomy scar and the fat and muscle are fashioned into a mound. The new breast is stitched into place and the incision in the back is closed.

Rectus abdominis flap

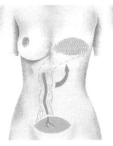

Flap is tunnelled into new position

Gluteus maximus flap (own tissue implant)

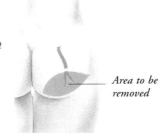

Area to be removed

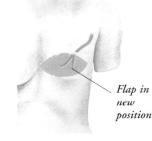

Flap in new position

Own tissue implant
A flap is taken from the rectus abdominis muscle, keeping its blood supply intact (the blood vessels are not cut). The flap is tunnelled under the skin to its new position. The incision in the abdomen is closed after the new breast mound has been stitched into place.

1 A flap of skin, muscle and fat is removed from the gluteus maximus muscle in the buttocks. Its feeding artery is severed so that the flap can simply be placed in position without having to be tunnelled under the skin as for other procedures.

2 The flap is transferred to the mastectomy scar site and microsurgery is used to connect its blood vessels to those behind the muscles in the chest. The new breast mound is then stitched into place and the incision in the buttocks is closed.

THE IMPACT OF TREATMENT

A diagnosis of breast cancer and its treatment – especially if it involves the loss of a breast – still brings havoc in its wake. Despite the advent of surgical techniques that aim to conserve the breast, rates of anxiety and depression are still high. Women are just as anxious about having cancer as they are about the potential loss of a breast.

Nor are the psychological problems necessarily less if you have a lumpectomy rather than a mastectomy. For doctors to believe that your fears are minor compared with those of a woman facing a mastectomy could cause problems that may continue throughout your treatment, even into the follow-up period. Your feeling that you shouldn't bother your doctors with your fears may also reflect the popular expectation that women should be unreasonably stoical in the face of both physical and emotional pain.

A woman with breast cancer who's had a lumpectomy shouldn't have to handle the disease with cheerfulness and fortitude. Nor should just having a "little lump" removed create the feeling that, since treatment was comparatively trivial, you should quickly return to a normal psychological state; if you can't, you could end up feeling worthless and depressed. A pre-operative psychological test can identify 90 percent of women who'll become anxious and depressed in the year after surgery, enabling proper follow-up and help to be offered. If you feel vulnerable, ask for a test using the HAD (Hospital Anxiety and Depression) scale.

"My husband was just great, really supportive. I know that he was far more worried that I had a life-threatening disease than about the loss of my breast. But our sex life has changed, of course it has. I can't rid myself of the idea that really he hates my scar but is just trying to pretend that he doesn't mind."

Cheryl, 36, Musician

RADIOTHERAPY

Radiotherapy can involve daily treatment for up to six weeks. The greater the amount of radiation, the greater the chance of side-effects, which can be draining. If you are pre-menopausal, you may be worried that radiation will prevent you from having children; this isn't true. When doctors try to help with comments like "it's an insurance policy just to be sure we've got all the cancer", they can create doubts in your mind rather than reassuring you. Just the thought of having radiotherapy can sometimes be enough to produce side-effects. The more you understand the rationale behind your treatment and how it works, the less anxious you will be.

CHEMOTHERAPY

Chemotherapy has the worst reputation of all breast-cancer treatments because it's nearly always accompanied by some side-effects, including increased risk of infection.

For a woman who is feeling emotionally and physically bruised, the prospect of going through several courses of chemotherapy can cause a mixture of fear and suspicion. As with radiotherapy, the need for chemotherapy sometimes provokes fears that the cancer has not been totally removed.

Understandably you'll get more anxious and depressed if you have troublesome side-effects. It's a mistake to believe that a treatment must hurt to be effective, and it won't be stopped if you disclose your distress and discomfort to your doctors and care-givers. Tell them, and they will do all they can to give you the help and support you need.

SEXUAL RELATIONSHIPS

Powerful stereotyping in our society means that women's breasts have become symbolically linked to motherhood, femininity and sexuality. Don't feel inadequate if breast loss causes you severe sexual disturbance together with lowered self-esteem, loss of perceived attractiveness, embarrassment or inhibition and loss of sex drive. About one in five women has a loss of sexual interest a few months after mastectomy, and at two years the figure rises to one in three.

Interest in sex declines in over a quarter of sexually active women irrespective of the kind of surgical treatment they have. If you've had adjuvant therapy, you're particularly vulnerable and likely to express more concern about physical affection, sexual relationships and lost feelings of femininity or sexual attractiveness.

Following radiotherapy, you may lose a lot of sensation in the affected breast. If your breasts were an important source of sexual stimulation prior to surgery, you'll need help and counselling to find another means of enhancing your enjoyment of lovemaking. Your partner may worry about being exposed to radiation by touching your breast while you are undergoing radiotherapy. This is not a danger.

The psychological impact of the diagnosis of cancer and treatment may make you so overwhelmingly preoccupied with thoughts of survival that sexual desire is at the bottom of your list of priorities. For some couples, however, the trauma of breast cancer can bring them closer together.

BODY IMAGE

Decisions about treatment are too often based on assumptions that older or sexually inactive women won't mind losing a breast. In one study of 62 women, more than half of those who chose lumpectomy were over the age of 50 and more than a quarter were over 60, demonstrating that age is not an acceptable criterion for deciding treatment.

- *You may become extremely self-conscious after mastectomy. Some women feel sure that people can tell they have only one breast, and become so distressed that they withdraw from the company of others. Up to one-third of post-mastectomy patients are unhappy with their prosthesis.*

- *Although mastectomy clearly has the greatest impact on how you perceive your body, not every woman who has breast conservation is pleased with the cosmetic outcome.*

- *Some women feel that being told they would have only the lump removed was misleading, since they expected to be left with symmetrical breasts. Unfortunately the necessary surgical procedure (called wide local excision) does not always fulfil these ideals.*

CHOOSING BRAS

Once your permanent prosthesis has been fitted, there's no reason why you shouldn't wear a wide variety of bras. The exceptions include styles that are wide on the shoulders and low cut, such as a half-cup bra. It's best to choose a cotton bra so that sweat can evaporate and your skin doesn't get hot and sticky under the prosthesis.

There are many attractive bras available with specially fitted pockets to hold your prosthesis in place, ensuring that it does not slip. Extra support in the rib-band and wide, supportive shoulder straps are important for comfort and can help your posture, which can be affected by a mastectomy.

LIFE AFTER TREATMENT

When treatment for breast cancer is complete, the story doesn't simply end. Rigorous follow-up will be necessary to pick up any problems and to check for any recurrence of the cancer. Having a mastectomy means that there are adjustments to make: you have to get used to a prosthesis and exercises to make your arm muscles strong. Then you have to learn to live with your new body. Even when treatment is complete, you could have psychological difficulties. After months of intensive medical attention you may feel alone and fearful, especially knowing there is no guarantee of a cure. This is a time when a care network such as a local breast-cancer group can be invaluable.

LYMPHOEDEMA

Disfigurement caused by surgery is not the only possible trauma you may face. Lymphoedema – painful swelling of the arm caused by radical radiotherapy or surgery on the axilla – can occasionally arise after treatment.

Healthy lymph nodes act as filters for the body's lymph fluid. Surgery can cause scarring of the nodes and this results in a blockage of the drainage system. The fluid stagnates in the arm, causing swelling and stiffness, which may be accompanied by a painful shoulder and possibly by nerve pain. With modern surgical techniques, lymphoedema is now rare and only five percent of mastectomy patients suffer from it to any degree. Severe lymphoedema hardly ever occurs.

Prevention and treatment   After the removal of your lymph nodes, you become more susceptible to infection, so you should protect your arm from knocks and scrapes, and wear gloves for rough household chores, gardening or any other work where your skin could be chafed.

It's important for you to do your post-mastectomy exercises regularly, since this can help to reduce the swelling by encouraging lymph drainage. Whenever you can, keep your arm raised, even when you're in bed or sitting on a sofa. Put your arm on a pile of cushions to keep it at about the same level as your neck. This will reduce swelling in your arm and help to build on the good work started by your daily exercises. If you have problems overnight with tingling in the fingers, try wearing an elastic bandage to prevent your arm from swelling.

PROSTHESES

A prosthesis is a false breast without a nipple but with an axillary tail, which resembles the texture, fullness and shape of a natural breast. You can wear a lightweight, temporary one as soon as your scar is healed, and then can be fitted with a permanent one to fit comfortably into your bra.

Every woman has the right to a good prosthesis. With the help of your surgeon, breast-care nurse or specially trained counsellor, you should easily be able to obtain one and even try various types to find the one that feels right.

If at first you can't find your ideal prosthesis, don't be disheartened. No prosthesis can fully replace your breast, but there's a good one for every woman who has had a mastectomy. Many kinds let you wear a swimsuit and low necklines without anyone being any the wiser, and you'll soon feel quite confident with your new shape. (There's a range of quite discreet prostheses for women whose breasts are asymmetrical following conservative surgery.)

BREAST PROSTHESES

A permanent prosthesis is made from silicone. It "gives" to the touch and feels heavy, just like a natural breast. A lightweight foam prosthesis has a hollow back that allows air to circulate. It can be useful as a temporary measure, for night wear and sports, or for very hot days when a permanent prosthesis can feel sticky and uncomfortable.

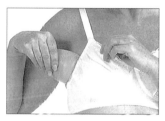

Fitting a prosthesis
Slip the prosthesis into the special pocket inside your bra. Make sure that it fills the cup and your underarm area.

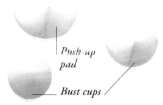

Push-up pad

Bust cups

Bra fillers
A variety of push up pads and bust cups is available to fill out your bra after partial mastectomy.

Silicone prosthesis
Soft to the touch, a silicone prosthesis has the weight and droop of a natural breast.

Silicone nipples adhere to the prosthesis when moistened

TINTED
PROSTHESIS

TRIANGULAR
FORM

UNDERARM
EXTENSION

TEARDROP
SHAPE

LIGHTWEIGHT
FORM

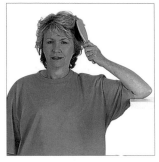

POST-MASTECTOMY EXERCISES

You may find that your shoulder movement is restricted immediately following your operation. Normal movement and flexibility should gradually return, however, with the help of a few simple exercises, which are shown here.

Hair brushing
Rest your arm on a firm surface. Keeping your head and shoulders upright, brush your hair upwards and sideways.

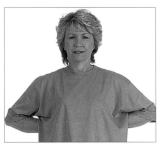

Bra fastening
Bend your arms at the elbows, keeping them at right angles to your body. Reach behind your back at bra level while slowly bringing your hands in towards your body. Relax from this position and begin again.

Arm circling
Stand as here, or sideways on to a firm table, leaning on it with your good arm. Bending slightly at the waist, let your affected arm hang loosely. Swing it forwards, backwards, left and right, and then in small circles.

Towelling
Hold a towel or scarf stretched diagonally behind your back. Move it up and down along the line of the diagonal as if you were drying your back. Repeat with the towel or scarf held the other way.

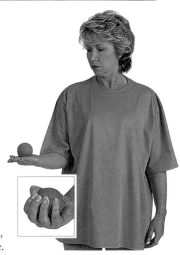

Lay your good arm on a flat surface

As your arm relaxes, slowly increase the size of the swings

Hand squeezing
Hold a rubber ball on your flat palm. It should be firm enough so you have to exert pressure to squeeze it, but "give" enough for you to notice any improvement in muscle strength. Forming a fist around the ball, gently squeeze, then release. Repeat, but stop if you begin to ache.

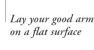

RECURRENCE AND RISK

Your age, menopausal status, the stage of the disease and the status of your axillary nodes will all have a profound affect on your initial chances of survival. In very general terms, women developing breast cancer under the age of 35 do less well than those whose breast cancer starts around the time of the menopause. Women between the ages of 35 and 50 who have not yet started the menopause do best. This means that many, many women have a good chance of surviving breast cancer, especially if it is detected early.

After successful treatment for breast cancer you will be concerned about how carefully you'll be followed up and how long it will be before you can be considered cured. The longer you live without a recurrence, the longer you will remain cancer-free, and the higher the chances of a cure. Because of this, most doctors believe that you should be carefully monitored for at least five years after treatment to detect possible recurrences or secondary spread.

You must be followed up for longer than five years before you can be said to be cured. Survival beyond ten years without any evidence of recurrence or spread would lead a doctor to be optimistic that you were cured, although women who have had breast cancer may still have a very small increased chance of dying from it, even 40 years after treatment, compared with healthy women of the same age.

TYPES OF RECURRENCE

There are three ways in which cancer can recur in the breast area. The most common recurrence is in the conserved breast in the region of the original cancer. This is not necessarily too serious; it's seen as cancer that is left over from the original treatment rather than as a secondary tumour. Since the cancer has not spread around the body, this type of recurrence is usually treated with a mastectomy.

Another kind of local recurrence concerns the lymph nodes (it affects only two percent of women). In general, it is not considered to be a sign of the cancer having spread and is therefore treated with further surgery or radiotherapy.

A recurrence of cancer in the scar or chest wall following a mastectomy is more serious. Because all your breast tissue has been removed, it is impossible for the cancer to be residual, and it must therefore have travelled from the lymphatic system or the bloodstream. Such recurrence, or

TREATMENT FOR RECURRENCE

Cancer can recur in the area of the treated breast regardless of the initial treatment. This happens in two or three cases out of ten, but is not a reason to be terrified or despondent.

Radiotherapy can cure any local recurrence, which is why follow-up schedules for patients must be strictly adhered to. A recurrence can then be detected so early that a relatively small dose of radiotherapy is all that is needed to eradicate it.

Bear in mind that mastectomy has a slightly lower risk of local recurrence than lumpectomy: mastectomy has a recurrence rate of 5–15 percent, whereas with lumpectomy the rate is 10–30 percent. In addition, radiotherapy following a lumpectomy is frequently given at the total body dose. This may mean that radiotherapy is no longer an option for treating a recurrence of breast cancer.

HOPE FOR THE FUTURE

In conclusion, bear in mind that one in three women who have treatment for early breast cancer can expect to live a normal life span.

For women who get local recurrences, radiotherapy can cure without the need for other treatment. Lastly, while breast cancer is predominantly a disease of older women, many women will die from causes other than their breast cancer.

recurrence in your other breast or elsewhere in your body, is considered a secondary tumour, and will certainly require rigorous attention to curb the spreading cancer.

PREVIOUS BREAST CANCER AND RISK

A woman who has already had cancer of one breast is at a higher than average risk of developing cancer of the other breast, and this is why women who have had breast cancer must be meticulous about doing BSE on their remaining breast. Tamoxifen seems to reduce the risk of a secondary cancer developing regardless of whether adjuvant treatment has been given, and in women with several risk factors tamoxifen might be considered as a preventive treatment. You should discuss this with your doctor.

As well as doing BSE, you should also have regular mammograms performed on your remaining breast, because about 7 out of 100 women may develop a second primary tumour at some time in the future. A reasonable schedule for follow-up mammography would be six-monthly for two years and every 12 months thereafter.

THE REMAINING BREAST

Doctors can't agree whether the opposite breast should be biopsied at the time of initial surgery or during follow-up. Performing these biopsies might detect a good number of in situ lesions that, if left alone, would cause no problems at all. On the other hand, since only a very small sample of breast tissue is taken during a biopsy, it's possible to miss some invasive cancers that are present.

An interesting study has been done on women under 65 with Stage I or II breast cancers – that is, early cancer. When the opposite breast was biopsied, nearly one in six women were found to have some cancerous changes at the time of finding the first tumour. The vast majority of them, however, proved to be cancers that might never have become symptomatic and certainly would not kill. So these findings are of doubtful significance and it's still not clear which patients need treatment for them.

Such obsessive searching for cancers can lead to intense and unnecessary anxiety, and a wise course to pursue seems to be to monitor the remaining breast during follow-up sessions and reserve biopsy for any suspicious physical or mammographic findings. Do not hesitate to discuss with your doctor any uncertainties or worries you may have.

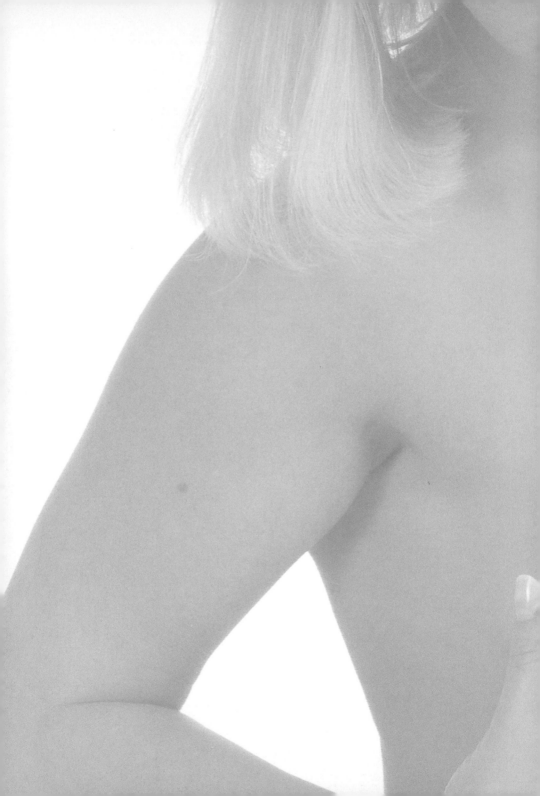

HEALTHY SEX

INTRODUCTION

Sex expresses something that nothing else can, and it is the main way that human beings show their love for each other. It has a place in your life that is as much as, or more important than, any other aspect of your relationships, be they long or short term. Beyond desire and procreation, sex is the time, place, means and language of knowing someone else on a level different from all others.

At the heart of sex is also the importance men and women hold for each other, something that many people have lost sight of. Loving partners give the kind of support that no-one else can; very often they are the only havens in the storms of life. They provide emotional back-up; they help you to feel worthwhile, useful and desirable. A loving partner makes you recognize yourself as a well-rounded and mature individual with every chance of happiness, and every right to it. And in this context, sex is of prime importance, because only a loving partner can give it. It is, therefore, the responsibility of every partner to do it well, because in the end, it is the one way of ensuring that a beloved companion will stay, and a loving relationship – with all its rewards – will endure.

But having a good sex life is not about sexual athletics, physical prowess or just learning a series of sexual skills. This is why many sex manuals simply don't work; they emphasize the technical skills related to sexuality instead of the people involved. Experimenting with different techniques and positions doesn't guarantee to make you a better or more sophisticated lover. Good lovers are aware of the importance of closeness and caring; they desire to give love, to give pleasure and to give themselves completely to their partners. The best lovers discover their partners' preferences through sharing the intimacy of mutual trust. The best sex is attained only in a truly loving, stable relationship that is nurtured, pursued and withstands the test of time.

THE TWO SEXES

Many men and women are successful in their voyages
of sexual discovery. They're helped by sympathetic partners
who are open about their sexual needs, who are prepared to
initiate and experiment and who understand their bodies
and feel comfortable with their own sexuality.
For many others, however, sex is still a matter of just
"doing it"; they've never known, or have forgotten, the
considerable joys of giving and receiving love.
Practical information about male and female sexual
anatomy and how it works can help to rescue people from
ignorance about sex, setting their sexual experiences on the
road to becoming the ultimate expression of intimacy.

SEXUAL DEVELOPMENT

Both scientific research and personal observation have convinced me that men and women are more anatomically similar than are the males and females of most other species. Any two men or two women are likely to differ more in stature, size and shape than does the average couple. Particularly distinctive in men and women are their reproductive organs and the developmental changes apparent in their mature shapes that are caused by sex hormones.

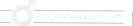

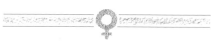

BOY INTO MAN

The changes that mark a boy's physical development into a mature man begin in the pre-teen and early teen years and are completed when he is between 14 and 18. These changes – when boys become taller and more muscular, with wider shoulders, more developed genital organs and with hair appearing on their genitals, underarms, faces, chests, arms and legs – are caused mainly by the male hormone, testosterone. As well as having the characteristics set out below, the adult male has experienced his voice "breaking", caused by the larynx enlarging and the vocal cords becoming longer and thicker so that the pitch of the voice drops, and an increase in sweat and sebaceous gland activity.

After testicular activity is established at puberty it normally continues for the rest of life with only slight impairment in later years. In old age there is a slight reduction in the production of sperm and androgen. This is associated with some degenerative changes in the testes, but there is no abrupt testicular decline comparable to the female climacteric.

The "average" man is approximately 173 centimetres (5 feet 9 inches) tall and weighs 74 kilos (162 pounds); his chest, waist and hip measurements are 98, 80, 93 centimetres (39, 32, 37 inches).

GIRL INTO WOMAN

In the latter part of adolescence, usually well after menstruation has begun, a girl's body begins to take up its female shape. (Prior to puberty, girls and boys, except for their external genitalia, are very similar.) The changes that a girl experiences are directly related to the secretion of female hormones, oestrogen and progesterone. She becomes taller, her hips and thighs get fleshier, and she is more rounded and curvier. Her breasts begin to swell and hair grows under her arms and between her legs. Her internal and external genital organs grow and develop, and the vaginal wall starts to thicken. Vaginal secretions may appear.

A woman's ultimate shape is dependent on two things: the amount of hormones she produces, and the sensitivity of her body in reacting to these hormones.

At around the age of 45, ovarian function gradually wanes, and levels of oestrogen and progesterone decline, resulting in cessation of menstruation and the loss of fertility, the thinning of the vaginal walls and, very often, bone changes that result in a loss of height.

The "average" mature woman is 158 centimetres (5 feet 3½ inches) tall and weighs 61 kilos (135 pounds); her bust, waist and hip measurements are 90, 75, 95 centimetres (36, 30, 38 inches).

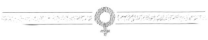

A MAN'S BODY

Skeleton Beginning at about age two, boys grow approximately 5 centimetres (2 inches) per year until the age of 13 or 14, when the sex organs begin to develop. Adolescence brings with it a rapid gain in both height and strength. The growth spurt that accompanies puberty may last for a few years, and during that time most boys gain approximately 9 centimetres (3½ inches) yearly. At the end of this period of growth, the bones have grown harder, more brittle, and have changed in proportion. Once the shoulders broaden, the hips look narrower by comparison – a characteristic of the adult male.

Body hair Early in puberty, pubic hair appears at the base of the penis, and after a while, it starts growing on the scrotum as well. It may also grow around the anal area. Pubic hair normally grows in an upside-down triangle on the lower part of the belly, though it may reach the navel, and may grow outwards towards the thighs. About one or two years later, hair will appear in the armpits and on the upper lip. Pubic hair is longer, coarser and curlier than hair that has been on the body since birth. It may be a lighter or darker colour than that on the head. With age, it may turn grey.

In addition to curly pubic hair, hair appears on the arms, thighs and lower legs. Hair may appear also on the chest, shoulders and back, and back of the hands. Facial hair becomes thicker and darker as a man matures. The beard and moustache may be the same colour as the hair on the head, or different.

The amount of body hair depends on racial or ethnic background and family history. Caucasian men generally have more body hair than oriental or black men; and "hairiness" runs in families.

A WOMAN'S BODY

Skeleton Starting around age two, a girl grows at the average rate of 5 centimetres (2 inches) per year. At around the age of ten, she experiences a growth spurt and begins to grow at a faster rate, gaining approximately 10 centimetres (4 inches) or more in a single year, but then slows down again until she reaches her final height, approximately one to three years after the onset of menstruation. While her bones are growing longer, not all grow at the same rate. Arm, leg and feet bones grow at a faster rate than, say, spinal bones, and the pelvic bones take on a characteristically wide shape.

A woman has a wider pelvis than a man, in order to accommodate a growing baby, and her thigh bones are set wider apart. The thighs have to slant quite steeply inwards for the knees to come near the centre of gravity, so most women have a degree of knock knees.

Body hair Sexual body hair usually appears around the eleventh or twelfth year, just after the breasts have begun to grow. Pubic hair is longer, coarser, darker in colour, and curlier than one's normal childhood hair, which has been present on the body since birth. Pubic hair first appears on the vulva and gradually spreads over the mons and vaginal lips, forming an upside-down triangle. In some women, pubic hair grows up toward the navel and out onto the thighs.

Women differ in the amount of pubic hair that grows. Some have a lot; for others it is sparse. It can be any colour and does not have to match the head hair. As a woman ages, her pubic hair may go grey. Almost two years after the appearance of pubic hair, further hair starts growing in the armpits.

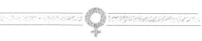

A MAN'S BODY

Muscles The thighs, calves, shoulders and upper arms begin to grow broader during adolescence, and strength increases, too. A grown man's muscles are 40 times those at birth. The main determinant of body strength is body size, and muscle itself accounts for 40 percent of total body weight.

The genitals The testes grow very slowly until about the age of 10 or 11, following which there is a considerable acceleration in growth rate and growth of the external genital organs. In the fully grown male, the testicles are usually about 3.8 centimetres (1½ inches) long, between 16 and 27 millilitres (½–1 fluid ounce) in volume, and are duskily coloured. One testicle, usually the left one, hangs lower than the other. This is to keep the testicles from crushing each other when you walk. In most men, testicles are the same size, but in a few, one may be larger than the other.

Changes to the penis begin at a later stage than for the testicles. During a growth spurt, the penis gets larger (both longer and wider) and the glans, or head, of the penis becomes more developed. A grown man's penis is usually between 7.5 and 10 centimetres (3–4 inches) long when flaccid.

Under certain conditions, for instance coming into contact with cold water or being out during cold weather, or if the man is feeling afraid or tired, the penis can temporarily shrivel somewhat. Old age, however, can cause it to become permanently a bit smaller in size.

A WOMAN'S BODY

Muscles and fat Fat begins to be deposited on the breasts, hips, thighs and buttocks when a girl is about nine to ten. Later on, when she is about 15 to 17, more fat appears in the same areas. While her hips become rounded and swelling, the waist becomes curved and well-defined. Some women develop stretch marks – faint purplish or white lines – on their skin at this time. This happens when the skin is stretched too much during this period of rapid growth.

The genitals A man's genitals lie on the surface of his body where they are easily seen and handled. A woman's genitals, however, are relatively inaccessible, more numerous and fairly complex in design. Just as in other areas of human anatomy, the genitals of women are individual; they come in a variety of shapes, sizes, colours and textures.

Breasts The breasts are a symbol of feminine identity, forming part of the body image. Initially designed to nourish an infant, they are often far more highly regarded by society as a principal source of eroticism, a symbol of femininity, a determinant of fashion and a measure of a woman's beauty.

The breasts, or mammary glands, are modified sweat glands. Each woman's breasts are unique in their size, shape and appearance, and this variation not only occurs between women but in the same woman at different times of her life, that is during the menstrual cycle, pregnancy and lactation. One breast is very often larger than the other.

In the centre of the breast is a ring of skin called the areola; the nipple sits in its centre. The nipple and areola can range in colour from a light pink to a brownish-black.

SEXUAL ANATOMY

There's no doubt that an awareness of and familiarity with sexual anatomy can make you a better lover. Knowing where your partner's most sensitive areas are, how they are likely to respond to stimulation and touch – and what happens when they do – means that you will be able to give him or her maximum pleasure. And, if you realize that your partner is an individual who certainly will respond to particular caresses, perhaps in a very individual way, your lovemaking will become much more effective and mutually satisfying.

YOUR GENITALS ARE UNIQUE

Men find it somewhat easier to understand their own sexual anatomy since their sexual organs hang outside the body and are clearly and constantly visible. But both women and men are less familiar with female anatomy, and this is because so many of the important parts lie hidden within a woman's body.

Just as in other areas of anatomy, the genitals of men and women are individual; they come in a range of shapes and sizes. Normal variation means that a few women have exceptionally large or small vaginas, just as the occasional man has an exceptionally large or small penis. Women rarely express dissatisfaction with the size and shape of their external genitals – maybe because comparison with those of other women is not usual, so ignorance is bliss. However, the vast majority of men are dissatisfied with the quality of their sex organs, and many feel that a small or average penis is a drawback to their sexual value.

Fortunately, there are many women who couldn't care less or who hardly notice the size of their partner's penis. Indeed, some women are physically uncomfortable with a big penis; a smaller penis is easier for a woman to take when it comes to oral sex, for instance. Furthermore, many of a woman's sensations from intercourse come from the clitoris and from the nerve endings that are mainly in the first couple of inches of the vagina, so the length of the penis really is irrelevant. It is a man's skill and patience as a lover, not the size of his penis, that is responsible for giving his partner sexual satisfaction.

On the other hand, many women are dissatisfied with their breasts and it may be that some of the dissatisfaction that both sexes have regarding their visible anatomy is the result of foreshortened viewing; both penises and breasts are normally viewed by their owners from the top down. What really matters, though, is taking pride and delight in your own individuality, and not worrying about what your genitals look like compared with others, and that everything functions normally.

A MAN'S SEX ORGANS

THE PENIS

There is no organ about which more myths have been perpetrated than the penis. It has been praised, blamed and misrepresented in art, literature and legend since time immemorial. These phallic fallacies have become firmly fixed in our culture, thereby influencing our attitudes and behaviour.

The penis has two functions – the passing of urine and the depositing of semen in the vagina – but it is the role of the penis as the organ responsible for orgasm in both men and women that has achieved mythical status.

Although they vary in length, the average penis measures 9.5 centimetres (3¾ inches) in its flaccid state. It is composed of erectile tissue arranged in three cylindrical columns. The column underneath expands at the end of the penis to form the glans. Through the centre of this column runs the urethra, a narrow tube carrying semen (and urine) out of the body through an opening at the tip of the glans. When a man has an erection, and for a few minutes after he has ejaculated, the urethra becomes compressed so that he can't urinate, although semen can get through.

The penis is covered by muscles and filled with a rich network of blood vessels and blood spaces; the latter remain empty when the penis is flaccid but have the potential to fill and expand with blood during erection.

The expanded glans is demarcated from the main shaft of the penis by an indentation that runs around its head, and the skin on the shaft of the penis forms a fold (the foreskin) that extends to cover the glans. On its lower side, the fold is tethered to the inner surface of the glans by the frenulum. For many men, this tiny band of skin is their most sensitive part and, if stimulated, may quickly arouse them.

At birth, the foreskin is attached to the glans; starting in infancy, it gradually separates. The foreskin may be removed by circumcision. There is no truth in the notion that an uncircumcised man can control ejaculation more effectively than a man who is circumcised. This myth is founded on the widespread misconception that the glans of the circumcised penis is more sensitive to touch than the glans covered most of the time by a foreskin. During intercourse, the foreskin retracts exposing the glans exactly as for a circumcised glans.

The skin of the penis is thin, stretchy, without fat and loosely attached to the underlying tissues. The penis is richly supplied with sensory nerves and nerves from the autonomic nervous system.

CHANGES TO PENIS SIZE

When a man is sexually aroused, the penis normally increases in size – an additional 7–8 centimetres (2¾–3¼ inches) – and stiffness. Erection may take place in a few seconds, and is due to a very great increase in blood flow into the penis. The blood spaces fill with blood, which is prevented from draining away into the veins by swollen arteries that compress them; the erection is thus maintained until after ejaculation.

It is widely accepted that the larger the penis, the more effective a man is as a sexual partner. This delusion, for delusion it is, that penile size is related to sexual potency, is based on yet another phallic fallacy: that when a larger penis becomes erect it achieves a bigger size than does erection of a smaller penis. But this is not the case. In the laboratory of researchers Masters and Johnson, men whose penises were 7.5–9 centimetres (3–3½ inches) long in the flaccid state increased by an average of 7.5–8 centimetres (3–3¼ inches) when fully erect, which essentially doubled the smaller organs in length over flaccid size standards. In contrast, in the men whose organs were significantly larger in the flaccid state – 10–11.5 centimetres (4–4¾ inches) – penile length increased by an average of only 7–7.5 centimetres (2¾–3 inches) when fully erect.

THE SCROTUM

The scrotum is the pouch of skin situated below the root of the penis that houses the testes. It's divided by a fibrous sheet and this division can be seen on the surface of the scrotum as a ridge. The skin of the scrotum is dark and thin and contains numerous sebaceous glands and sparse hairs. Under the skin is a smooth muscle that contracts in response to cold, or vigorous exercise; its contraction makes the scrotum smaller and its skin wrinkled.

THE TESTES

The testes are smooth, oval structures that are compressed from side to side like broad beans. The left testis may be slightly lower than the right. Each testis is inside a sac and has four coverings that correspond to the various layers of the abdominal wall; these are carried down into the scrotal sac when the testis migrates from inside the abdomen just before birth. Small muscles control the height of the testes. The position of the testes may change according to a man's level of sexual arousal, his emotions and

the temperature of the scrotum, among other things. If sperm are to develop normally, they must be produced at a temperature two or three degrees lower than the rest of the body. That is why the testes are "outside" the body.

The two functions of the testis are to produce sperm and male hormones or androgens, primarily testosterone. A fine tube carries sperm developed in the testis to the epididymis where it is stored. This comma-shaped structure is stuck to the rear surface of the testis and is, in effect, an extensively coiled duct.

The vas deferens carries sperm via the spermatic cord into the pelvis, where it joins the back of the bladder with the seminal vesicle. Each duct (see above) then continues downwards and, joined by the duct of the seminal vesicle, forms the ejaculatory duct, which runs on through the body of the prostate and enters the urethra inside the prostate gland. Each seminal vesicle contains a small quantity of sticky fluid in which the sperm are supported and nourished, and which forms the ejaculate.

THE PROSTATE

The prostate is a fibrous, muscular and glandular organ shaped like a chestnut. It produces secretions that form part of the seminal fluid during ejaculation. It's contained in a fibrous capsule and sits just below the neck of the bladder. The male urethra passes right through the centre of the prostate. If the prostate gland enlarges, the urethral outlet may be narrowed. This leads to difficulty in urinating, dribbling and poor stream (a not uncommon condition in men over the age of 55). Beyond the prostate are a pair of glands that also add lubricant to the seminal fluid prior to ejaculation.

A WOMAN'S SEX ORGANS

THE VULVA

A woman's external and visible genitalia are known as the vulva or pudendum. It is a very erotic, sensitive area, which also serves to protect the vaginal and urethral openings. The fatty tissue and skin at the front of the vulva is the mons pubis, or mound of Venus; it covers where the pelvic bones join at the front, and acts as a cushion during intercourse. In the mature female, it is covered by hair.

The most superficial structures of the vulva, the labia majora, extend forward from the anus and fuse at the front in the mons pubis. These "lips" are two-fold and usually lie together and conceal the other external genital organs. They comprise fibrous and fatty tissue, and carry hair follicles as well as sebaceous and apocrine glands. The latter give rise to a special form of odorous sweat, which is a sexual chemical attractant.

The labia minora are folds of skin that lie between the labia majora. They have many sebaceous glands that produce sebum that lubricates the skin and, combined with the secretions from the vagina and sweat glands, forms a waterproof protective covering against urine, bacteria and menstrual blood.

The size and shape of these lips vary greatly and, like the labia majora, one is usually larger than the other. They may be hidden by the labia majora or project forward. During sexual excitement they become engorged, change colour and increase in thickness – sometimes even two to three times their normal size.

THE CLITORIS

The clitoris (the most sensitive organ of the vulva) is the female equivalent of the penis, with the same component parts but in miniature. In anatomical and physiological terms, the clitoris is a unique organ. There is no organ in the human male that acts solely as a receptor and transmitter of sensual stimuli, purely to initiate or elevate levels of sexual tension.

The body of the clitoris is 2 to 3 centimetres (¾ to 1¼ inches) long and is acutely bent back on itself. The top of the clitoris is covered by a sensitive membrane that contains many receptive nerve endings. During intercourse, the clitoris doubles in size and becomes erect – in exactly the same way as the penis. The length of the whole clitoris, including the shaft and glans, varies greatly depending on stimulation by hormones during puberty.

THE HYMEN

In childhood, a thin membrane, the hymen, guards the opening to the vagina. It is normally perforated and so allows the escape of menstrual blood. Its thickness and stiffness vary from woman to woman; in rare cases it is so strong and resistant that intercourse is difficult; the hymen must then be cut under local anaesthetic. Usually, however, it is torn during various childhood activities such as cycling or horseback riding, or by the use of tampons. Even if intact, it is rarely as painful during first penetration as literature would have us believe.

THE VAGINA

The vagina is a potential, rather than an actual space. It is a fibromuscular tube about 8 centimetres (3¼ inches) long, but its size is variable, and so capable of distortion that any normal vagina can accommodate any size of penis with

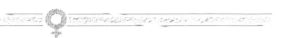

ease. If penetration happens before expansion of the vagina in length and diameter has fully developed, a woman may experience initial difficulty in accommodating the erect penis. But vaginal expansion continues rapidly so that the penis – regardless of its size – is accommodated within a few thrusts.

As excitement increases, the vagina normally overextends in circumference and also length. This elliptical vaginal expansion accounts for some loss of stimulation for the penis, and reduces vaginal sensation for the woman.

INSIDE THE VAGINA

The projection of the cervix allows the space of the vaginal vault to be divided into front, back and lateral fornices. The cervix enters the vault through the upper part of the front vaginal wall and as a result, the front wall is shorter than the rear wall and the rear fornix is much deeper than the one in front. This arrangement favours the passage of sperm into the cervix during intercourse because when a woman lies on her back, the opening of the cervix is not only directly exposed to semen, but is bathed by the pool of ejaculate that forms in the rear fornix in which it rests. During intercourse, it is this rear fornix that takes the brunt of penile thrusting and so protects the cervix from injury.

The lining of the vagina is thick and is thrown into prominent folds. The lining cells of the vagina contain glycogen, a kind of starch. The fermentation action of bacteria, which normally live in the vagina, on the glycogen produces lactic acid that renders the fluid in the vagina on the acid side of normal. This acid environment is necessary to maintain the health of the vagina and deters

bacterial growth. Any interference with the delicate ecological balance, for instance vaginal douches, can cause irritation, inflammation, discharge and allergic reactions.

The lining of the vagina does not contain glands, even though the vagina lubricates itself with a kind of sweat when a woman becomes sexually aroused. Under normal circumstances, cells that are routinely shed from the lining of the vagina, plus mucus secreted from the cervix, plus vaginal sweating, combine to form the normal colourless and odourless vaginal discharge.

Inside the top of the vagina, lying directly behind the pubic bone, is said to be an area of erectile tissue that, when stimulated, produces a different type of orgasm. This area, called the "G" spot, is discussed in more detail on page 200.

THE GREATER VESTIBULAR GLANDS AND URETHRA

The greater vestibular glands, also called Bartholin's glands, lie behind and slightly to the side of the vagina. The ducts of these glands open into the angle between the labia minora and the ring of the hymen and carry lubricating mucus to the vaginal opening and the vulva's inner parts.

The urethra is embedded within the substance of the lower half of the front vaginal wall. Bruising of this wall can therefore result in inflammation of the urethra and an ascending infection of the bladder (cystitis). The middle third of the rear wall of the vagina is closely related to the rectum, and the muscles that form the pelvic floor, called the levatores, blend with the middle part of the sides of the vagina to form the most crucial support of the vaginal structure.

SEXUAL RESPONSE

If you are attuned to your body, you know that your sexual responses have identifiable stages – desire, arousal, climax and resolution – and that these are accompanied by bodily changes. What is less well known is that although these stages occur in men and women in the same order, and in much the same way, there are vital differences. For women the changes

A WOMAN'S RESPONSE TO SEX

Exciting a woman brings about visible changes in many different parts of the body. As she becomes sexually aroused, a woman's breathing becomes more rapid, and her heart beats more quickly. Her lips become pink, the pupils of her eyes dilate and her nipples become erect and stiffen. As excitement climbs, her skin becomes pink and flushed, it begins to sweat and her breasts swell as they become engorged with blood.

THE VAGINA BECOMES MOIST

A woman's first response to sexual stimulation, which invariably must be touch, is vaginal lubrication, which can appear within 10–30 seconds of her becoming excited. Individual droplets of mucus-like material appear at intervals throughout the folds of the vaginal walls – a form of sweating. While the clitoris is the main focus of a woman's sexual response, its reaction is slower, and nowhere near as fast as a penile erection.

As sexual excitement increases, the droplets fuse together to form a smooth, lubricating coat over the entire barrel of the vagina, making penetration by a penis extremely easy. This lubricating mucus can appear in the most copious amounts, and it is thought to originate from an enormously increased blood supply, which is almost simultaneous with the onset of sexual excitement. No

other source has been discovered. The response is almost certainly not a hormonal one, as it occurs in women who have had a complete hysterectomy.

THE CLITORIS RESPONDS

The speed of response by the clitoris depends on whether it is stimulated directly or indirectly. The most rapid response depends on direct stimulation of the clitoral body or the mons area. Indirect stimulation, which includes manipulation of other erogenous zones such as the breasts or vagina, without direct clitoral contact, has a definite but certainly slower response.

The only form of direct stimulation is touch – by the fingers, mouth or erect penis – and most women require touch in addition to penetration to achieve orgasm. Because of its position, the clitoris is not stimulated directly during intercourse, so movements of the penis on its own are often insufficient to excite the clitoris to orgasm. However, indirect stimulation of the clitoris does develop with penile thrusting, the body being pulled downwards and then the hood being released.

THE VAGINA CHANGES

As sexual excitement increases, the shape of the vagina changes in readiness for penetration. The inner two-thirds of are usually initiated by different stimuli, take a longer time to occur, but they last longer, and can be repeated more quickly. The changes are reversible if either party is distracted.

Desire begins in the brain, which then sends messages to the body that result in a variety of changes indicating arousal. Arousal, if prolonged sufficiently, leads to climax, and with orgasm, muscular tension is released and the flow of blood to the pelvis is reversed.

the vaginal barrel lengthens and distends; in highly excited women, this distension is quite marked. The cervix and uterus are pulled backwards and upwards into the pelvis, further expanding the upper end of the vagina.

At the same time, the colour of the vaginal walls changes. Normally, the vagina is a deep pink, but this colour slowly alters to a darker purplish hue as the blood supply to the vagina increases.

In the pre-orgasmic state, the vagina is so distended that all the folds of the wall are stretched and flattened, and the lining becomes thin. In the plateau phase, the outer third of the vagina swells with blood, and this distension may be so great that the lower part of the vagina is reduced by at least one-third. In addition, an increase in blood supply results in enlarged labia minora and majora, which become separated, elevated and turned out.

ORGASM OCCURS

It has never been possible to study the orgasmic changes in the clitoris due to its retraction beneath the hood formed by the labia minora. The changes in the vagina, however, are much easier to study. The outer one-third contracts regularly during orgasm, with normally three to five, up to a maximum of 10 to 15, contractions at 0.8 second intervals. After the initial three to six contractions,

the space between them lengthens. Each contraction is intensely pleasurable; these fantastic sensations fall away as the contractions lessen.

How long orgasmic contractions last, their degree and the interval between them, varies among women and from one orgasm to another. Occasionally, with the highest tension levels, orgasm may start with a single deep contraction that lasts two to four seconds before muscle spasm develops into the regular contraction lasting less than a second.

During orgasm, the uterine muscle contracts, and the fornices expand, forming a tent to receive the sperm.

A RETURN TO NORMAL

After orgasm it can take a considerable time for the vagina to return to its normal appearance. As long as 10 to 15 minutes may elapse before the basic coloration returns to the vagina, and for the folds to reappear.

The clitoris returns to its normal overhanging position within five to ten seconds after orgasmic contractions have ceased, and the discoloration of the labia minora disappears just as quickly. Detumescence of the clitoral glans is a relatively slow process and may last five to ten minutes; in some women, it may take as long as 30 minutes. If orgasm isn't reached, swelling of the clitoris may last for several hours after sexual activity.

A MAN'S RESPONSE TO SEX

When a man becomes excited, his reactions, just like a woman's, are not confined solely to his sex organs. Excitement begins in the brain, when a man becomes aroused by something either real or imagined. A man is aroused by mainly visual stimuli; clothing and make-up, as well as the sight of naked or semi-naked female bodies, turn him on. A man readily becomes conditioned by his experiences; objects or circumstances associated with sex may elicit arousal, also. In this way, without any physical contact, male arousal occurs frequently and rapidly.

THE PENIS BECOMES ERECT

Messages from the brain travel down the spinal cord to the genitals and shut off the outflow of blood from the penis, and this brings about an erection. A man's usually limp, downward-hanging organ becomes a rigid, upward-pointing, dusky coloured, throbbing one with prominent veins.

By carefully controlling the variation and intensity of stimulative techniques, erection can be maintained for extended periods; it can be partially lost and rapidly regained many times during a long period of stimulation.

Erection can be easily interrupted by non-sexual stimuli, even though sexual stimulation is continued. Any form of mental distraction, a sudden loud noise, or a change in temperature or lighting, may result in partial, or even complete, loss of erection.

BODILY CHANGES OCCUR

As well as causing the penis to become erect, the increased blood supply leads also to reddening and mottling of the skin in about a quarter of all men. This "sex flush" starts in the lower abdomen and spreads over the skin of the chest, neck and face. It may appear on the shoulders, forearms and thighs and, when fully developed, may even look like measles. Its appearance is always evidence of high levels of sexual excitement. After ejaculation, the sex flush disappears very rapidly.

A man's breast, like a woman's breast, is very responsive to sexual stimulation. Though the pattern is inconsistent, nipple swelling and erection, which may develop without direct contact and can last for an hour after ejaculation, occurs frequently. Many women are not aware that a man's nipples, and even his chest, can become erogenous zones if they are given enough stimulation.

A man's heart rate increases with sexual excitement, and his respiratory rate and blood pressure also rise. His scrotum thickens and his testes will be drawn closer to his body. Many men sweat involuntarily immediately after ejaculation, but this is not proportional to the amount of physical exertion during intercourse. Sweating is usually confined to the soles of the feet and the palms of the hands but may appear on the trunk, head, face and neck.

PRIOR TO ORGASM

Right before orgasm there is a sense of ejaculatory inevitability for an instant. Many men have described the onset of this sensation as "feeling the ejaculation coming". From the onset of this sensation there is a brief interval, two to three seconds at the most, during which a man feels the ejaculation coming but is no longer able to prevent, delay, or in any way control the process. This experience of inevitability develops as seminal fluid is collecting in the prostatic urethra, just before the actual emission of seminal fluid begins. While a woman's orgasm can be interrupted by extraneous stimuli, once initiated, a man's orgasm cannot be delayed until emission has been completed.

Just prior to ejaculation, the glans may change colour; its mottled, reddish-purple colour may become darker. (This is reminiscent of the pre-orgasmic discoloration of the labia minora in a woman.) A drop of fluid may form at the urethral opening of the penis prior to ejaculation. This is not seminal fluid but secretions from Cowper's glands. The size of the testes increases slightly and they also become elevated. At this point, it is increasingly difficult for the penis to return to its resting state without ejaculation.

Muscle contractions occur at a late stage of sexual excitement and may be involuntary or voluntary, depending on body position. Spasms of a man's hands and feet can occur – rarely if the man is on top – but more commonly when he is supine.

ORGASM OCCURS

Regularly recurring contractions of both the urethra and the deep muscles of the penis result inevitably in ejaculation and the exquisitely pleasant sensations of orgasm. The entire length of the penile urethra contracts rhythmically, forcing seminal fluid from the full length of the penis under pressure, often from some distance away. When ejaculation occurs, contractions of the rectal sphincter are experienced at the same time as the expulsive contractions of the urethra.

The penis contracts similarly to the vagina during orgasm: the contractions start at intervals of 0.8 seconds and, after three or four major expulsions, they are rapidly reduced in frequency and expulsive force. Minor contractions of the penile urethra may continue for several seconds in an irregular manner, projecting a minimal amount of seminal fluid under little, if any, force.

If a man has not had intercourse for several days he usually ejaculates a larger volume of seminal fluid than when he is more sexually active. A larger volume can be more pleasurable than a lower volume, and this may account for a man's greater pleasure after a significant period of continence than after repeated orgasms. This pattern is the opposite to that reported by women who, as a rule, enjoy the second or third orgasm most.

Orgasm and ejaculation are two separate processes and may, or may not, occur at the same time. One can occur without the other. Orgasm involves the sudden pleasurable sensations and release of tension, which usually occur in the genital area and elsewhere in the body; ejaculation involves the discharge of seminal fluid from the penis. A man may ejaculate as the result of sexual stimulation but not experience the sensation of orgasm. Less frequently, a man may have an orgasm but not ejaculate. Most men who experience multiple orgasms ejaculate only once.

Normally, the penis becomes flaccid following intercourse and a man will not get another erection for some while, particularly if a man removes his penis from his partner's vagina immediately following ejaculation. Once the penis returns to its normal size, the man will relax and very often feels sleepy.

ORGASM

Orgasm, the climax of sensation, is a uniquely human experience. For men, orgasm depends almost entirely on the stimulation of the penis, either by hand or mouth, as well as the vaginal walls, and is usually, though not always, accompanied by ejaculation of seminal fluid. For women, clitoral stimulation and movement of the penis within the vagina, prolonged through skill and experience, produce these intense feelings, although they can reach orgasm in other ways, for instance by manual or oral stimulation of the clitoris, vagina or "G" spot. About one woman in ten experiences the emission of fluid from the urethra with orgasm. It is thought that this fluid comes from the Skene's glands, which run alongside the urethra, since it is not urine or vaginal mucus.

Orgasms vary: mood, level of energy or fatigue, amount and type of loveplay, the level of mutual trust, and what is happening in either partner's life, all have their effects on the sensation. And not every sexual experience can, nor should, end in orgasm; there are times when orgasms are a natural outcome of sexual activities and others where lovers will have orgasms only if they really work at them.

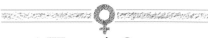

A MAN'S ORGASM

Physical response As the engorged reproductive glands spurt out their contents into the part of the urethra that runs through the prostate, expanding it as they do so, exquisitely pleasant sensations are produced. A series of four or five contractions, at the rate of one every 0.8 seconds, follows as the man ejaculates the semen in store.

Some men tend to have extremely powerful physical reactions during their orgasms: they may moan and groan, contort their faces and bodies and sometimes even scare their partners by their cataclysmic reactions. On the other hand, there are men who have very tranquil, quiet orgasms, leaving their partners wondering whether they have come at all. Most men probably experience a range of intensities between these two extreme reactions.

A WOMAN'S ORGASM

Physical response How long orgasmic contractions last, their level of intensity and the space between them, varies from woman to woman and from one orgasm to another. Some women experience a high peak of pleasure that fades away rapidly, while others feel orgasm as a more widespread, warm, internal sensation; some arrive at a peak, which subsides gradually into a series of pleasurable plateaus.

In response to orgasm, a woman may arch her body, tense her muscles, and her face may be pulled into a grimace. She may scream, cry out, or bite her lips. Alternatively, she may be silent and you may simply observe a quickening of excitement, feel some involuntary hip movements, muscle contractions in the genital area, and a general release of tension as the orgasm subsides.

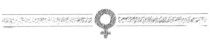

A MAN'S ORGASM

Types We're just beginning to discover that like women, men have a variety of orgasms with the added differences that different patterns of ejaculation can provide. There is no right way for a man to ejaculate or to have an orgasm.

Often the main source of pleasure is a powerful ejaculation. On the other hand, the sensations of orgasm may be felt for a long time with the ejaculation experience almost as an anti-climax. On other occasions a man may experience several continued orgasmic sensations long after he has ejaculated, or he may experience a pattern similar to the multiple orgasms of women – a series of fairly closely spaced mini-orgasms with ejaculation occurring at the last.

Multiple orgasm After a major orgasm most men experience a refractory period during which further sexual stimulation will not lead to an erection. Many males below the age of 30, however, have the ability to ejaculate frequently with only short resting periods. While men are resistant to sexual stimuli immediately after ejaculation, with practice and learned control, many men can extend their sexual cycles and enjoy several mini-orgasms before a final climax.

After experiencing orgasm a man's emotional reactions generally tend to reflect the relationship that he has with his partner. Feelings of satisfaction, contentment and happiness usually result from a loving relationship, while sadness, depression and a drained feeling frequently follow where intimacy and understanding are lacking, as in one-night stands. The majority of men, too, often feel mentally exhausted after orgasm, with the common result that sleep readily ensues.

A WOMAN'S ORGASM

Types Masters and Johnson declared categorically that the female orgasm originates in the clitoris and that there is not a second kind of orgasm that originates in the vagina. Research into the personal experience of many women does, however, suggest at the very least, that there is a type of orgasm that starts in the clitoris and spreads down into the vagina resulting in a more powerful climax than when the orgasm involves the clitoris alone. This kind of orgasm is said to result from stimulation of the "G" spot and is reputed to be a deep, powerful, prolonged sensation that is accompanied by contractions of the vagina, uterus and pelvic organs. Women state that it is truly transporting and brings them in closer union with their partners than any other.

Multiple orgasm A major difference between the sexes is that many more women are capable of experiencing more than one orgasm during a single sexual act. By holding back from the brink or preventing themselves from ever reaching orgasm, men should be able to prolong coitus and give more than one orgasm to their partners. Instead of moving to the resolution stage, those women able to have multiple orgasms remain at the plateau phase in a highly aroused state, and from there they can be stimulated to orgasm quickly and repeatedly.

After orgasm, women are less prone to the slightly depressed feelings that men often experience, and the majority welcome further loving attentions from their partners. A very few women experience a drifting into a mild form of unconsciousness, poetically known as the "little death", after orgasm.

MAN'S SEXUAL RESPONSE

After only a few minutes of stimulation, excitement increases quickly until the man reaches the plateau phase, where he can remain for any length of time according to his desires. Most men have to remain here for several minutes, sometimes 30, but on average about 15, until their partners catch up and penetration becomes mutually desirable. Once inside, a man's sexual pleasure increases markedly, especially as thrusting movements bring him step-like to the point of no return, and an intensely pleasurable moment with orgasm and ejaculation. After this, excitement drops steeply, the penis becomes flaccid, and he enters the refractory period, a variable time during which an erection is no longer possible.

MAN'S EXPERIENCE

ORGASM

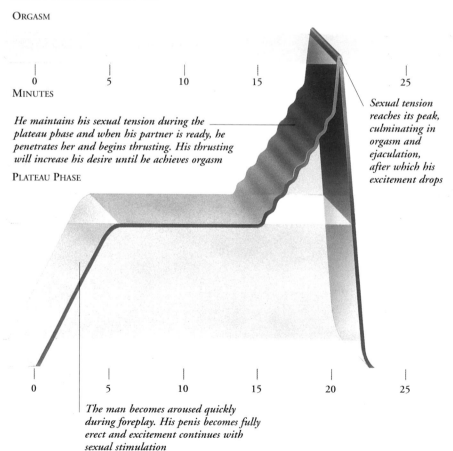

MINUTES

0   5   10   15   25

He maintains his sexual tension during the plateau phase and when his partner is ready, he penetrates her and begins thrusting. His thrusting will increase his desire until he achieves orgasm

PLATEAU PHASE

Sexual tension reaches its peak, culminating in orgasm and ejaculation, after which his excitement drops

0   5   10   15   20   25

The man becomes aroused quickly during foreplay. His penis becomes fully erect and excitement continues with sexual stimulation

WOMAN'S SEXUAL RESPONSE

Sexual tension in the initial stage increases more slowly in women than men, frequently taking 20 or 25 minutes but, on average, 15 minutes. The more varied and stimulating the foreplay, the more rapidly a woman passes through this initial arousal phase. Her pleasure then rises in a parallel and step-wise fashion with the thrusting of the penis within her vagina. If direct stimulation of the clitoris is maintained simultaneously throughout this period, a woman can proceed quickly to the point of orgasm. After orgasm there is a slow and gradual return to normality often extending up to half an hour. During this resolution phase, the breasts return to their normal size and the swelling of the labia diminishes.

WOMAN'S EXPERIENCE

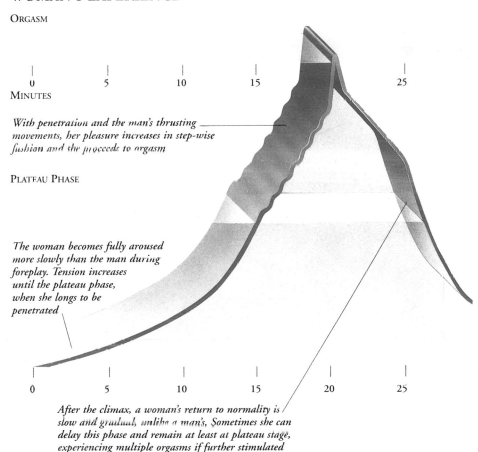

ORGASM

MINUTES

With penetration and the man's thrusting movements, her pleasure increases in step-wise fashion and she proceeds to orgasm

PLATEAU PHASE

The woman becomes fully aroused more slowly than the man during foreplay. Tension increases until the plateau phase, when she longs to be penetrated

After the climax, a woman's return to normality is slow and gradual, unlike a man's. Sometimes she can delay this phase and remain at least at plateau stage, experiencing multiple orgasms if further stimulated

199

THE "G" SPOT

In Germany in the 1940s an obstetrician and gynaecologist called Ernst Grafenburg, researching new methods of birth control, claimed to have discovered a new, internal zone of erogenous feeling in the women he was studying. This sparked a controversy, which has become more prevalent in recent years, concerning whether or not these male and female "G" (Grafenburg) spots in fact exist.

There seems to be little doubt that there is a hidden area, at least in some men and women, which when stimulated, produces intense excitement and orgasm; in women this has become known as the "G" spot, and in men has been identified as the prostate gland. While it is

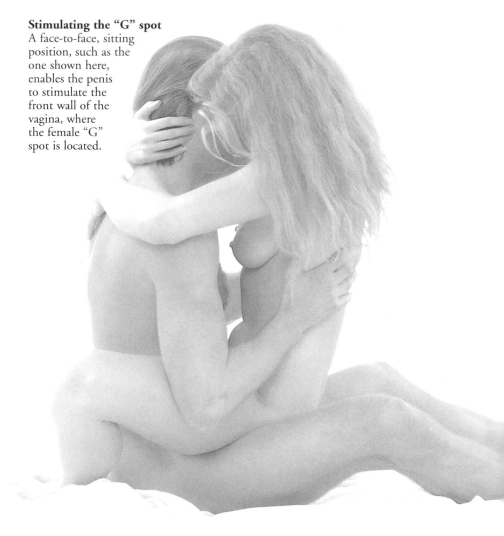

Stimulating the "G" spot
A face-to-face, sitting position, such as the one shown here, enables the penis to stimulate the front wall of the vagina, where the female "G" spot is located.

physiologically undeniable that men have a prostate gland, pathologists have failed to find the "G" spot (which feels like a small bean when stimulated), when performing post-mortems on females. Several experts believe that it is possible that the "G" spot exists only in some women; others believe simply that the front wall of the vagina is extremely sensitive and when stimulated can produce an orgasm in some women; others dismiss the whole notion as complete nonsense and claim that the entire controversy causes unnecessary feelings of inadequacy and anxiety among both men and women.

Self-discovery is really the only way you can find out if the "G" spot can produce intense pleasure for you or whether, as for some people, it is a complete waste of time.

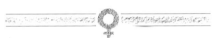

THE MALE "G" SPOT

The male "G" spot has been identified as the prostate gland. It is situated (like the female "G" spot) around the urethra at the neck of the bladder. The prostate gland has an organic function helping to produce the fluid that carries sperm into the vagina during intercourse. Many men discover that stimulation of the prostate before or during intercourse can result in an extremely intense orgasm, during which they ejaculate in a gentle stream rather than in spurts.

It is very difficult for a man to find his own "G" spot, or prostate gland. The best position for discovering the gland yourself is to lie on your back with your knees bent and your feet flat on the floor, or with your knees drawn up to your chest. Insert your thumb into the anus and press against the front wall. Your prostate should feel like a firm mass about the size of a walnut, and when it is stimulated, it should produce feelings of intense sexual excitement.

THE FEMALE "G" SPOT

The "G" spot appears to be a small cluster of nerve endings, glands, ducts and blood vessels sited around a woman's urethra, or urinary tract. This area cannot normally be felt when the woman is unaroused, only becoming distinguishable as a specific area during deep vaginal stimulation. When this happens it swells, sometimes very rapidly, and a small mass with distinct edges stands out from the vaginal wall. As it seems to have no organic function other than helping a woman achieve a high degree of sexual fulfilment and, at orgasm, can appear to "ejaculate" a clear liquid similar in composition to that created by the prostate, some experts think that the "G" spot is a rudimentary form of the male prostate gland.

The easiest way for a woman to find her "G" spot is to sit or squat, because lying down positions the relevant spot further away. First stimulating your "G" spot can feel like wanting to urinate, so it is a good idea to start your explorations while sitting on the toilet. Once your bladder is empty, you will know that the sensation is caused by the "G" spot, and not by having a full bladder.

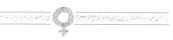

THE MALE "G" SPOT

The anus is delicate, unused to having things inserted into it, and is not a naturally lubricating organ. Ensure that fingernails are short and that fingers are well lubricated with KY jelly or a similar substance so as not to cause damage.

If you want your partner to stimulate you, lie down on your back and have her gently insert a finger into your anus. Allow yourself enough time to become accustomed to having her finger there, then have her feel up the front rectal wall until she finds your prostate and massages it firmly. Then she can stroke the gland in a downward direction. This can be tiring to both partners but is made a little easier for yourself if you pull your knees back towards your chest. Without her even touching your penis you will probably become erect and have an orgasm.

This manoeuvre is not as "messy" as a woman may perhaps think, since unless you are constipated, there are no stools in your lower rectum. Your partner must, however, wash her fingers at once and must not touch inside her vagina, or bacteria could be transferred to her from your anus. Some women feel better if they use a disposable plastic glove, especially since it gives some protection against transmitting the AIDS virus.

Some women like to fellate their partners at the same time as massaging the prostate, and you might suggest this to your partner as well.

THE FEMALE "G" SPOT

Using your fingers, apply firm upward pressure on the front of the internal vaginal wall, perhaps pressing down simultaneously with the other hand on the outside of the abdomen. As it becomes stimulated, the spot should start to swell and will feel like a lump between the fingers inside and outside your vagina. Extremely pleasurable contractions may sweep through the uterus and you may experience a deep, satisfying orgasm, which will feel totally different from a clitoral orgasm.

At this point you may also find that you ejaculate a small amount of clear fluid from the urethra. This is not urine, despite its appearance.

Since your partner can reach the spot more easily, it may be more effective if he stimulates you. Lie down on a bed with two firm pillows underneath your hips, with your legs slightly apart and your bottom a little in the air. Your partner can lie down, lean close against you, gently insert two fingers (palm down) and stroke the front vaginal wall.

Sexual positions that produce "G" spot stimulation are the woman-on-top and the rear-entry positions. When a woman is on top of a man, she can control the depth and direction of her partner's penis, and can move forward or from side-to-side to guide it to the place that feels best for her. In rear-entry positions, the penis is rubbing directly on the front wall of the vagina in which the "G" spot is located.

A man can help by moving his own body and pressing the base of his penis to make sure that its head makes full contact with the "G" spot. The result of these movements can be a series of intense orgasms for both partners.

ATTRACTION AND DESIRE

Although many myths exist as to what men and
women find attractive in each other, scientists believe that
many of the associations we form in infancy help
to determine whom we choose as sexual partners, or soul
mates, and that patterns laying down tendencies
for love relationships are etched into our brains.
The infinite range of human experience through holding,
touching, feeling, stimulating, trusting, talking and
listening is involved in the sexual attraction of
a loving couple and their desire for each other.

ATTRACTING A PARTNER

Both our ability to love, and our style of loving, begin to develop from the moment we're born. Scientists believe that many of the associations we form in infancy help determine whom we choose as sexual partners, or soul mates, and that patterns which lay down tendencies for love relations are etched into our brains.

I can show you how this might be so by looking at how just one of the five senses – smell – predetermines a particular choice. Each of us, even in our highly deodorized society, has a unique odour that is the sum of our glandular secretions – a "smell signature". Whether our smell signature is attractive to other people – for instance, because it reminds them happily of their mothers – or is off-putting because it reminds them of detested ex-spouses, say, depends on those people's own associations. Associations are linked to smell because the olfactory bulb involved with smell reception feeds into the part of the brain that is intimately linked with emotion and affective memory.

In the same way, we can learn to like the smells of our loved ones. Studies have shown that lovers can pick each other out of a group solely by their unique aromatic signatures (and that is how babies first bond with their mothers). If we lose our ability to smell, we normally suffer a pronounced slump in sex drive.

THE CHOICE OF A PARTNER

Highly personal patterns, like our individual smell associations, make it extremely difficult to generalize about attraction. Men and women, in general, are attracted to the sexual characteristics that separate them – for example, women's larger breasts, men's broader shoulders. Cultural expectations, too, have a large role to play; a man to whom an English woman would be attracted is probably very different from a Chinese woman's ideal partner. Age, social class, personality and the qualities we are looking for in a particular partner also very much determine whether or not we find a person attractive.

Many myths exist as to what men and women find attractive in each other. There is no proof, for example, that gentlemen prefer blondes as studies have shown that dark-haired men prefer brunettes, and fair-haired men like brunettes and blondes equally. And, while men think women like men with hairy chests and large penises, most women mention attributes such as tenderness, affection, respect, sensuality and kindness as a man's most attractive qualities. If pressed, women will admit generally to preferring dark-haired men of average build, with small buttocks, and a tall, slim physique; penis size is rarely mentioned.

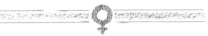

WHAT WOMEN LOOK FOR IN MEN

The choice of a sexual partner is still determined very much by evolutionary patterns whereby women first looked for mates who could be relied upon. For that reason, physical appearance appears to be less important to women than personal qualities.

Age is also not such an important factor in a woman's choice of a man. Unlike men, who have a tendency to look for younger women, women can be attracted to men of all age groups.

Personality Confidence, assertiveness, independence and dominance tend to be found appealing, as are reliability and faithfulness, and qualities that suggest warmth, intimacy and attentiveness. Men who try to get on with women and talk freely and openly about what interests them, and use a soothing voice, are more successful with women.

Prowess Men who are successful at work or sports, and have the visible proofs, are more likely than less able men to attract women.

Physical qualities A man who is fit and healthy, with a fairly lean, well-muscled body that is not weedy, and who may have some surprising feminine characteristic such as long eyelashes, is considered more attractive than a stereotyped muscle man. Women prefer men taller than themselves.

Personal characteristics Attractive features to women are a body cleansed of the sweat of the day and free of body odour; a genital area whose scent is not too pungent; well-cared-for hands; well-washed feet, and a clean pair of socks daily; clean hair; a face that is clean-shaven or with a shapely beard, and without a rash.

WHAT MEN LOOK FOR IN WOMEN

Men generally place a higher premium on physical appearance than women do. In surveys, physical attractiveness is top of the list. Women's bodies are often on display in advertising and magazines, and men have been conditioned to find certain attributes especially stimulating. Legs, for example, tend to be powerful attractants because they indicate the state of a woman's maturity; high-heeled shoes, stockings and skin-tight pants emphasize their allure and reinforce their sexual imagery. A woman's more pronounced female buttocks, narrow waist, bare shoulders, and lips all act as sexual signals, but her breasts are her most obvious turn-on. Men, however, differ in what precisely they find attractive. Some men even describe themselves as leg, buttock or breast men. By and large, men are attracted to women younger than themselves – perhaps a subconscious recognition of their child-bearing capacity.

Personality Desirable qualities cited by men are sympathy, gentleness, warmth, kindness and cheerfulness. Erotic ability rates higher than domesticity.

Physical qualities A lean but still curvaceous outline is desired rather than thinness, or a more maternal figure. A narrow waist and long legs are admired by the majority of men; breast size and shape are individual tastes.

Personal characteristics Attractive qualities to men are a genital area that is not too pungent or whose natural smell is not masked by strong deodorants or other synthetic smells; shapely polished fingernails and well-cared for hands; not too much body hair; clean soft hair; clean-smelling breath.

MAKING ADVANCES

Sending out sexual messages requires directness as well as a certain degree of vulnerability. It nearly always requires self-esteem to take the knocks and rejections that we might possibly receive when we make an advance. We need to have a mixture of arrogance and humility to assume that someone would want to know us better, while remembering that many people might rather have nothing to do with us. We ask ourselves the questions: "Do I remember taking this risk before and was it comfortable or uncomfortable?" and "Am I prepared to take this risk again?". An encouraging thought is that it is rare for someone that you are very interested in to be entirely indifferent to you.

WHERE AND HOW TO MEET

Many people think that there are only certain social situations where sex can be on the agenda. However, this is not true; any situation can lend itself to sexual advances. Of course, in some situations, advances need to be subtle and very low-key; in fact, rather difficult to pick up unless the other person is sexually aware and alert.

Only someone with a closed mind would limit his or her horizons to parties, dinners and social occasions. Sexual interest can be revealed at any time. For instance, a working business meeting between two sexually interested people, when each may be thrilled by the other's professional performance, can be an exciting and intriguing prelude to more open sexual overtures. Here, the enjoyment of a common task can greatly enhance sexual interest. Indeed, sexual interest grows more often in the day-to-day working environment than almost anywhere else.

While women rate discos and parties as the most likely way of meeting men with whom they would like a sexual relationship, reality is, in fact, quite different. Most people meet potential sexual partners through friends, and like any other form of friendship, most happy sexual relationships are based on friendship and on working or studying together. You can get to know someone better at work than in a disco. Furthermore, when looking very glamorous and affected by drink, we don't necessarily give a realistic picture of ourselves, nor are we able to get a true insight into a partner.

A less obvious advance could occur when you have lunch with or talk to someone over a period of time in a quiet spot. Glances are often exchanged and conversations may include messages with a double meaning, testing how interested the other person is. These interactions may just be in the form of play, but all of us do engage in them and establish brief, "mini" bonds with many people.

SENDING OUT MESSAGES

The truth is we cannot help but communicate. Even if we are not actually speaking, we are giving out signals through the body. People are perceived as being friendly or unfriendly without a word being spoken. Body gestures give messages about subconscious emotions and are, therefore, a very direct form of communication. You can use them to see what others are thinking. They often belie what we are saying; probably, non-verbal gestures are more accurate in many situations than words themselves. And, as we gain awareness of non-verbal behaviour and an interest in interpreting the body language of others, we become aware of our own bodily gestures, resulting in more effective outward communication.

EYE CONTACT

By far the most common initial sexual advance is eye contact. Our eyes meet with interest, with approbation; a very brief fantasy may occur – "I'm sure I would like to have a relationship with you. I will never talk to you but I think we could do something together" – and we may think about this anonymous message later. These encounters may take place in the street, walking down the hall at work, on the stairs, in a lift, or at a traffic light, and they happen often. We do this every day of our lives, even if we are very happy with a partner. We seem to keep practising attraction by sending at least mini-messages to test our abilities.

Eye contact is one of the simplest and most direct ways of showing someone that you are sexually interested in him or her, and by making eye contact, you make it easier for that person to respond to you.

Always look at the person you are talking to, not over his or her shoulder or down at the floor. To show interest in another, hold your glance longer than you would do in an ordinary social situation but don't overdo it. Most people find intermittent eye contact – about five seconds out of every 30 – most comfortable and will probably drop their gaze if you look at them directly for too long. A person expresses interest if he or she returns your gaze steadily.

VERBAL COMMUNICATION

Conversation, too, whether at a casual encounter, an intimate dinner, or during the course of work, can be a huge sexual turn-on. Glances are often exchanged and conversations may include messages with a double meaning that test the interest of the other person.

Expressing ideas, motivations, goals and aims can bring two people closer together than can many other activities. And, where there are areas in common – similar interests, ambitions and plans – this is very thrilling to both partners. The exchange of thoughts and ideas along these lines between a couple who are sexually aware of one another is, in my opinion, one of the most pleasant ways of initiating a sexual relationship, and also it will solidify the relationship once it has begun.

FACIAL EXPRESSIONS AND GESTURES

Another thing to look out for in order to make certain you are sending out the right signals is to keep your facial expressions pleasant. Smiling is especially important as it is a direct way of telling someone that you find him or her attractive. Using hand and head movements are also ways of encouraging people, as they indicate interest. Make sure you stand the right distance away – proximity indicates attraction and is a cue for greater intimacy, while standing far away points to mistrust and aloofness.

Finally, learning to use touch to communicate can step up the pace of any relationship. To give a positive response in the early stages, touch your partner's arm while talking to him or her or, if you come up from behind, put a hand on his or her shoulder in greeting. Bear in mind that you should keep it subtle. You don't want to overstep the line between showing interest and being too pushy or pawing. Remember, too, that skin-to-skin contact – touching a bare forearm with your finger, for instance – is always much more intimate than skin-to-clothing contact.

When you want to increase the pace further, move on to more prolonged and frequent touching – holding hands, for instance – and from purely social gestures like brushing hands as you pass something over to more overtly sexual ones, like lingering pressure on the palm.

JUDGING RESPONSES

By paying attention to body language and other signals, you should be able to see if you are having a positive effect on the other person. Encouraging responses include raised eyebrows, wide-open eyes and dilated pupils. A definite "come-on" signal is if you are looking into each other's eyes for longer and longer periods, and if you are standing close as you do so. You can test this by moving slightly closer and seeing whether the other person draws away (negative) or not (positive). Watch the gestures the person makes; if he or she nods the head in enthusiastic agreement at what you are saying, or if he or she touches you to emphasize a point when talking to you, you are making progress!

RESPONDING TO AN ADVANCE

Responding to a message requires a lowering of defences, and some risk taking. Acknowledging that an invitation is being sent out to you is one of the riskiest steps. Most of us find ourselves thinking the following,

"How well can I trust my senses, even my own ears?", "Have I interpreted the intonation of what is being said correctly; does that person really mean what he or she is saying?", "Why should that person be interested in me?", "Maybe it is just a joke, a tease; will I look a fool if I take this seriously? But (and it is a big but) will I hate to miss the chance just in case it is serious and I would like to go further?". When an invitation is perceived, all of these thoughts can occur almost simultaneously to the person receiving the advance.

Once an encouraging message is sent, received and acknowledged, each person is on his or her best behaviour and projects the kind of person that they think would please the other. It is only later that partners begin to show their true colours and test how their relationship might work in everyday life with its stresses and strains.

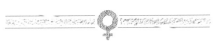

SOME POINTERS FOR MEN

Social responsiveness is not the same as sexual encouragement. And invitations can be misunderstood. For instance, when you're invited to a lady's home for the first time and told to make yourself comfortable, do you remove your jacket, loosen your tie and lounge on the sofa? Do you allow your anticipation to show and then, when the lady returns in jeans and an old shirt, do you feel an absolute fool when she says, "What do you think you're doing, moving in? I've got to finish putting up my bookshelves. You can get yourself a drink before letting yourself out."

Nor should you expect every single encounter to lead to great romance or sex. If you get too serious or expect a woman to give you more than she is prepared to, you will probably make her retreat. Many women prefer a softer approach to an overtly sexual come-on, and it is not a good idea to be familiar too soon. Express your admiration and interest but stay away from endearments or physical caresses at first.

SOME POINTERS FOR WOMEN

Sexual relationships usually progress in small steps, with each of you giving and responding to signs of encouragement. Picking up on and responding to the other's cues correctly will minimize any risk of your social responsiveness being interpreted as sexual encouragement.

It is important, too, to know exactly what you want out of a relationship. Many women are shy about admitting that they just want sex, not a long-term loving relationship. Some women even will go so far as to generate feelings of love in order to have sex, and this, in the long-term, will prove unsatisfactory for both you and your partner.

Do not expect every encounter with a man to lead to great romance or sex. If you get too serious or expect a man to give more than he is prepared to, you will probably make him retreat. It is not usually a good idea to be familiar with him too soon. Express admiration and interest in him, but stay away from endearments or physical caresses in the early stages of the relationship.

AROUSAL

When we are attracted to or aroused by someone sexually, all our senses, but particularly sight, touch and hearing, come into play. Our sense of smell, while important, plays a much smaller part than it does in other species. Traditionally, it has been the woman who attracts with visual displays of gestures and apparel, and the man who responds with sexual arousal, but changing patterns of sexual behaviour has led to a somewhat greater equality of roles. For example, today both sexes wear clothes explicitly to attract the opposite sex – men wear tight trousers and form-fitting tops, and women wear low-cut necklines and slim, short skirts.

In terms of the stimuli that excite them, men and women differ markedly. Men, generally, are stimulated by what they see. Women, on the other hand, are very different; as a general rule, they respond very little and very slowly to visual stimuli. Women are more interested in men in the context of their personalities.

WHAT TURNS US ON?

Sight This plays a greater role in arousing men than women, but a woman may take advantage of this by making herself as visually attractive as possible, with a properly made-up face, flattering clothes, and by ensuring that her movements – such as when undressing – are pleasing to watch. The eyes are supposed to be the windows of the soul, so it is very common to see lovers gazing intently into each other's eyes, oblivious of everything else around them.

Hearing This contributes much, too, which is why music, played quietly and at the right moment, can be highly exciting for both men and women. We become excited when we hear our beloved approaching, his or her laugh and particularly his or her voice. Some men and some women have very beautiful voices, and are aware of their seductive effects. A man may have a warm, velvety voice whose every modulation has the power to move a woman's heart. A good voice used well is a caress. A telephone call may simulate an act of love and be as potent as any form of foreplay. The opposite pertains, too, of course, and some women's voices literally drive men mad.

Touch Small touches, even accidental touches, have an enormous effect on everyone. We all need touch very badly. We find it relaxing and reassuring, and it helps us to loosen up our inhibitions. Sometimes the greatest intimacy and the most acute closeness can come from simply touching and holding. Most of us have had experiences where dancing has been highly erotic, involving the rhythmical contact of two bodies. Dancing can be pure foreplay – try dancing cheek to cheek, hand in hand, breasts against a man's chest, pelvis against pelvis, legs slightly apart, thighs brushing each other, sexual organs pressed together – all of which simulate sexual contact. The potent mixture of sight and sound created by movement, light and music only adds to the effect.

Taste A delicious meal accompanied by fine wine often puts a couple in a good mood and lowers their inhibitions so they are more inclined to make love. Talk over a meal, soft lighting, and the ritual of eating, can be very seductive, and lovers feel that there is a metaphor between eating and deriving emotional nourishment from a partner's body.

Smell Women like wearing scent and men like smelling it but it can have a much greater effect than a woman ever thinks – especially when her body is warm; the scent evaporates and body smells mingle with the perfume, acting as a powerful stimulant. Coco Chanel once said that a woman should scent her body wherever she expects to be kissed, and with the array of scents available, both partners would delight in this. Women probably have the strongest preference for the unadulterated smell of a man's skin, which in itself is very exciting, but as a way of showing interest, most wouldn't mind if their partners used some aftershave.

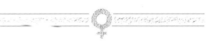

WHAT MEN LIKE

Bare flesh This is rated very highly by men. Exposed bodies and expressions of a "come hither" variety are extremely arousing to most males.

Make-up Bright red lips are a sexual turn-on, as are other things connected with physical appearance, such as hair style and colour.

Sexually explicit material Men find "girlie" magazines, soft-porn videos and pin-up photos very arousing: they use them to feed their fantasies and to enhance masturbation. The majority of men, however, would not be particularly aroused by their own partner appearing in a girlie magazine; it is the fact that such a woman belongs to somebody else that is part of her attraction.

Sexy clothing Black, lacy underwear and scanty nightclothes are particularly pleasing to most men, hence models posing in suspender belts and stockings.

WHAT WOMEN LIKE

Physical attractiveness Even though physical appearance is not necessarily at the top of the list of qualities women consider important, most women will confess to being attracted to certain aspects of their partner's body, though not normally their genitals.

Power and wealth Visible evidence of dominance, which is expressed in today's world by being in possession of money and status, are turn-ons for the majority of women.

Romance and intimacy Expressions and manifestations of an intimate or romantic interlude such as champagne, moonlight and flowers, are also arousing to most women.

Erotic literature Though women will confess to enjoyment of erotic literature in the form of romantic novels, sexually explicit material, however, has been found also to excite many women.

THE FIRST SEXUAL EXPERIENCE

The driving force behind your first sexual experience may be love, but it could also be lust, or even curiosity. It is quite usual for most people to be a little apprehensive and tense, and also to feel a little disappointed with the outcome – first-time sex not proving to be the ecstatic experience they might have imagined. Like most things, sex improves with practice and familiarity with a partner. While for most men, orgasm is fairly automatic even on the first occasion, women rarely achieve orgasm with early intercourse; this is something that has to be learned.

MAKING IT BETTER

It will certainly help, however, if you choose the right setting and make sure you have complete privacy with no fear of interruptions. You should decide beforehand whether you will be spending the whole night together or leaving before morning. If the former, you not only need to think about bringing along a change of clothes (and personal toiletry items), but how you feel about waking up in bed with someone you might not know very well.

Allow yourselves plenty of time so that your lovemaking can proceed unhurried, and in a relaxed manner. With the first time this is especially important, since any nervousness that one or both partners feel must be completely dispelled if arousal is to take place. The man particularly should not be in too much of a rush.

Make sure that a reliable form of contraception is used. Lovers should bear in mind, too, that since AIDS and other sexually transmitted diseases – such as genital herpes and chlamydia – can be caught or spread the first time sexual intercourse takes place, the man also should wear a condom (see opposite).

Virgins (both men and women) should declare themselves. This is particularly important for the woman, since she needs to inform her partner to be gentle and not to thrust too deeply at first. The man should always make certain the woman is aroused by caressing and stimulating her for a minimum of ten minutes before penetration. This way she will have enough natural lubrication to make things easier. Saliva or artificial lubricants can also be used to make things more comfortable. Do not use petroleum jelly (such as Vaseline); it may be irritating to the vagina.

Choose a man-on-top position; putting a pillow beneath the woman's hips also may make it more comfortable for her. Penetration should be gentle but firm, and thrusts should be light. A woman can help her man by guiding his penis into her vagina, and bearing down slightly as he enters to relax the pelvic muscles.

SAFE SEX

The notion of "safe sex" was initially promoted in the 1980s as a response to the spread of AIDS, but practising safe sex will help to protect you against sexually transmitted diseases in general and not just against AIDS. Safe sex is a matter of commonsense combined with an awareness of the risks involved in different kinds of sexual activity.

High-risk Sexual Activities
• Any sexual act that draws blood, whether intentionally or accidentally.
• Anal intercourse without the use of a condom.
• Vaginal intercourse without the use of a condom.
• Insertion of fingers or a hand into the anus.
• Sharing penetrative sex aids.

Medium-risk Sexual Activities
• Anal intercourse with a condom.
• Vaginal intercourse with a condom.
• Cunnilingus.
• Fellatio, especially to climax.
• Anal kissing or licking.
• Sexual activities involving urination.
• Wet (tongue-to-tongue) kissing.

Low-risk Sexual Activities
• Mutual masturbation (except cunnilingus and fellatio).
• Rubbing of genitals against a partner's body.
• Dry kissing.

No-risk Sexual Activities
• Non genital massage.
• Self-masturbation.

USING A CONDOM
One of the chief weapons in combating the spread of sexual disease is the more widespread use of the condom. Though it does not guarantee complete protection, it does reduce the risks substantially.

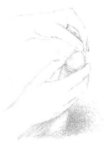

1 The penis needs to be fully erect and the condom must be in place before vaginal or anal penetration, or oral sex, takes place.

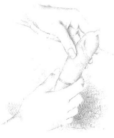

2 Squeeze the teat end free of air and unroll the condom fully over the penis. Do not stretch it tightly or it may burst.

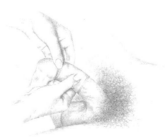

3 During withdrawal, hold the base of the condom to prevent semen from spilling into the vagina. Always use a new condom for each act of intercourse.

INITIATING SEX

While a few individuals believe that one-night stands are one of the most satisfactory forms of human relationships, the majority of people feel that, in addition to physical attraction, there has to be love, and love involves knowing someone intimately. In fact, sex is the ultimate act of knowing. But in order to know someone, you have to show yourself to them. For the majority of people knowing is not easy; you feel vulnerable and open to the possibility of being rejected, which can be extremely painful. Sex can rarely be fulfilling without knowing your partner and showing yourself. No relationship can thrive where these two basic ingredients are missing.

Right from the outset, you must tell the truth and nothing but the truth. Any other form of

Becoming intimate
Sex is our primary way of showing love. With a sympathetic, loving and open partner, it can be a magical voyage of discovery.

behaviour is distancing and hypocritical; you must represent yourself honestly. In a loving relationship, even a white lie is an insult and extremely damaging. Honesty in itself is arousing; it can be a stimulant. Truth is probably the best aphrodisiac.

Everyone is vulnerable, both emotionally and romantically, so in a relationship that will involve love and sex, you should declare your vulnerability. Don't forget that having sex is a decision as well as an impulse, and it doesn't mean that you have to lose control. It means letting your partner know that the basic reason for your being there is that you are looking for love; you are looking for someone to bond with. When you decide to have sex with someone you are being intimate with all they are; so declare all you are.

The myth of romanticized women and eroticized men distorts the natural interaction that takes place between the two sexes. The infinite range of human experiences through holding, touching, feeling, stimulating, trusting, talking and listening to one another is involved in sexual interaction, and it is a distortion of the male and female personality to say that love and sex is the sole prerogative of either gender.

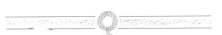

SOME POINTERS FOR MEN

• Take care over your appearance and cleanliness; never fall into bed unshaven and unwashed.
• Have something nice planned; almost all women appreciate thoughtfulness in the form of a bouquet of flowers or a candlelit dinner, for instance.
• Compliment your partner on her appearance, tell her she smells nice, hold her hand, give her light, affectionate kisses and catch her eye and smile whenever you can.
• Be attentive, whether you're at home, out together or at a party; for example, don't ignore her for the television.
• Once you're in bed be attentive to her wishes and indulge in as much loving foreplay as you can.
• Try not to fall asleep immediately you've climaxed; talk to her for a while afterwards and hold her in your arms.

SOME POINTERS FOR WOMEN

• In matters of love, go for it; don't dissemble and deceive. Nothing works as well as going full tilt after someone you want, and to keep on working at it once you are together. Going after someone means giving yourself.
• Take some care over your appearance; clean, well-cut, sweet-smelling, freely moving hair and an attractively made-up face can be very appealing.
• Be free with your compliments, like telling your partner he's handsome.
• Avoid behaving in an overly critical and unromantic manner, or acting too aggressively about having sex.
• Encourage your partner in his efforts; let him know what you find exciting in nice ways that will please him.
• Sexy underwear, subtle perfume and a readiness to cuddle and be close can all be terrific come-ons.

YOUR APPEARANCE

While there may be many ways of enjoying sex, most people will enjoy sex more if they are sure of themselves, not simply sure of what they are doing, but sure of their attractiveness and desirability.

Attractiveness or sex appeal is hard to define but sexuality has more to do with your attitude towards yourself, your partner and your lifestyle than with anything else, and certainly more than with obvious physical attributes. We have all met rather plain, unassuming people who have great charm and attraction, which is difficult to pin down but often has to do with having a positive attitude towards life, a ready smile, a subtle sense of humour and enthusiasm. Other people are attractive because of their eccentricity and uniqueness – how they speak or express themselves, mannerisms, surprising candour, or individualistic presentation.

Such qualities are probably more important than your actual appearance, and while it is worth spending some time on how you look, you should maintain a sense of balance by not becoming obsessive about your physical appearance. Too many men and women feel dissatisfied because they compare themselves to an exaggerated image of what is good looking. Responding to your partner and being willing to share pleasure are the qualities that ultimately make a person attractive.

Although over-attention to appearance is not necessary, some relationships can founder if either partner neglects his or her appearance and hygiene. The best possible reason for taking trouble over your appearance is for your own self-esteem, but you should also do so for the sake of your partner, otherwise he or she could interpret neglect as a sign of not caring. This does not imply that one has to spend hours on preparation but an unclean and/or smelly body, dowdy, ill-kempt clothes, an unshaven face, curlers in the hair and an ill-tempered face all imprint themselves on the memory and become difficult to erase at times of intimacy. A sloppy appearance invites comparison with the time when you first met, and the inevitable thought arises that love is on the wane.

LOOKING AT YOURSELF POSITIVELY

Many people find it worthwhile to take a good, hard look at themselves as a way of getting in touch with and appreciating their bodies. Most of us are far too hard on ourselves. It will buck up your feelings quite a lot if you concentrate on your good points rather than emphasizing the bad.

Doing the following should help to lessen self-consciousness and make you more comfortable with yourself and with your body as a source of sexual pleasure. It is best to do these "exercises" in private, when you have plenty of time and feel as relaxed as possible.

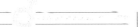
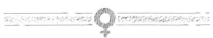

— MAN'S SELF APPRAISAL —

1 Undress and stand in front of a full-length mirror. Examine your naked body carefully, from head to toe. Imagine you are seeing yourself for the first time. Look at yourself from every angle.

2 Stand, kneel, bend and then move around. Sit with your legs apart and then together. Look over your shoulder to see the curve of your back and the set of your buttocks.

3 Focus attention on your best points; everybody has some. They might be the breadth of your chest, the flatness of your stomach, the fullness of your hair, or your height.

4 Then pay attention to the features that you dislike and try to see them in a more positive way. For instance, while you may think yourself shorter than you would like, you may be trim and perfectly proportioned.

5 Now study your genitals. Feel your testes; one, usually the left, will hang slightly below the other. Your flaccid penis will probably be between 5 and 10 centimetres (2 and 4 inches) long and, when you touch it, you will find the most sensitive area is the head and, in particular, the ridge on the underside.

6 Finish by taking a warm bath. Soap your hands and explore your body with them, noticing all the different sensations you experience by changes in touch and pressure. Explore your penis and testicles again, too, if you like, but try to become aware of sensations throughout your whole body.

— WOMAN'S SELF APPRAISAL —

1 Stand naked in front of a full-length mirror and take the time to examine your body carefully, from head to toe as though you were seeing yourself for the first time. Use another mirror to see yourself from the side or back.

2 Move around. Kneel, bend and sit with your legs apart, then together.

3 Concentrate on your best points; you are bound to have some. The shapeliness of your legs, the length of your neck, high cheekbones, or dainty feet, for example.

4 Reconsider the features that you dislike and try to see them in a more positive light. For instance, although you may think that you are fatter than the ideal, you may have a Rubenesque physique that is attractive to men.

5 Using a hand mirror, and in the best possible light, examine your vagina. Identify your different parts. In order to see and touch the clitoris properly, you will need to pull back the hood of skin covering it. You can run your fingers along the inner and outer vaginal lips and back along the area between the anus and vagina to find the more sensitive areas. Separate the inner lips in order to explore the entrance to the vagina and inside.

6 When you have finished, take a warm bath. Soap your hands and explore your body with them, noticing the different sensations you experience in all your body areas by changes in touch and pressure.

THE SEXUAL REPERTOIRE

The activities described here are practised by most people. There are more bizarre practices, but these aren't included since they occur rarely and may not be embraced whole-heartedly by both partners. Your sexual experience may include some or all of the activities listed below; if the former, you might like to try out the new ones. Remember that for truly satisfying experiences, partners must learn how to receive as well as give.

—— WHAT MEN CAN DO ——

- You talk warmly or sexually to your partner to arouse her.
- You hold or rub your body against your partner's body.
- You kiss your partner passionately.
- You kiss with your tongues in each other's mouths.
- You fondle your partner's body when she is clothed.
- You undress your partner and see her naked body.
- You caress your partner's naked body.
- You kiss your partner's breasts and lick, suck, or gently take her nipples into your mouth.
- With your hands you explore and stroke your partner's vaginal area.
- You lick and kiss around and inside your partner's vagina.
- You bring your partner to orgasm by stimulating her clitoris and vaginal area with your hands and fingers.
- You bring your partner to orgasm by stimulating her clitoris and vaginal area with your mouth.
- You reach orgasm by intercourse in any of the following positions: with you on top; lying side-by-side; with you approaching behind; with your partner on top; both sitting; both kneeling; both standing.
- You fondle or kiss your partner's buttocks and anal area.

—— WHAT WOMEN CAN DO ——

- You use sexual terms in your conversation and speak intimately to your partner.
- You take your partner's body and hold it or rub it against yours.
- You offer him a variety of kisses.
- You engage in open-mouthed kissing, with your tongues inside each other's mouths.
- While he is clothed, you fondle your partner's body.
- You take off your partner's clothes and look at his naked body.
- On your partner's naked body, you bestow a variety of caresses.
- You lick or gently suck your partner's nipples.
- Using your hands, you explore and stroke your partner's penis and testicles.
- You lick and kiss your partner's penis and testicles.
- While stimulating his penis with your hands, you enable your partner to reach orgasm.
- Using your mouth on his penis, you bring your partner to orgasm.
- You reach orgasm by intercourse in the following positions: your partner on top; lying side-by-side; with you on top; with your partner approaching from behind; sitting; kneeling; standing.
- You caress or kiss your partner's buttocks and anus.

CHAPTER 3

FOREPLAY

Satisfying lovemaking takes time, and can never take too long. On rare occasions, you may become so aroused during foreplay that you immediately move on to actual intercourse, but usually a couple enjoys the gradual intimacies that leisurely kissing, undressing, petting, massage, oral sex and the sharing of fantasies – among others – provide. Foreplay should be savoured as an integral part of lovemaking. Learn to excite each other slowly but surely, discovering and exploring your partner's erogenous zones and whole body in a loving, caring, thoughtful, and not simply mechanical, way.

BECOMING AROUSED

Satisfying lovemaking takes time, and can never take too long. There are numerous activities for lovers to indulge in that do not involve actual sexual intercourse. On rare occasions, you may be so aroused that you immediately proceed to penetration and an orgasm, but usually a couple enjoys the gradual intimacies that leisurely kissing, undressing, petting and oral sex, among others, provide.

The variety of techniques that can be used to pleasure each other can be enjoyed as activities in their own right, or as delightful prologues to sexual intercourse. The longer, more refined and attentive the foreplay is, the more receptive you and your body will become, and the better, more magical and more fulfilling the ultimate pleasure will be.

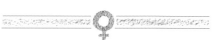

A MAN'S NEED FOR FOREPLAY

Contrary to popular belief, men too need and enjoy foreplay. It offers them the necessary stimulation to build up a good, firm erection and prepare the penis for intercourse. In fact, numerous cases of impotence could be prevented if foreplay was long and exciting enough.

There are, however, a few situations where the length and type of foreplay needs to be carefully discussed, and that is where a man experiences premature ejaculation or where he has trouble maintaining an erection. In those cases, if he is undergoing therapy, he may want to keep foreplay to a minimum.

Some men see foreplay as a variety of things they have to go through in order to prepare their partners for intercourse. Others want their partners to touch their genitals straight away. Encourage your man to appreciate the delights foreplay offers by being enthusiastic about trying new sensual experiences so that he learns that joy in sexual activities comes in a large part from the affection expressed between you.

A WOMAN'S NEED FOR FOREPLAY

A woman's body requires prolonged stimulation if she is to become fully aroused. Arousal is brought on by a complex blend of mental and physical stimuli when the emotional atmosphere is sufficiently encouraging.

Some women need a particularly long time, and a considerate lover must therefore be patient. As you arouse your partner, you will feel intense pleasure as well, and she will not only be more receptive but also more helpful during intercourse, so that the experience will be equally pleasurable for both of you. Men who kiss and cuddle a lot, and indulge in sensitive foreplay, are much more likely to see their partners reach orgasm frequently and easily.

Don't be in a hurry to undress your partner and proceed immediately to touching her breasts and vagina. Hold her close, and keep early caresses non-genital. Concentrate on your partner. Let the resulting feelings range all over your body, and avoid thinking solely about what is happening to your penis.

UNDRESSING

Removing your clothes, and/or those of your partner, can be a very exciting and important part of foreplay. Undressing not only results in general arousal, but the wearing of and/or the removal of particular items of clothing can strike a much more resonant chord in a susceptible lover, particularly a man.

A good lover will seek to discover which garments and their removal will act as turn-ons, and will make use of them to increase a partner's pleasure. You may have to practise removing your partner's clothes with one hand, and without clumsiness or hold-ups, if undressing is to be a truly exciting aspect of foreplay.

Nudity may become routine and boring, particularly in marriage, so some subtlety in undressing is worth retaining. Even after years of living together, undressing each other will be highly arousing; each partner should feel increasingly excited as one garment after another is removed.

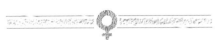

WHAT A MAN FINDS EXCITING

Many men prefer a hint of nudity to total nudity as it allows the imagination to run riot. Lovely, lacy, fine lingerie is attractive to and exciting for men, both the sight of it and its removal. Your man may well enjoy making love particularly when you keep on an undergarment such as a slip, stockings, suspender belt, panties, bra or camisole.

The removal of certain clothes, especially garments that emphasize a woman's breasts, buttocks and genitals, is almost universally a turn-on. Women who take time about getting undressed, and who "accidentally" reveal parts of themselves are certain to excite their men. If a woman strips off in front of her partner, this active display of herself has an impact which no man can fail to find erotic. The memory of his partner undressing may prove irresistible, and he will want to recreate this scene over and over again in his mind.

WHAT A WOMAN FINDS EXCITING

Wearing lovely, lacy, fine lingerie is attractive to and exciting for women. Many like to retain an undergarment such as a slip, stockings, suspender belt, panties, bra or camisole during the early stages of foreplay. Many women also like their men occasionally to retain some of their garments during sex, though not their socks. A hint of nudity allows the imagination to run riot.

A lot of women prefer to have their partners undress them because it allows them to show off their bodies passively without being sexually overt. Other women may feel sufficiently confident to strip off in front of their partners. If done with artistry (something that may require a bit of enjoyable practice in front of a mirror), it will be highly erotic, mainly because the woman's role is no longer passive. She is actively displaying herself in an attempt to arouse her partner, and he knows this.

221

KISSING

A kiss is very often the first expression of love, and no matter in what other sexual activities a person may indulge, kissing remains one of the most voluptuous of all caresses. The mouth is highly responsive and mobile, and can offer a great variety of sensual pleasures. Through it you are able to experience touch and taste at the same time.

Kisses can be tender, light and lingering or passionate, deep, burning and even rough. Between couples who are strongly attracted to one another, kissing can mimic intercourse; the tongue penetrates the mouth with the same rhythmical intensity of the penis in the woman's body.

There is an infinite variety to kisses, with lips closed or open, dry or moist, still or moving, explorative or quietly tender. What lends variety to kissing, too, is that it can be done to any part of the body. It should not be restricted to mouth-to-mouth contact; kissing should be used on every crease and in every crevice. Kissing your lover's erogenous zones, particularly the genital parts, can be the most intimate and stimulating part of foreplay, and here kisses can result in the most profound reactions. For some people, kissing is a necessary accompaniment to orgasm and lends passion and depth to their climaxes.

Heightened sexual response
A kiss can be highly arousing.
A woman can feel it
in the breasts and
genital area, and
often by itself, it
can result in
orgasm.

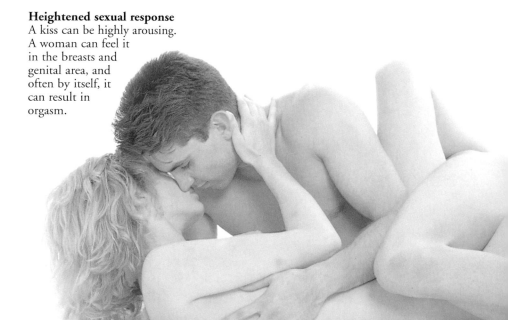

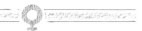

—— WHAT A MAN LIKES ——

Although the notion persists in a few men that kissing may be "soft", the vast majority enjoy the physical closeness and body contact that it brings. Few men, however, would be content to stop at kissing, especially if there was any possibility of intercourse, and often kisses that a woman means to be simply affectionate, without further promise, can be misunderstood as an invitation to greater intimacy.

Men love to be kissed passionately, and you will be almost certain to arouse your partner by kissing and caressing certain areas such as the back of his neck, his ears and eyelids. Use deep, sensuous kisses to stimulate his lips, tongue and the inside of his mouth. Flick your tongue in and out of his mouth and try to have your tongues touching.

Gentle biting and nibbling can be highly erotic as well, but it's best to avoid "love bites" on the genitals, which are highly sensitive and may be easily damaged or caused excessive pain. While some men particularly enjoy having their nipples kissed, nibbled, licked and sucked, what most men love above all is having their penises kissed.

—— WHAT A WOMAN LIKES ——

Women enjoy kissing very much, and most complain that they don't get enough of it – too many men proceed to genital touching far too soon. Women enjoy a rather gradual progression to the genitals, and like having their ears, necks, shoulders, breasts, stomachs, inner thighs, knees and feet kissed along the way. Women also use kissing as a way of initiating sex and stimulating interest in their partners.

Simple kisses on the lips can be quite delicious but many women enjoy deep tongue-to-tongue kisses and hard, prolonged kisses on the lips. You will be almost certain to arouse your partner by kissing and caressing certain areas such as the back of her neck, her hair, ears, cheeks and eyelids. Use deep, sensuous kisses to stimulate your partner's lips and tongue and the inside of her mouth. Tantalize her by flicking your tongue in and out of her mouth and try to have your tongues touching.

Gentle biting and nibbling can be highly erotic as well, but it's best to avoid "love bites" on the genitals, which are highly sensitive and may be damaged or caused excessive pain, and on the breasts, where gentle sucking is more widely preferred. Some women can even reach orgasm this way. And for many women, kissing can be an end in itself.

EROGENOUS ZONES

Discovering and exploring your partner's erogenous zones should be loving, caring and thoughtful, not simply mechanical. Every woman should try to discover as much as possible about her man's body, and every man should experiment to find out what exactly will please his partner. Couples should learn to excite each other slowly but surely, and gradually find out which certain parts of the body will provide pleasure and stimulation when touched.

As you kiss and stroke various parts of your partner's body, he or she should always let you know immediately what effect your touch has, and you should always express the rising excitement that you feel. Mutual feedback is necessary for successful lovemaking.

For both men and women, stimulation of the erogenous zones begins with the hands and fingers but, of course, all these areas respond even more intensely to touches from the mouth, lips and tongue. In addition to gentle stroking, patting and rubbing, occasional gentle slaps should be used also to bring variety to sensation and love-making techniques. Men will also enjoy their partners using their breasts and nipples to caress them; women find the most potent touch is from the penis, particularly the glans penis, which to them is a miracle of softness and hardness.

——— DISCOVERING A MAN'S EROGENOUS ZONES ———

In common with those erogenous zones enjoyed by women such as the lips, any area of the face and the fingertips, there are certain general areas of a man's body that are very pleasurable for him when touched, for instance the shoulders, the palms of the hands, the back, the chest and the nipples. Stroking and sucking your partner's nipples gives pleasure and they will become erect, a sign of arousal.

The whole of a man's genital area responds to the slightest touch; within this area there are many specific points to be explored. The area just behind the root of the penis, between the penis and the anus that overlies the prostate gland, can be exceptionally sensitive to touch, both in arousal and in reaching orgasm.

The testicles are very sensitive and must be handled gently, as excessive or clumsy handling can hurt. Unquestionably, the penis is a man's most sensitive erogenous zone and the place where he experiences the most intense feelings. The whole shaft of the penis is very sensitive but the glans at the tip is particularly rich in nerve endings, especially on its crown. The frenulum is also extremely sensitive in all men, as is the area lying just behind the opening.

The buttocks are a sexually arousable area; most men find pleasure in having their buttocks caressed, and some men also like having them gently slapped or spanked. The anus is also very sensitive to caresses of all types.

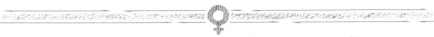

—— DISCOVERING A WOMAN'S EROGENOUS ZONES ——

In contrast with a man, the whole of a woman's skin is an erogenous zone and all of it will respond to touches, caresses and kisses. However, there are certain areas where stimulation results in more intense arousal. These erogenous zones vary from woman to woman.

GENERAL BODY AREAS

A woman's face has several erogenous zones including her hairline, forehead, temples, eyebrows, eyelids and cheeks. In general, women prefer light facial caresses. The mouth for most women is one of their most erogenous zones, and it can be stimulated readily with the fingertips and kisses. Stimulating a woman's mouth can set alight her whole body, and has a direct effect in arousing her genital organs. On the other hand, erogenous stimulation of any other part of a woman's body often produces a reaction in her mouth, in her breasts, and in her genital organs as well.

The earlobes are extremely sensitive to stimulation and can be caressed gently; some women even can have an orgasm after such a simple caress. The neck, particularly at the back and down the sides, is a very sensitive area. The arms, armpits, hands and back, hips and the whole of the lower abdomen can also be stimulated erotically.

An extremely sensitive zone is the area around the navel. Most women relish caresses with the fingertips, lips or penis over the whole length of their legs, particularly on the inner thighs.

THE MOST RESPONSIVE SITES

For most women the breasts are highly erotic and play a vital part in sexual excitement. Sucking, nibbling, licking, stroking and gentle squeezing will cause the nipples to become erect, a certain sign of arousal. However, women do differ greatly here in their reactions to stimulation so it's important to find out what exactly she likes and doesn't like.

The most highly erogenous area of a woman's body includes the perineum, an area of skin between the vagina and the anus. If you put your whole hand on this area, with the outer lips of the vagina closed, and press hard or massage, a woman can be aroused extremely quickly because of the dense network of nerve endings.

Both the inner and outer lips of the perineal area are extremely rich in nerve endings also, and are a highly erogenous zone. The inner lips, however, are much more sensitive than the outer ones, especially if stroked along their inner surfaces along the cleft of the vulva. If you press both lips together and firmly massage with your fingers all the sensitive parts of the vulva, high levels of excitement should result. The clitoris is the most sexually sensitive part of a woman's body, and the easiest part to stimulate if a man can only learn to do it gently and skilfully, without haste. Stimulation of the clitoris with the tip of the erect penis is particularly pleasurable to many women.

As with the mouth, the entrance to the vagina is rich in nerve endings and reacts intensely to all sorts of caresses (the ultimate being from the glans penis), but it can be ecstatic for some women to be caressed there by a man's lips and his tongue.

The buttocks are another erogenous zone and they are easily stimulated by patting, rubbing or gentle slaps.

PETTING

Whether sexual intercourse is on the agenda or not, a man's generalized kissing and cuddling will sooner or later lead to his touching, caressing and kissing a woman's breasts, nipples and clitoris, and a woman will be encouraged to do the same for a man's scrotum and penis. Petting, or love play using fingers, is more than just romantic. It is vital to the escalating spiral of sexual excitement necessary for satisfying sexual intercourse.

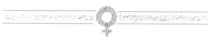

—— WHAT A MAN LIKES ——

Kissing should lead into and blend with caresses over the man's whole body. Passionate kissing, sucking and stroking are all pleasurable. Vivid sensations can be produced in a man, too, by slowly and seductively rubbing your hands or other body parts on his bare skin.

Men are easily aroused by having their genitals stimulated (though it is in a woman's interest to prolong foreplay and delay genital caressing until nearer to penetration), and many men also enjoy having their buttocks stroked, kneaded or smacked. Many men also take great pleasure in having their scrotums and testes held or squeezed. The crescendo reached in such ascending sexual activity can frequently bring a man to orgasm without penetrative sex taking place.

Petting is extremely powerful. Sexual excitement begins with some stimulus that orders the pituitary gland in the brain to send out a hormone that travels through the bloodstream in order to stimulate the testicles into releasing more hormone, and this makes a man feel sexy and aroused. The hormones themselves push the hypothalamus into producing more of its hormone. This process is an escalating spiral in which the sexier a man feels, the more sexy he will be. It is in a woman's interest to maintain this high level of arousal.

—— WHAT A WOMAN LIKES ——

One of the reasons why petting is so potent and so enjoyed by women is that it arouses and prepares them for sexual intercourse. For women, intercourse is welcome only when they have had enough stimulation so that the vagina lubricates and unfolds, ready to receive the penis. Without the chance to build up the level of sex hormones through kissing, caressing and petting, intercourse can be very uncomfortable for a woman. Most men underestimate how long this takes, since their own erections occur much more quickly.

Kissing should lead into and blend with caresses all over a woman's body. Most women prefer initial caresses to be in areas other than the breasts and genitals, but once they have begun to feel aroused, they do enjoy having their breasts and bottoms stimulated. Breasts, however, need careful stroking until a woman is more highly aroused, then more passionate kissing, sucking and stroking are pleasurable. Most women like their buttocks caressed or squeezed; some enjoy gentle smacking. Only when a woman is sufficiently aroused does she want her partner to move on to genital caresses. Women differ in their tastes, but most prefer initial genital caresses to be gentle, with harder, more vigorous movements as they near orgasm.

MASSAGE

Mastering the techniques of sexual and non-sexual touching is very important to a satisfactory sexual relationship. For people who already enjoy a good sex life, massage can enhance enjoyment; for most of us, there is plenty of room for improvement.

Massage is important because not only does it have the general effect of relaxing you and giving you the opportunity to really think about and enjoy touching, but it allows you to focus your senses acutely and deeply on the responses that are aroused in your body, and in this way increases your sex drive. During massage some people experience this "sensate focusing" for the very first time.

Massage can be particularly important for women because it can have exactly the same effect as kissing, caressing and other forms of foreplay, in that it allows a woman's sex hormones to build up and to arouse and prepare her body for intercourse. It is helpful also for men who have difficulty in arousal or suffer from impotence.

One of the aims of massage is to give you the opportunity to discover for yourself what gives you pleasure, and you should approach it with a completely open mind. Men and women are often surprised how sexy it feels to have certain parts of their bodies – which they had never thought of as remotely erotic – caressed.

GETTING THE MAXIMUM PLEASURE

Getting to know every inch of your lover's body is among the most pleasurable shared experiences, and it is worth taking the time and trouble to set the scene properly. You should alternate between being the passive or pleasure-giving partner. Choose a time when you won't be interrupted, and a place that is warm and private. Soft lighting and background music also can contribute. You can use a bed that isn't too soft, or the floor with sufficient cushions.

Both partners should adopt comfortable positions and should be undressed to get the maximum benefit. The person giving the massage should make certain his or her hands are warm and preferably oiled. If you are the pleasure-giving partner, concentrate on what you are doing and how your partner is responding. If it is your turn to be on the receiving end, lie back and enjoy every minute.

Start with a gentle, exploratory massage, going over all parts of your partner's body except the genitals and breasts, as this will make the process much more sensual and relaxed. You can, if you like of course, go on to touching the breasts and genitals, and this may prove so arousing that sexual intercourse or an orgasm cannot be avoided.

MASTURBATION

The majority of both men and women come to know about their own sexuality through masturbation, which usually starts around age 10 or 11. Of course, boys and girls do play with themselves long before this, particularly boys, who may grasp their penises in their first year of life, but only because it is an appendage that juts out from their body.

As a pleasurable sensation, though not a sexual one, infants fondle themselves around the ages of three and four, and may explore each other around the ages of five and six, but it is not until adolescence, when sex hormones are being produced, that masturbation for sexual pleasure starts. Age 10 or 11 is the earliest, but it can start much later; for some, masturbation is not experienced until the late teens or early 20s.

It is only through personal experimentation that people come to understand their preferences and develop techniques that they find most pleasing. But it is essential that these preferences are expressed to a partner, and that the techniques are candidly shared.

In the majority of people, auto-erotic experience is highly private and masturbation is one of the most difficult of all topics for couples to discuss. Perhaps religious orientation forbids it, or it still may be an area they feel unable to discuss because it is so highly private. Many people find masturbation a difficult subject to approach because they think they have to share what they actually do. This isn't at all necessary, but you should try to share with your partner how you feel.

Auto-eroticism, of course, is not limited to self-stimulation of the genital organs; there are many other experiences in life that are auto-erotic, such as taking a long, luxurious, sensuous bath, or simply feeling the wind in your hair and the sun on your skin. Don't limit your view of auto-eroticism entirely to sex; allow yourself to be stimulated by the many naturally occurring, everyday experiences such as a crisp, sunny winter morning, a walk along the beach on a fine day, or swimming in the sea.

ATTITUDES TOWARDS MASTURBATION

Many women think of masturbation as unnatural and disgusting and a complete waste of time, and don't understand why anybody does it and are unsympathetic to the view that people might continue to do it even though they have sexual partners. The majority of men, though they may keep their feelings to themselves, don't agree.

For most people, once it is faced, masturbation in front of, or with a partner, and particularly if it is mutual, can be an extremely enjoyable and exciting way of making love, especially if it comes at the end of an extended period of foreplay. Differences in attitudes can be ironed out only if you are candid with your partner and voice your feelings about masturbation. You may get a shock; you may find that you are both mutually attracted to the idea.

There are many myths about masturbation, but it is important to realize that masturbation cannot cause any trouble for anyone unless it is against one's own moral sanctions. View it as an excellent opportunity for self-education. You should be open and comfortable with it; it should never end up leaving impressions of hurriedness, guilt or secretiveness about sex. More importantly, masturbation can lead to intense orgasms, and it is the one way to develop sexual comfort, security and self-esteem.

Above all, masturbation is not something that means sex with your partner is not as good as it should be, or even that your partner cannot stimulate your genital organs in the way that you like. Many partners have their best sexual experiences when masturbation or mutual masturbation is engaged in prior to or during sexual intercourse.

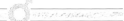

—— WHAT A MAN LIKES ——

Male masturbation has always been a secret from which women have been excluded. Even in marriage, few women are given the opportunity to witness it. But without knowledge of how your partner gives himself pleasure, it is difficult for you to know how to. There is no better way to learn about what he likes than to look and talk.

A man's sexual focus is the head of his penis; this is in contrast to women who have a far greater range of sensation-producing apparatus. (In addition to the high level of response concentrated on the clitoral shaft and glans, women can be excited by stimulation of the labia, the opening into the vagina and the vagina itself.) Touching the scrotal sac and the testes is not as exciting for men as stimulation of the labial area or the vaginal entrance is for women.

A man concentrates his efforts on the glans and frenulum; the shaft is relatively insensitive and allows him to move his hand up and down rhythmically.

—— WHAT A WOMAN LIKES——

The easiest way for a man to find out how a woman likes to be stimulated, and how much stimulation is necessary, is to study how women masturbate. Some women, however, especially those who may have guilty feelings about self-pleasuring, prefer to be masturbated by their partners. Many women do it at particular times, such as while they are menstruating, and keep it secret from their partners. Others may indulge in it routinely as a way of relieving sexual tension. Because direct and continued genital stimulation is so necessary to a woman's orgasm, some women use self-masturbation as a way of guaranteeing that they reach a climax while having sexual intercourse.

In fact, since only about 30 percent of women achieve orgasm with intercourse but over 80 percent experience a climax with masturbation, orgasm by means of masturbation, rather than by sexual intercourse, should be regarded as the normal experience.

MASTURBATION CAN BE FUN

Masturbation is an option, a way of mutually enhancing a couple's sexual enjoyment. Masturbation is generally helpful to sexuality in all areas of your life. That doesn't mean to say that if you don't masturbate you're abnormal; you're not inadequate or deficient.

Remember that masturbation does not reflect badly on your marital sex; in fact, there is some evidence showing that people who masturbate without guilt are freer in expressing their sexuality, more aware of the nature of their own sexual response, and therefore enjoy sex more than those who are guilt-ridden. Moreover, masturbation is a good alternative to intercourse for women in late pregnancy or just after childbirth, or following gynaecological surgery; also, when a man can't get an erection.

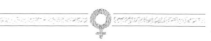

CAN A MAN MASTURBATE TOO MUCH?

Men commonly report masturbatory frequency ranging from once a month to two or three times a day. Nearly every man is concerned about the supposed mental effects of excessive masturbation, but every man considers excessive levels of masturbation to consist of a higher frequency than he practises himself. A man who masturbates once a month sees once or twice a week as excessive, with mental illness as a quite possible complication of such frequency. A man who masturbates two or three times a day thinks five or six times a day is excessive. No man, however, has the fear that his particular masturbatory pattern is excessive, regardless of frequency.

There is no medical evidence to suggest that masturbation, regardless of frequency, leads to any form of mental illness. In fact, it may be the case that men masturbate too little – both in time spent and in number of occasions. More pleasure, more sensuality and greater control can be positive results of masturbatory activity.

CAN A WOMAN MASTURBATE TOO MUCH?

For most women, masturbation is the introduction to sex. Few women have a clear idea of their own sexual anatomy, and so wouldn't know where they like stimulation unless they'd masturbated. Masturbation helps a girl to know how she functions sexually, and it helps her to form preferences. It almost certainly gives her the first orgasm.

Women can often find it harder than men to achieve orgasm, and the ability to discover what feels good and exciting, what arouses them and what makes them less inhibited, less fearful and more willing to let go is most often discovered through masturbation. Once a woman has achieved orgasm by this means, it becomes easier to repeat.

Masturbation is important for older women too. It increases lubrication and reduces vaginal pain due to dryness. Whether it has been continual, or taken up again on the loss of a partner, it is an ideal sexual activity – an easy way of achieving orgasm – and one guaranteed to prolong your sexually active life.

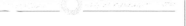

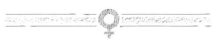

WHAT MEN DO

It is only through experimentation that each man discovers how best he likes to be stimulated. Some men use only the lightest of touches on the upper surface of the penis; some use strong, gripping and stroking movements over the whole organ that for many other individuals could be painful. Often, men prefer to stimulate the glans alone; they either confine their manipulation to the upper surface of the penis on or close to the frenulum, or pull to stimulate the entire area of the glans. Most men, however, manipulate the penile shaft with stroking movements that encompass the entire organ; rapidity, length of movement and tightness vary from man to man.

Many men masturbate incorrectly; they try to get it done as quickly as possible and much of their technique and timing is wrong. This may result in problems later, since many men come to associate masturbation and ejaculation with getting rid of tension quickly.

As ejaculation approaches, most men increase their actions until they are stroking the penile shaft as rapidly as possible. During ejaculation, most men either ease completely or markedly slow the movements along the shaft. This is because the glans is quite sensitive straight after ejaculation. (This is rarely appreciated by women, who often have very different preferences, see right.) It can be distressing for a man if a woman continues to carry out active manual stroking or pelvic thrusting immediately subsequent to ejaculation.

Some men find using a lubricant on their hands can enhance their pleasure. Petroleum jelly, hand or body lotions, and massage oils can all make the experience more pleasurable.

WHAT WOMEN DO

No two women masturbate in the same way, although they rarely manipulate the glans of the clitoris directly, as it often becomes overly sensitive to touch or pressure. This is particularly the case immediately after orgasm, and care has to be taken to avoid direct contact with the glans unless renewed stimulation is desired. Some women move their bodies to feel sensuous, others lie quite still and only let their hands work.

Most women who manipulate the clitoris do this through the shaft, manipulating the right side if right-handed, and vice versa. Many women change sides; concentrated manipulation can give rise to numbness if too much pressure is applied to any one area.

Very few women concentrate on the clitoris itself; most stimulate the mons area in general. Indeed, the entire perineal area becomes highly sensitive to touch; the labia minora may also be a main source of erotic arousal.

During masturbation, most women manipulate the shaft of the clitoris continuously right up to orgasm and through it without a break. This is the opposite of the usual man's reaction to orgasm, which is to stop rapid pelvic thrusting; stopping clitoral stimulation can account for the lack of a satisfactory orgasm in females during intercourse. Unlike a man, a woman who masturbates often is not content with a single orgasm but may well enjoy several subsequent orgasms until fatigue intervenes.

Some masturbation techniques, such as rolling on an object or climaxing by clenching the perineal muscles, are difficult to integrate with intercourse, and a woman may need to adjust her practices when a partner is involved.

STIMULATING A WOMAN

To provide the most satisfying sensations over the entire clitoral area, use the whole hand – all the fingers, palm or the heel of the hand – rather than just one or two fingers. Your fingers need to be well lubricated so use vaginal fluid, saliva or jellies. There are two major types of movement, circular and vibratory.

For circular movements, place your hand over the clitoral area. Apply light pressure with your palm or fingers, moving them gently round and round.

Move your hand up so that the heel is right over the clitoris at the top of the vulva and is resting partly on the pubic bone on either side, where you can press firmly as you rub.

Alternatively, you can press gently with your hand, palm downward over the pubic mound so that your fingers overhang the clitoris, and make firm, circular movements.

For vibratory movements, cup your hand over the pubic area and vibrate it rapidly, brushing your fingers to and fro across the clitoris. Then, keeping your hand still, put a finger each side of the vaginal lips and vibrate them from side to side. Pressing firmly through the fleshy folds, rub on each side of the inner vaginal lips at the base of the clitoris.

Most women also often enjoy being penetrated by a finger while their clitoris is being stimulated. Make sure that your fingernail is short and straight before slipping your middle finger into the vagina, keeping your other fingers bent forward so that the knuckles continue to press against the clitoris. You can move your finger in and out gently, applying pressure on the front wall of the vagina. Alternatively, rub the tip of your penis against the clitoris.

HOW TO STIMULATE A WOMAN
The clitoris is delicate and highly sensitive; most women find indirect pressure more comfortable than direct pressure.

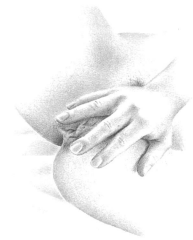

1 Placing your hand over your partner's entire perineum or vaginal area, while applying light pressure and gentle circular movements, will increase her arousal.

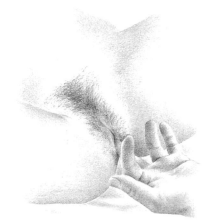

2 When your partner is sufficiently lubricated, insert your finger into her vagina and move it gently in and out, while keeping contact with the clitoris.

STIMULATING A MAN

To be a good lover, knowing how to stimulate the penis is one of the most valuable skills that a woman can possess. Older men especially may need direct stimulation to reach erection, but men of all ages enjoy the sensations they receive from manipulation. You can use these techniques both as an adjunct to, or as a replacement for intercourse, and vary your approach as much as you like, such as rolling the penis between your palms, stroking it with your fingers, alternately squeezing and letting it go, brushing your fingertips against the frenulum or caressing the penis between your breasts. To enhance his sensations, and especially if your partner has erection difficulties, use a lubricant.

Begin by positioning yourself beside your partner. Grip his penis firmly with your thumb nearest his navel. Move your hand up and down on the penis in a regular rhythm, keeping your grip steady and the firmest pressure on the sensitive area on the uppermost side. Try long and short strokes to see what he likes best. A slow rhythm prolongs pleasure, while a speeded-up one intensifies pleasure and will bring him to orgasm sooner.

Your partner's climax is imminent when his muscles, particularly those in his thighs, tense up and his breathing becomes more rapid. The testes will be drawn up to his body and may also be swollen. The head of the penis will darken in colour and increase slightly in size. One or two drops of pre-ejaculatory fluid may ooze from the tip of his penis.

Your partner will want you to carry on with the stimulation until ejaculation is completely over and his tension relaxes. Most men will want you to desist from further genital caresses for a while.

HOW TO STIMULATE A MAN
All men find genital caresses highly stimulating; however, after ejaculation most prefer the stroking to cease.

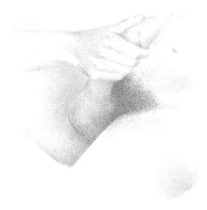

1 Hold the penis close to the head to ensure optimum stimulation of the underside of the penis, as well as the glans and frenulum.

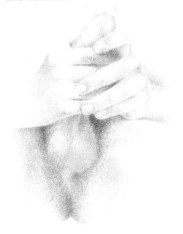

2 Your partner may want to control the rhythm. With his hand over yours, grasp the penis firmly, though gently, and move your hand rhythmically up and down the shaft, either quickly or slowly as your partner wishes.

ORAL SEX

Fellatio, sucking or otherwise stimulating a penis with the mouth, with or without ejaculation, is almost always the most powerful way of arousing a man, and all find it intensely exciting.

The mouth appears to men as similar to, but more exciting than, a vagina, particularly because the tongue is actively used to stimulate. In fact, the mouth is exceptionally well designed for sexual pleasure and is capable of a broad range of activities such as stroking, kissing, licking, probing and penetrating. The mouth is also the recipient of a wide variety of sensations including the many tastes of a lover's body parts.

Cunnilingus, using the tongue and mouth to lick and nuzzle the clitoris and vaginal area, is highly arousing to a great many women. The tongue is softer than the fingers so it provides gentler and more varied stimulation. Most men are willing, if not always keen, to perform cunnilingus on their partners.

There is no doubt that oral sex is an intensely intimate experience and that it demands a level of trust that is rarely found in other areas of lovemaking; for one thing, the act can be extremely painful if care isn't taken. This intimacy generally contributes to the participants' satisfaction since it implies total acceptance of each other. To some people, it is the ultimate expression of love.

MAKING IT FUN

A woman's fear of ejaculate in the mouth will be minimized if partners agree beforehand on what is to be done. If ejaculation in the mouth is to be avoided, the man should signal and withdraw in time so that his partner can continue with manual stimulation. Fear of choking is easily dealt with by the woman controlling how much of the penis she takes into her mouth, or by encircling the base of the penis with her hand to hold back his thrusting.

Worry about body odours can be dispelled by daily bathing – afterwards the healthy odour of sexual arousal will prove pleasant and exciting. A woman should not try to disguise her natural smells or flavours with sprays or deodorants, which can prove intrusive, and anyway, most men find the acid taste of vaginal juices pleasant.

Never get so carried away during sex play that you bite the sex organs. Don't blow into your lover's genitals, as this can be dangerous, and never indulge in oral sex if you have a cold sore or genital infection. It is also a good idea not to indulge in oral sex with a casual partner whose sexual history is unknown to you. There is some evidence that the AIDS virus can be transmitted this way.

PERFORMING CUNNILINGUS

While some men perform cunnilingus because they find it intensely exciting, others may do it more to please their partners. If you are in the latter group, you should never let your partner think that you find it a chore. This is a certain turn-off. Concentrate instead on the sure and certain knowledge that you will give her maximum pleasure. Remember, too, to use your hands to caress her breasts, thighs and buttocks at the same time to stimulate her further.

If your partner appears to be slightly reluctant, reassure her about how nice you find the experience, especially if you think she is worried about her genitals tasting or smelling bad. You shouldn't have difficulty sympathizing with her if you bear in mind that you have odours and tastes, too.

HOW BEST TO PLEASURE HER

Women need direct stimulation in order to reach orgasm, so the most important thing that a man can do for his partner sexually is to learn the areas, pressures and rhythms that excite her most. The clitoris is the most sensitive part of a woman's anatomy and it may easily become exquisitely tender. It is often better in the beginning to direct your attentions to the labia minora and the entrance of the vagina.

Start by kissing and licking her lower belly and the inner side of her thighs, working your way down to her pubic mound. Then, move your tongue over the genital area, flicking it along the fleshy folds up to the clitoris. Thrust your tongue in and out of your partner's vagina to see if she likes it.

Separate the vaginal lips with your hands and then, using your tongue, gently probe her clitoris – first nuzzle and suck it, then vibrate your tongue quickly against it. If given sufficient stimulation, your partner should be able to reach orgasm easily. Once she has climaxed, she will probably prefer not to be stimulated for some while.

It is important to take care with your teeth. Keep them protected by your lips and be careful not to graze or bite the sex organs, as this can be very painful. Make sure, too, that your fingernails are not too long.

Work your way down her abdomen, kissing and licking her skin

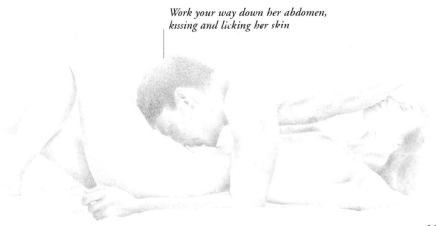

PERFORMING FELLATIO

First, find a comfortable position; it is relaxing for your partner if he lies down but you can kneel down in front of him while he stands or sits in a chair. He should always be immaculately clean. You can bathe together or wash him yourself, making this into more foreplay. While you are performing fellatio, caress the rest of his body with your hands to make it really exciting for him.

You can begin by kissing and licking his penis; then, holding the shaft in one hand, swirl your tongue gently around the tip. Stimulate the tip with your tongue and push the tip of your tongue into the slit. Next, explore the shaft, running your tongue around the ridge where it meets the head, and vibrate it gently against the frenulum.

When you feel ready to take his penis into your mouth, cover your teeth with your lips and take in the whole head of the penis. With your teeth well apart, move your mouth up and down, letting your partner guide your rhythm with his hands on your head. Maintain a steady rhythm and firm pressure. Make certain you don't bend the penis too far down when sucking; this can be painful. The penis should always point upwards.

Gradually increase your speed until he is about to climax. Then, if you don't want him to ejaculate in your mouth, withdraw and bring him to orgasm with your hand, or switch to intercourse.

As you come to enjoy performing fellatio, you can experiment with some other sensations. Whirl your tongue around the penis while it is deep in your mouth, push it in and out of your mouth, or try sucking on it. The scrotum is fairly sensitive, so you can use your tongue and mouth there as well.

HOW TO PERFORM FELLATIO

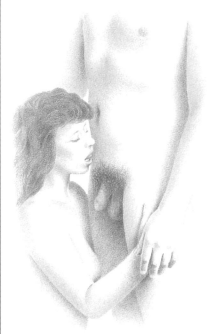

1 A woman can stimulate her partner initially by kissing and caressing his abdomen, thighs and buttocks, as well as the penis and scrotum.

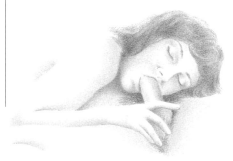

2 Keeping one hand on the penile shaft or scrotum, a woman can use her lips and tongue to stimulate the head of the penis with a variety of movements.

ANAL STIMULATION

For numerous people, the anus and its surrounding area are very sensitive sexually, and for some it is their most erogenous zone. The anal region is well supplied with nerves that follow a similar pathway to the nerves supplying the penis and vagina. Anal stimulation, therefore, gives deep feelings of sexual pleasure unobtainable in other ways, and adds variety to lovemaking. Orgasm that occurs as a result of anal penetration is thought by many to be exceptionally exquisite.

The most basic form of anal stimulation is merely touching your partner's anus during intercourse or oral sex. This is an activity known as "postillionage". More sensation can be produced by inserting a finger into the rectum. When doing this, always lubricate your finger first, and make sure your nail isn't jagged or you could cause harm. Never do this if you have any infection on your finger or hand.

Another technique, gluteal sex, involves the man using the crease of the woman's buttocks as an alternative to the vagina. If the woman contracts her gluteal muscles and rotates her pelvis, the man can thrust into there and reach orgasm this way.

Anal penetration carries with it the risk of AIDS, and if performed over a long time, can lead to stretching of the anal sphincter, which could lead to incontinence. However, the illicit overtones of the act (it is illegal in many parts of the world), the dominant and submissive qualities inherent in it, and the particular sensations it inspires are, to its practitioners, alluring and attractive reasons for indulging in it, and quite a few heterosexuals do.

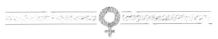

— STIMULATING A MAN —

The prostate gland and back passage, when stimulated, can provide intense sensations; this is a useful technique, particularly when a man's virility is flagging. Making certain your finger, or fingers, are well lubricated (lack of a lubricant will be very uncomfortable), insert them approximately 5 centimetres (2 inches) into the rectum. To stimulate the prostate gland, press against the front wall of the rectum with a slight downward pressure. At the same time, apply firm pressure behind the scrotum with the heel of your hand.

— STIMULATING A WOMAN —

Using very gentle pressure, insert a well-lubricated finger into the rectum or move it gently in and out. Keep the heel of your hand pressed firmly between the anus and the vulva. As you apply pressure from the outside, ask your partner to bear down on your finger. This may help to tighten up the anal sphincter deliberately, and then let it relax.

For reasons of hygiene, once you have inserted your finger into the rectum, keep it well away from the vagina, and make sure that you wash it thoroughly immediately afterwards.

SEXUAL AIDS

Men and women respond romantically and erotically to environment, ambience and atmosphere. There is little question that soft lighting, subdued colours, gentle background music, pleasing scents, melodious voices, and soft and sexy clothes all help to reduce inhibitions and increase the possibility of intimacy. There are, however, a variety of other devices and techniques that add to sexual pleasure and which, for some people, may even be a necessity.

VIBRATORS

The first vibrators were fashioned on the dildo, an artificial penis that has been used by both sexes for many thousands of years. The most recent variation on the traditional dildo is the battery-operated vibrator, which

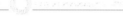

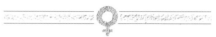

—— MEN AND VIBRATORS ——

It is unlikely that a vibrator will have the explosive effect on a man that it has on a women, though it is able to heighten pleasure enormously in sensitive spots.

The area just behind the root of the penis and in front of the anus is highly sensitive to deep vibration: a vibrator used there will increase sexual pleasure enormously. Almost all of the shaft of the penis, particularly the undersurface, is sensitive to vibration, too, and this rises as the tip is approached. Sensation is exquisite around the frenulum and so arousing when vibration is felt over the tip that a vibrator can sometimes be used as a cure for impotence.

— WOMEN AND VIBRATORS —

A woman who can't reach orgasm during intercourse often wonders if there is something physically wrong with her that prevents her from reaching orgasm. A self-induced orgasm answers that question in a few minutes, and it is here that a vibrator may be truly useful. There is certainly nothing wrong with, and virtually no difference between, an orgasm reached with a vibrator and one reached during sexual intercourse. More importantly, a self-induced orgasm gives the emotional and physical foundation for having orgasms during intercourse.

A vibrator, therefore, can tear down the barriers of guilt, shame and prudery that prevent so many women from finding the sexual fulfilment that they deserve. Some women have for years subconsciously imposed the same kind of paralysis on their sex organs as on their minds. A vibrator provides intense sexual excitement, which is sufficient to overwhelm emotional obstacles, and makes the brain and the genital organs respond explosively in unison.

is widely available in sex shops. Vibrators are used mostly to stimulate a woman's clitoris, and they can be a great help in cases when a woman otherwise has difficulty reaching orgasm during sexual intercourse.

The vibrator works by stimulating the millions of sensory nerve endings in the skin of the woman's labia and the clitoris. A man can also benefit from a vibrator, applying it to his penis and surrounding area to heighten his sensations there.

During intercourse, the penis pushes and pulls against the labia and clitoris and, so to speak, flicks on millions of tiny switches that fire off electric impulses to the brain. In a basic sense, the more sensors the penis stimulates, the greater the sexual sensations. Sad though it may be, a vibrator is better than most penises; in a given moment it can trigger at least a million more sensors than the most educated penis, and that means orgasm is virtually inevitable. This does not mean that a vibrator is necessary, or that the penis is redundant. The whole idea of self-produced orgasm is simply to pave the way for satisfying sexual intercourse.

CREAMS AND LUBRICANTS

The vagina produces a natural lubricating fluid within a few seconds of effective sexual stimulation. This normally makes penetration by the penis easier and pleasurable. However, if a man does not persist with foreplay long enough, the vagina won't be given the chance to produce lubrication. Some women, too, do not produce enough lubricant and most, at different times in their lives, for instance after childbirth and the menopause, will produce less secretions than usual. At these times, an artificial lubricant may be used, and creams and jellies that are water soluble are widely sold. (Take care when using petroleum jelly such as Vaseline, which may irritate the vagina.)

Creams and lubricants come in handy, too, when anal stimulation or intercourse is contemplated, and when manually stimulating your partner. Many men use them during masturbation to ease friction and enhance their pleasure. During massage, too, scented oils or creams can add to the pleasure.

Many women feel pressured not just by society or their partners but also by their own feelings about the presence or absence of lubrication as a sign of arousal. It is comforting to remember that erection of the clitoris and lubrication of the vagina, even erection of the penis, are merely reflexes that do not always accurately reflect our emotional or aroused state. Women can be intensely aroused without being well lubricated, and similarly men can be intensely aroused without an erection. It is an untenable sexist view of things to think that a well-lubricated vagina is solely an opening for an erect penis.

APHRODISIACS

An aphrodisiac is a drug or substance that increases sexual desire. Despite powerful folklore and considerable effort to find such a substance, no proven, reliable aphrodisiacal drug has ever been found, though a wide variety of chemical products, animal and plant extracts and foodstuffs have their devotees. Such substances only leave a temporary impression of well-being, which may well be due to the person's faith in them. Spanish Fly or cantharides, if taken internally, causes excruciating irritation to the intestine and the gastric-urinary tract, especially of the mucous membranes of the urethra. The resulting irritation can cause death in both sexes.

Pornographic pictures, love potions made from bits of animals, narcotics and amulets in phallic form have all been used in an attempt to stimulate sexual desire artificially. So far, no universal aphrodisiac has been discovered and, in view of the diversity and complexity of individual tastes, it is highly unlikely that one ever will be. Real aphrodisiacs are the subtle physical and emotional factors that will revive sexual desire when it is low; these include intense love fantasies, erotic dreams or a particularly attractive quality in a partner.

EROTIC MATERIAL

Reading or watching sexually explicit material can produce genital sensations in both women and men, and can have an effect on sexual behaviour. Many men use pornography as an aid to masturbation, and many women find that racy material increases their interest in having sex, though few will admit to it.

If you are open and talk to your partner about your reactions to erotic stimuli, you will discover that you have many areas in common, including those things that turn you both on or off. If we only can free ourselves from the social customs of the past, the emphasis on the mechanical in early sex books and our own ingrained perspectives, we can find that we are always in a situation to be turned on. It is reassuring to realize that in any situation we can control our sexual response, through our own selection of stimuli, by sharing with our partners and by being aware of the different needs we have for love. In realizing this we liberate ourselves.

If, however, you pressurize your partner to watch material she or he finds offensive, or you force your partner to join in sexual activities that she or he doesn't enjoy, then the problems involved go far beyond your sex life. What is at stake is more likely to be whether either of you actually wants to continue in a relationship in which one person's views and preferences are given unequal weight, and whether the other is willing to change his or her attitude.

FANTASIES

Everyone fantasizes. It would be very odd if we didn't, because fantasy is a form of sexual rehearsal along paths that are familiar and also some that are entirely new and imaginary. We all respond to fantasies because the brain is the most important organ of sexual pleasure. As the seat of emotions, it can be responsible for turning us on or off sex. If we are full of resentment, grief-stricken, angry, anxious or miserable, the most

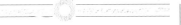

MEN'S FANTASIES

- Being involved in group sex.
- Watching others having sex.
- Making love in public.
- Having sex with a woman other than one's regular partner; she can be a celebrity, neighbour, previous lover, or friend.
- Watching two women you know making love together; one could be one's partner, the other a relative, friend or neighbour.
- Being forced by a woman to have sex.
- Forcing a woman to have intercourse against her will.
- Forcing a woman to have oral sex against her will.
- Making love in an unusual place.
- Being part of a threesome with another man and a woman.
- Being part of a threesome with two women.
- Having a homosexual encounter.
- Watching one or more men having sex with other women.
- Being sexually abused by a woman.
- Making love to a virgin.
- Having sex with a woman with enormous breasts.
- Making love outdoors, on a famous monument, for instance.
- Having a woman urinate on you.
- Having a woman use a dildo on you in order to have anal sex.

WOMEN'S FANTASIES

- Making love with one's partner.
- Making love with a former lover or someone other than one's partner.
- Having sex in an exotic location.
- Being made by a man to have sex against one's will.
- Having sex in public while being watched by others.
- Taking part in group sex.
- Making love with a total stranger.
- Having sex with a partner of a different colour.
- Making love to another woman.
- Being taken from behind by a stranger and never seeing the man's face.
- Stripping in public.
- Sexual activities involving an animal, particularly a horse or dog.
- Watching others having sex.
- Watching your regular partner having sex with another woman, or another man.
- Having a male slave.
- Taking part in a threesome, either with another man or with another woman, and one's usual partner.
- Having sex in unusual and unexpected places or circumstances, for example in a courtroom.
- Working as a prostitute and having a large number of clients to satisfy.
- Being tied down and taken forcibly against your will.

attractive person in the world will not seem so, and any amount of foreplay will not arouse us. On the other hand, being sexually aware, being interested in sex, thinking about it and fantasizing about it will all be arousing. In this sense, it would seem that the brain is the most crucial sex organ because it can override our sexual urges in any direction, either by turning them off, or by turning them on. Fantasies, therefore, are one of the cheapest and most effective sexual aids.

The best sexual fantasies, the ones that offer maximum pleasure, usually centre around ideal situations – ones that are, for practical purposes, unobtainable in "real life". And, also unlike real life, they can be turned on and off at will, either to accelerate or calm sexual activity. Often, we use fantasy to concentrate our minds on what is actually happening to us during our own lovemaking. We "see" what is happening as well as experiencing it. This helps to focus our attention on our own sexual responses, and encourages the brain to respond even more enthusiastically to the signals of arousal it is receiving. It then sends out hormones that increase the excitement in our genital organs.

Many people don't fantasize in terms of stories but in terms of sexual images and, while some people would have difficulty confessing their fantasies, others are willing to discuss a particular set of mental images.

In rare cases, a person can become so fixed on a particular fantasy that they cannot become aroused without it. While a fantasy that exercises such a strong hold over your imagination can be very useful during masturbation, it can get in the way of shared sexual activities. Instead of concentrating on how your partner is reacting, and what you can do to please him or her, you can become fixed on bringing your fantasy to life, and thus seem remote and non-responsive.

Sharing fantasies is another way of personalizing your relationship, and can be introduced into a long-term sexual relationship to add new excitement and rekindle arousal. Some people are happy to join in a fantasy once it has been recounted; however, others may find that they cannot cope with the desires expressed, and may take their partner's fantasy as a criticism of their lovemaking, which can put a considerable pressure on the relationship. If you are in doubt about what to share, bide your time until you see the situation more clearly.

MAKING LOVE

While a large part of being a good lover is to make and keep a relationship exciting, which depends on exploring and mastering a range of sexual activities, to my mind the most important thing is to satisfy each other's emotional needs. Real sexual happiness means having positive feelings about your own sexuality and that of your partner.

Sex is our primary way of showing love. The best sex happens in the best relationships. Partners should explore and develop their sexuality with honesty and trust: honesty is in itself arousing. Sharing the wonder of sex with a sympathetic, loving and caring partner can be a magical voyage of intimacy and discovery.

BEING A GOOD LOVER

While a large part of being a good lover is to make and keep a relationship exciting, which depends on exploring and mastering a range of sexual activities, the primary task is surely to satisfy each other's emotional needs. Real sexual happiness is not the direct result of technical ability or athleticism but depends on your having positive feelings about your own sexuality, and that of your partner. The best sex happens in the best relationships. True sexual chemistry can develop only when partners are attracted to each other as individuals, not just as representatives of the opposite sex. With affection, honesty and trust, partners should explore and develop their sexuality together, bearing in mind the likes and dislikes they each have.

A man often forgets that a woman is both sentimental and sensual, so that her idea of lovemaking includes a prologue of emotions tenderly exchanged. In order to recapture these feelings, it helps to look back to the time when you first fell in love with each other, when just sitting together talking or in companionable silence was enough. I'm sure you will agree there was pleasure in every treasured sign of affection – touches, looks, nuzzles, gentle caresses and kisses. You will have greater pleasure and satisfaction if you remember these earlier emotions when the time comes to arouse one another intensely.

COMMUNICATION IS IMPORTANT

No-one can know instinctively what his or her partner enjoys. It is up to each of us to talk about our likes and dislikes; it is not unnecessary, and it is not at all insulting. It is almost impossible to have a good sexual relationship without clear communication.

We should all let our partners know which caresses are pleasurable and which are not. We should always say if something is particularly arousing or painful. Lovers should be bold enough to suggest a different way of making love, and should ask each other questions and make requests. Exchanging of these confidences will help to build up a better physical relationship, while not doing so may make matters irrevocably worse. This can be achieved by saying that something is pleasant or it is not, making encouraging noises, or by moving a hand to a spot where the sensation is more pleasurable.

What is appropriate and enjoyable varies from occasion to occasion, so simply because you have expressed a preference once does not mean to say that you do not have to express it again, or that you might express a different preference on a different occasion. Good lovers should never take each other for granted.

Ideally when conflicting desires are expressed, or when differing degrees of arousal are experienced, a couple should engage in a process of negotiation. If not, you will find yourselves falling into habitual, routine sexual activities. The best of partners may eventually become bored after years of exactly the same activity in the same sequence, in the same position, in the same bed. Boring sex is rarely rewarding to either partner, and there is a vast range of sexual activities that people find appealing and stimulating. Communication does not mean that everything said has to be negative; say what pleases you, and at the same time listen to what your partner is telling you.

And if you want to get more enjoyment out of your sexual relationship, you need a partner's full involvement and participation. For two people to enjoy their sexual relationship fully, both must be able to accept the pleasure a partner gives, and both must be able to enjoy the process of giving a partner pleasure. The most satisfying sexual relationships have the joint commitment and sharing of the two people involved. The more pleasure you give your partner, the more they will want to give you pleasure in return. A good sexual relationship is always a giving relationship, not a taking one.

TALKING OPENLY ABOUT DESIRES

An amazing number of people find it extremely difficult to talk directly and honestly with their partners about their sexual desires, fears and problems. Many people have been trained to perceive discussions about sex as being so private, so embarrassing and so revealing, that they hesitate to talk about their own feelings and wishes even with the person they've been married to for years.

In this context it is absolutely essential for partners to talk to each other about sex, so that their bodies can adjust mutually and their pleasures increase. Despite this, in my experience, most couples never talk to each other about what they do in bed, whether it is good or bad, or whether it gives them any satisfaction. I, for one, find it hard to believe that during the most intense moments of a couple's relationship, neither partner knows what the other is thinking; their minds remain separate whereas their bodies are striving to get as close as two bodies can.

Many women talk freely to their friends about unfulfilled desires, disappointments and frustrations, but men generally keep their sex lives secret. I'm convinced that there would be far fewer misunderstandings, arguments and conflicts if both partners would talk openly about their physical and emotional expectations. I believe that nothing but good would come of sharing these innermost desires, however strange and fantastic they might appear to be.

Men as Lovers

Many men, no matter what else they may be, are not skilful lovers. Research has shown that the most consistent complaint made by women is that their partners do not take enough time over foreplay. Most sexual relationships tend to develop on a friendly basis for some time, and then gradually evolve into physical intimacy, stopping at petting. During this time, both partners are keen to please each other and usually find that they communicate extremely well. This gradual exploration and steady development means that couples are sexually relaxed the first time they try intercourse. But over time, with many men seeing penetration as the goal to be achieved as quickly as possible, talking and foreplay dwindle, much to the universal disappointment of women.

Meeting Women's Needs

What the majority of men don't seem to understand is that during foreplay the progress from kissing and cuddling to caressing the breasts, nipples and clitoris is not only very exciting and pleasurable for a woman, and incidentally to most men, it is absolutely necessary for a woman's arousal, and crucial to her pleasure and satisfaction. Without it, a woman is not sexually aroused or an uninhibited participant, and is not even physiologically ready. But, worse, after sexual intercourse she is unsatisfied and resentful and remains wide awake while her partner turns over and goes to sleep. Men and women are mismatched in this respect because a man is much more easily and quickly aroused, and reaches orgasm in a very short time in almost any situation. Is it any wonder that sex can end up being a battleground, very often of unspoken resentments and hostilities, and becomes more and more uninteresting and infrequent.

Perfecting your Technique

Some of the things women say about men indicate what they would like to see changed.

"I'd like him to touch me all over a lot more – more foreplay, more heavy petting, more kissing everywhere and more oral sex."

"I love my breasts and nipples to be fondled and caressed, and I've always wondered if I could have a climax just by simply being played with, but my partner is too impatient."

"My partner thinks it's 'soft' to kiss." Men should be sensual as well as sexual and many feel uneasy about engaging in purely pleasurable activities. To overcome this, when giving caresses, think of the pleasure you are providing to a loved one. Most women find foreplay hugely enjoyable, and see hugs and kisses as the true signs of affection. Try to find your partner's most sensitive areas and the kind of stimulation she prefers.

Don't be afraid to relax and let your partner take the initiative. Let her know, either in words or gestures, what feels especially good and, if necessary, guide her hand with yours. Try to concentrate on what you feel and the proximity of her body as she touches you. Respond to your feelings by breathing more heavily, moving, or expressing pleasure verbally. Most women find a responsive man very exciting. Don't feel that you have to be successful at every sexual encounter. Most women are quite sympathetic to an occasional failure, and may even view it as an opportunity to show their love.

WOMEN AS LOVERS

While we know that men are easily aroused and reach orgasm more quickly and easily than women, not all are quite as sexually straightforward as many women believe.

MEETING MEN'S NEEDS

I have no doubt that men also require the excitement and gratification derived from an emotional involvement in love-making. There is hardly a man who does not need to feel loved, admired and physically cherished if he is to experience the true depths of sexual pleasure with his partner. Yet far too many women tend to place the entire responsibility of initiating and orchestrating sex on their men. Traditionally, the man suggests sex and the woman either accepts or rejects him, and in this way the man usually determines how much sex a couple has. This amounts to a great deal of pressure, and many sensitive men do not really relish having such a burden. Better sex and happier couples ensue when partners feel equally free to suggest or refuse sex, and do so equally often.

Taking responsibility for suggesting sex also means that lovemaking will result more from inclination rather than obligation. Women can easily say "yes" to sex but are uninvolved. For a man, a compliant but unresponsive woman will never be as exciting or as satisfying as a woman who is involved and skilful.

PERFECTING YOUR TECHNIQUE

To be a good sexual partner means that you should keep sex interesting, not only by regarding it as the best means of expressing your affection towards your man, but also by experimenting with a variety of techniques and practices. You always should be willing to take the initiative. Men want to feel that they are accepted by their partners, and are worth making an effort to arouse and delight. Try some seduction occasionally; tell your man to lie back and enjoy your caresses as you take the active part.

Remember always to communicate your enjoyment of what you are doing or what is being done to you. Don't be embarrassed about the way you look or sound while making love. Almost all men find expressions of desire and signs of growing sexual excitement in women extremely stimulating. Far too many women give their partners too little feedback so that their men tend to feel discouraged and unappreciated for what they are doing and will, in future, pay less attention to foreplay.

Use your imagination as much as possible. This is especially important in long-term relationships when boredom can easily set in. In addition to picking and choosing among the entire range of the normal sexual repertoire, introduce activities that will bring novelty into your relationship. Suggest taking a bath or shower together; make love outdoors in a private place; plan lunch at home but make love instead; abandon your bed in favour of the floor, sofa or a rug; use a mirror to watch yourselves making love; view a sexy video together; or indulge in a sexual banquet of both partners' choosing.

Show enthusiasm towards your partner if he suggests ways of enlivening your sex life. Unless something is painful or distressing, it is always worth finding out whether or not it gives you pleasure. In sex, as in all things, let your instincts be your guide.

VARYING EXPERIENCES

Earlier we looked at the individual experiences of men and women in achieving orgasm. But, as with all the best love-play, orgasms should be a shared experience. That doesn't mean to say, however, that they must occur necessarily at the same time.

Some couples feel erroneously that only a simultaneous orgasm is the perfect one. This is a romantic notion that doesn't necessarily work for all lovers. At the moment of climax, you move to an entirely different level of consciousness, and you become totally absorbed in the experience. If you are prevented from doing so, because you need to know where your partner is, you may not be able to manage a climax at all, or manage it less well. And, for many lovers, watching the other experiencing his or her orgasm is the greatest of sexual turn-ons.

For most couples, the attainment of simultaneous orgasms only happens now and then, and sex is no less enjoyable for that. Seeking simultaneous orgasms should not become obsessive. There are many patterns of successful lovemaking that exclude simultaneous orgasms (and some that exclude all orgasms), but nonetheless draw couples very close and have infinite positive effects on everyday experiences as well as on social and family life.

And then there are the exceptional circumstances – prolonged and multiple orgasms – that are quite rare unless both partners are aware of each other's sexual needs, and are generous enough to look after them. Most couples find these forms of sexual intercourse the most exciting and sexually satisfying, but they take quite a lot of practice and are most often found within long-term relationships. Partners must be very familiar with each other and have worked to reach a state of sexual sophistication.

PROLONGED ORGASM

This can be practised only if a man is able to control his ejaculatory reflex at will. It is a form of sexual union indulged in usually by partners who have been making love together for some time, who know each other well and who have learned how to adjust to each other's needs. This can be one of the most exciting forms of sexual union, and it is one of the most treasured aspects of a long-term loving relationship.

For it to occur, the woman must be highly aroused during foreplay and then the sexual tension of both partners must be maintained by intermittent thrusting movements, punctuated by pauses from time to time for as long as each partner wishes. When sensation reaches a peak and can't be put off further, both partners enjoy orgasm in a mutually agreed, final burst of lovemaking.

MULTIPLE ORGASMS

Until recently, we believed that only women were capable of multiple orgasms, but new research has shown that some men are able to have them, too. Since orgasm is not necessarily synonymous with ejaculation, but is more accurately defined as the intense and diffuse pleasurable sensations the man feels, it is perfectly possible for a man to have several climaxes in fairly quick succession.

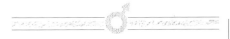

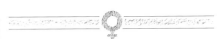

—— MAN'S EXPERIENCE ——

American doctors have documented the experiences of multi-orgasmic men who had from two to nine orgasms per session. Some ejaculated at the first orgasm, some at the last and the rest somewhere in between; some even ejaculated more than once. Many of the men first experienced multiple orgasms in middle age.

Probably, more men could become multi-orgasmic if they overcome the conditioning that says they will only ejaculate and then detumesce. A non-demanding atmosphere, combined with emotional closeness and the opportunity for leisurely sex, will improve a man's chances of enjoying multiple orgasms, as will having a partner who is sexually responsive and does not easily tire of prolonged intercourse.

However, just as with multi-orgasmic women, men who are capable of more than one orgasm will not be able to experience them every time.

A man can practise becoming multi-orgasmic by coming to the brink of orgasm yet inhibiting ejaculation until he can separate the two sensations. In the positive, relaxed atmosphere of a loving relationship, some men will find that they don't necessarily lose their erections, and they will be able to carry on achieving further climaxes.

—— WOMAN'S EXPERIENCE ——

For a woman to enjoy multiple orgasms, her man must exercise careful control to avoid ejaculating, yet give her sufficient deep and rapid thrusting for her to achieve orgasm. Or, a woman may use a vibrator, or she or her partner may masturbate her. After each orgasm, both partners rest for a while and then the cycle can begin again. In this way, a woman can enjoy two, three or many more orgasms. Ideally, her partner will climax simultaneously with her last one, but often the rigid control needed means he experiences his own orgasm only when his partner is fully satisfied.

Most women find that they can build up their level of sexual arousal with practice; the more frequently a woman masturbates, the more pleasure she gets from it, and the more she will want to do so. Most women can improve their chances of multiple orgasm by keeping their pelvic muscles in good condition, and sharing fantasies, but above all, they need to encourage their partners to help them. If you are trying to have multiple orgasms, your partner needs to know; and you should encourage him to carry on stimulating you even after you've had an initial climax. Because a man's experience of orgasm is so different, your partner may think you have had enough of love-play just because he has.

POSITIONS FOR MAKING LOVE

Often, when couples whose sex life has gone off the boil consult me about making improvements, one of the first questions I ask is whether they vary the way they make love. Many of these couples have tied themselves to a single position for lovemaking, and it has simply become boring. The missionary position with the man on top and the woman underneath is most commonly used and, for some couples, never varied. (It is so-named because it was forcibly advocated by missionaries who took their faith to "heathen" or "uncivilized" peoples.) For many years the church tolerated this position and no other, since it was thought to be the one in which the woman would almost certainly be fertilized. This rigidly adhered-to tradition allowed the man always to adopt the dominant role during sexual intercourse and to experience most or all of the pleasure of sex.

But between consenting lovers, all coital positions are perfectly normal and legitimate, and everyone's sex lives will certainly be enlivened by a little adventure and experimentation.

CHOOSING A POSITION

There's no such thing as the best position; each couple should experiment and find their own most favourable positions, which will depend on the shape and size of the couple's bodies, both partners' strength and stamina, and any special situations such as a pregnancy, disability or illness. Couples who are making love and exploring each other for the first time very often experiment with a variety of positions in quick succession in an attempt to satisfy their curiosities.

At the same time, partners should try to find out as much as they can about the other's body so that they can adjust to each other physically. One of the purposes that a book like this serves is to enlighten couples who know little or nothing about loving sex, or who are lacking in imagination, and who cannot believe that there are other positions apart from those they happen to have come across by chance. Remember that expertise can't be attained in a day; it may take months of enjoyable experimentation before a couple finds the several positions that for them are wholly satisfying and fulfilling in every sense.

The following pages illustrate a number of positions. For a variety of reasons, each position has particular benefits for one or both partners. Set out opposite, in no special order, are some of the considerations that each partner in a couple looks for, and that the positions they choose take into account. Both partners should take notice of the preferences of the other, which means that each partner has the responsibility for expressing his or her predilections in the first instance. To enjoy intercourse to the maximum, however, any position in which it is tried should be comfortable and allow freedom of movement, and must accommodate the abilities of the less athletic partner.

Certain positions are uncomfortable or even painful for one partner, some are better for the man than for the woman, and vice versa, while others can increase the feeling of pleasure and enhance sexual arousal so that the chances of an orgasm for both partners, but particularly the woman, are increased. This is not to say that any one position is better than another. Each position may have its own advantages in any given situation and on any given occasion, taking account of how each partner feels physically and emotionally.

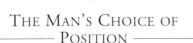

THE MAN'S CHOICE OF POSITION

- Does it allow good penetration (shallow or deep, as desired)?
- Will he be able to see his partner's vulva clearly?
- Will he have good access to his partner's clitoris?
- Can he reach her breasts with his hands or mouth?
- Can he move easily?
- Will it prolong intercourse or, if desired, is it good for a quick getaway?
- Is it tiring?
- Can his partner move?
- Does it allow for his unusually small or large penis?
- Does it allow full stroke movement?
- If he has erection difficulties, can the position and penetration be achieved without a firm erection?
- Can he kiss his partner and hug and cuddle her?
- Is it good if his partner is much heavier or lighter than he is?
- Does it need a lot of undressing?
- Does it allow him to take the dominant (or passive) role?
- Can he stimulate his partner's buttocks and anal area?
- Is it possible during pregnancy?

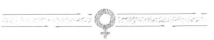

THE WOMAN'S CHOICE OF POSITION

- Can she move so that stimulation remains good?
- Does it allow her to see her partner?
- Is it comfortable during the latter stages of pregnancy?
- Can she or her partner reach her clitoris easily?
- Does it allow her to kiss her partner and hold him close?
- Will it stimulate her G-spot?
- Is it comfortable?
- Does it allow her partner to reach her breasts?
- When in the position, can she reach down and touch her partner's scrotum?
- Is it good for cuddling?
- Does it allow good skin contact?
- Is it good for conception?
- What sort of penetration does it allow – shallow or deep – and is it the sort she wants?
- Is it good for learning sex with a new or shy partner?
- Does it stimulate the back or front vaginal wall?
- Does it allow her to take a dominant (or submissive) role?
- Can she look into her partner's eyes and speak to him?

MAN-ON-TOP POSITIONS 1

Man-on-top positions, in particular the "missionary" position, where the man lies between the woman's thighs, are probably the most widely used of all the sexual positions. They give the man almost total control over intercourse, but the woman is allowed very little freedom of movement.

Man-on-top positions are particularly good for couples who are just beginning to have sex with each other, as there is full eye contact and the opportunity to communicate with each other so that preferences and responses can be noted. The other advantages these positions offer are plenty of scope for kissing, deep penetration and manual stimulation, plus access to the male posterior. They are also good if conception is desirable.

2 If the woman brings her leg up to apply pressure to her partner's back, she can control the depth and angle of his thrusts, perhaps so that he presses on the front wall of her vagina, the site of her "G" spot.

1 The man enters his partner straight on so that his penis is parallel to her vaginal walls. If she spreads her legs wide, the stretchy feeling is quite sensuous.

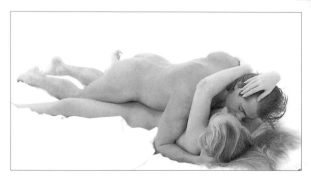

Face-to-face the couple have full eye contact and can kiss passionately

He can take his weight on his elbows, allowing his partner to move her pelvis more freely

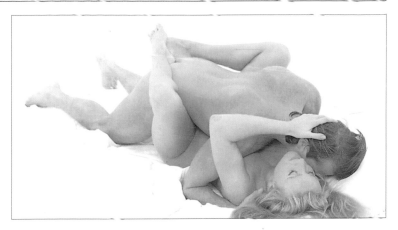

She can use her leg to apply pressure to his back and buttocks, and for some control over his thrusting

3 By bringing up both legs to wrap them around her partner, a fit and supple woman alters the tilt of her pelvis, which can produce pleasing new sensations for both her and her partner, and increases genital contact.

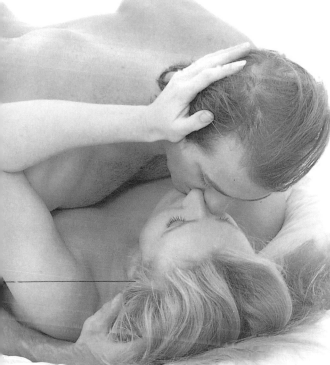

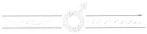

MAN

The man has wide access to his partner for kissing and caressing her upper body and breasts, and he can control his thrusting, speeding up or slowing down, as necessary.

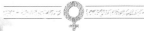

WOMAN

Man-on-top positions are very good for kissing and caressing, and feed a woman's romantic needs. She is being made love to, and can lie back and enjoy the sensations.

MAN-ON-TOP POSITIONS 2

Man-on-top positions feed a man's need to dominate by allowing him to penetrate his partner deeply, and a woman's desire to be dominated because in them she takes the passive role. Most men enjoy penetrating a woman's body as deeply as possible, and women like it too, especially when they are particularly aroused and want to be "filled up". And, when a woman opens herself completely to her partner, it makes him feel very wanted. In these positions, the man can move freely to control the intensity and depth of his thrusts; the woman can add to his sensations by contracting and relaxing her pelvis to "milk" her partner's penis.

1 As a variation from entering his partner from above, the man can kneel and approach her from a vertical position. He can thus push off against the bed into his partner. She helps increase contact by wrapping her legs around him tightly.

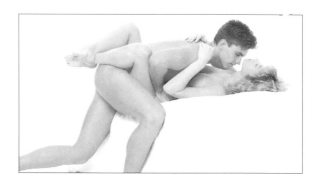

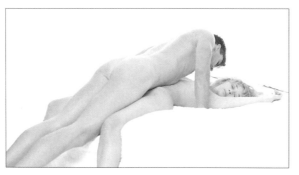

When highly aroused, spreading her legs widely will make deep penetration easier

2 By sliding his partner down the side of the bed, the man can lean forward on her body, taking most of his weight on his forearms while she relaxes and lets herself be taken completely. Movement and penetration are limited so that arousal can be controlled.

MAN

Using these positions the man is able to control his thrusting, and thus the speed at which he achieves orgasm. Control such as this is particularly beneficial if the man is at all worried about losing his erection, or if he wants to delay ejaculation.

WOMAN

Being on her back is relaxing and allows the woman free rein to lie back and enjoy the sensations of being taken or overpowered by her partner. It also "absolves" her from having to be responsible for what happens during sexual intercourse.

3 Finally, pushing them both up the bed, his knees thrusting her legs wide apart, the man can penetrate his partner quite deeply. For her, the sensation is increased by having her knees close to her chest and her bottom raised by a pillow.

Deeply entwined, she feels secure enough to open herself completely to her partner

He uses his thigh and knee to give added pressure to the tempo and depth of his thrusts

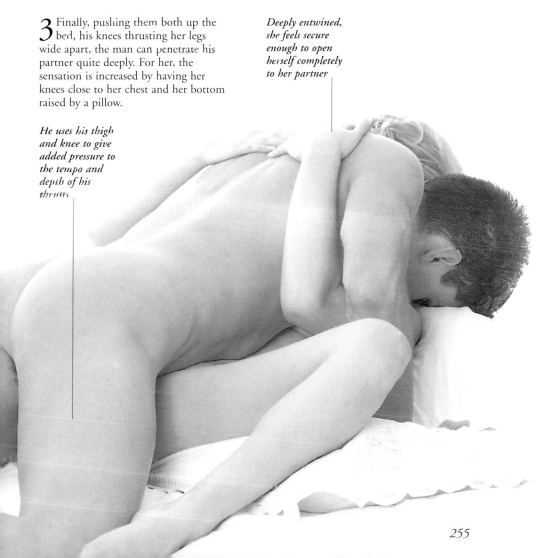

WOMAN-ON-TOP POSITIONS 1

Both men and women find the woman-on-top positions extremely satisfying. They enable a woman to take a more active role in controlling both the sensations she gives and those she receives. With her man underneath and relatively immobile, she can stimulate his penis easily by moving up and down, and more readily control the depth of penetration. For the man, such positions prove that his partner is taking the lead; with them, he can feel himself the object of her active seduction. Woman-on-top positions are also comfortable ones, particularly when the woman is much lighter than her partner or if she is pregnant.

He is the passive partner, feeling wanted and seduced, and can concentrate on his own arousal knowing that his partner is controlling her own stimulation

1 To get into the simplest position, where the woman lies on top of her partner with her legs outside, it is probably best to start from a side-on embrace. Then she needs to gently throw a leg across her partner's thighs, and climb gracefully on top. The man, of course, needs to have an erection, which the woman will have to guide inside her.

His hands can caress her back and buttocks, occasionally holding her to guide the angle of penetration

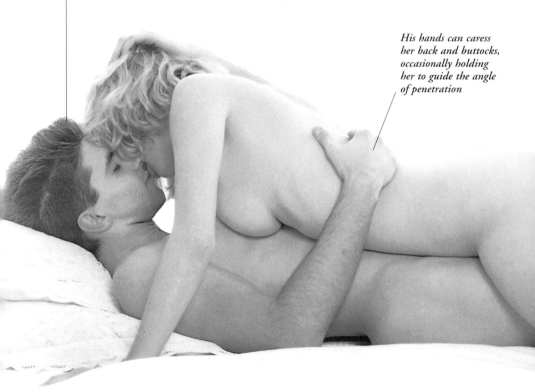

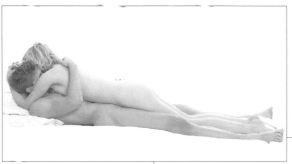

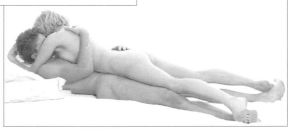

2 If the woman now brings her legs inside her partner's this results in a snugger fit between both genital areas. If she keeps her legs tightly closed, she heightens the friction between the vagina and pelvis. She can add to the sensation by contracting her pelvic muscles.

3 Finally, if the woman spreads her legs out widely to the side, the pubic regions are perfectly aligned. From here, she can press down on her partner's feet, which is highly arousing to him because she is obviously "using" her partner in order to satisfy herself.

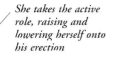

She takes the active role, raising and lowering herself onto his erection

She can push his legs apart or together with hers thus changing the sensations for both of them

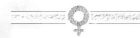

MAN

He can lie and enjoy the sensations she arouses. This is useful where he can't take the lead due to fatigue or illness.

WOMAN

As well as being ideal for a woman to please herself, this helps when a partner is large, or when she is pregnant.

WOMAN-ON-TOP POSITIONS 2

Woman-on-top positions where the woman is sitting up, have several advantages. The woman has full view of her man, and by taking all her weight on herself, she can more actively caress him while adjusting his penile movements to her liking. The man is free to fondle his partner's freely moving breasts, which are held tantalizingly close to him, and he can see his penis entering her vagina; both sights are very exciting to him.

1 The woman starts from lying straight on top of her man. She then lifts herself up, and gradually brings her legs forward and bends her knees. Initially, to avoid applying painful pressure on her partner, she will put most of her weight on her arms and knees.

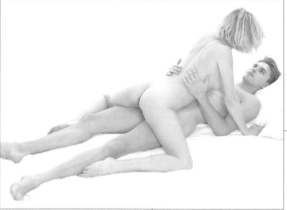

She can lean back on to his thighs to take some of her weight from his pelvis

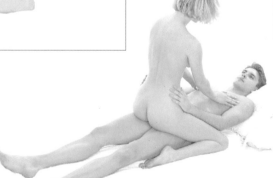

2 By taking all her weight on her knees, she is free to use her hands on her partner – caressing him or holding him down to add an extra element of control, if she so wishes.

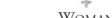

MAN

These positions can be very exciting. The man has a full view of both his and his partner's genitals, and good access to her breasts, and he is free to stimulate her and vice versa.

WOMAN

In these positions a woman's breasts and genitals are free to be caressed, and she can most easily control the position and depth of penetration of her partner's penis.

3 Or, she can lean backwards, taking her legs behind and pressing them close to or pushing them away from her partner's body as she chooses. She even can bring her legs forward, stretching them towards her partner's shoulders. In this way, she is free to make swaying or rotating movements.

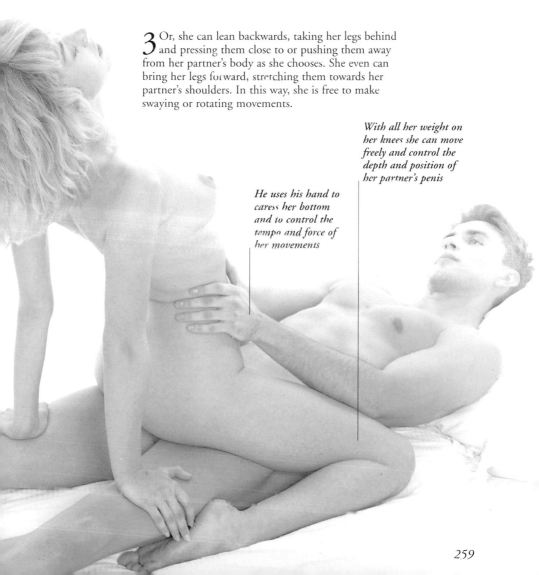

With all her weight on her knees she can move freely and control the depth and position of her partner's penis

He uses his hand to caress her bottom and to control the tempo and force of her movements

STANDING POSITIONS

Making love standing up is most achievable when both partners are about the same size. If the man is considerably larger than his partner, insertion and intercourse are possible only with a certain amount of difficulty and determination. Sexual intercourse standing up can be tiring if it is kept up for any length of time (particularly if there is an uncomfortable difference between the couple's sizes), but owing to the muscular exertion it necessitates, it can considerably increase sexual excitement.

If the man picks up his partner, the greatest amount of exertion is the initial lift. Once he has achieved this, the standing position is not particularly demanding because the weight is evenly distributed between the two partners. From here, making love can continue while standing up, walking or even dancing.

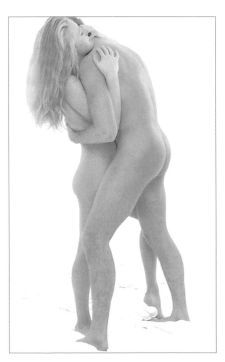

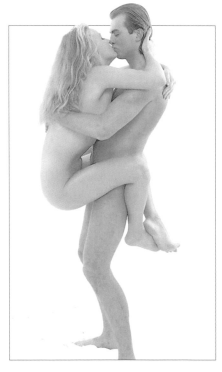

1 To facilitate insertion, the woman should lift one leg, turn it sideways so that her partner can introduce his penis, and then use both legs for support. The vagina then clasps the penis firmly; she can use her pelvis to make strong sexual movements.

2 Once the man is inside, he can lift his partner by placing his hands under her thighs while she firmly clasps her hands behind his neck and holds on to it. She should then cross her legs behind his back and press her thighs around his hips.

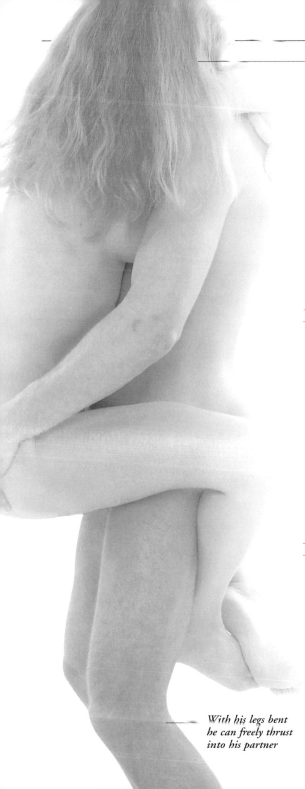

She can entwine herself around his body, gripping with her arms and thighs to distribute some of her weight. Her muscle tension can heighten sexual excitement for both of them

3 If both partners are agile, insertion can be achieved after the woman has been raised off the ground. Now the man can move his partner back and forth with his hands and alter tempo and motion.

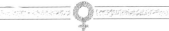

MAN
The main benefit of standing positions is the novelty factor, since a degree of agility and strength is required, but they are ideal when the man wishes to dispense with preliminaries. More vigorous thrusting can be achieved if the woman is pressed against a wall or door for extra support.

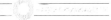

WOMAN
Standing positions are useful when the time and place for sex is limited, and when she wants to add some variety to her sex life. She can produce a very powerful stimulation on her vaginal lips and clitoris if she leans forward a little and bends her knees while her feet are on the floor.

With his legs bent he can freely thrust into his partner

SIDE-BY-SIDE POSITIONS 1

For relaxed, unhurried lovemaking, few positions beat side-by-side ones; it is not at all unusual for couples to fall asleep locked together after making love in this way. When both people are on their sides, rear entry is easy to achieve, and intercourse can be prolonged easily, too, without being too tiring. Such positions also provide maximum body contact and plenty of scope for affectionate caresses.

During pregnancy, and where a man is particularly large, side-by-side positions with the woman facing away are ideal, because he can't put pressure on her this way. These positions also make a relaxing change from more athletic sexual postures.

1 The "spoons" position, with the man cuddling up to the woman's back, is one of the most comfortable and affectionate of all sexual positions. If the woman draws her knees upwards, when her partner tucks up against her he can penetrate very easily.

Surrounding her body with his own, he can lovingly kiss and caress her back and neck, and reach around to stimulate her breasts and clitoris

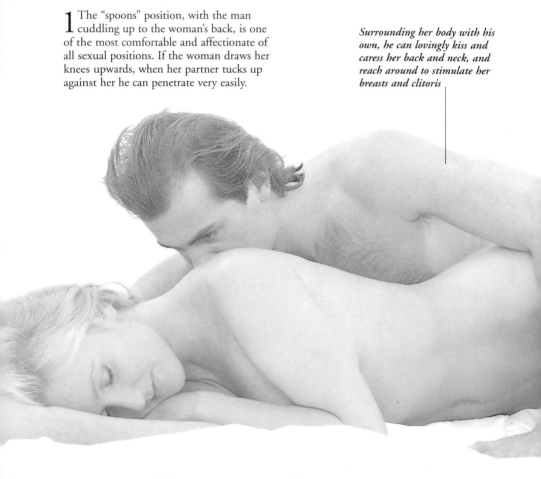

2 Moving on to her back a bit more and raising her bottom slightly lets the woman's partner thrust into her without restriction while having access to her breasts and vagina. There is a lot of skin contact, and the couple can kiss easily and passionately.

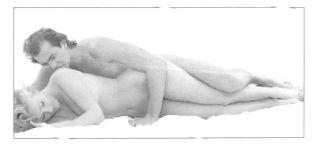

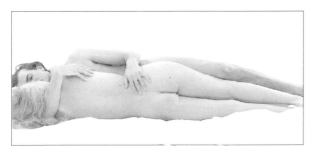

Facing variation
This can be achieved from a man-on-top position, without disturbance, if both partners slide onto their sides. Or, it can be initiated this way if the woman lifts or bends her leg to allow the man to insert his penis.

Raising her knee slightly allows easy penetration. Both partners are comfortable and can prolong their lovemaking for some time

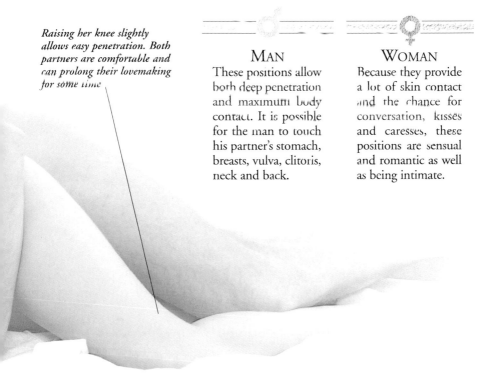

MAN
These positions allow both deep penetration and maximum body contact. It is possible for the man to touch his partner's stomach, breasts, vulva, clitoris, neck and back.

WOMAN
Because they provide a lot of skin contact and the chance for conversation, kisses and caresses, these positions are sensual and romantic as well as being intimate.

SIDE-BY-SIDE POSITIONS 2

By slight alterations in movement, side-by-side positions can produce a wide variety of new sensations. By rolling backwards a woman opens up her vulva considerably and leaves her clitoris free for herself or her partner to caress. Drawing her legs upwards increases penetration. By changing the position of his legs and thighs, the man can achieve different movements and control the pressure that the root of the penis directs against his partner's vulva.

Drawing her legs up along her partner's back and sides can increase penetration, particularly if she presses with her legs and feet, coaxing him to thrust further into her

1 The woman places her bent leg on top of her partner's hip as he pushes his thigh between hers. Then she should lie back and her partner can lean into her, keeping his legs stretched out straight. One of his hands is free to caress her, while she has both free to attend to him. He has more freedom to attempt some active movements while bestowing some caresses.

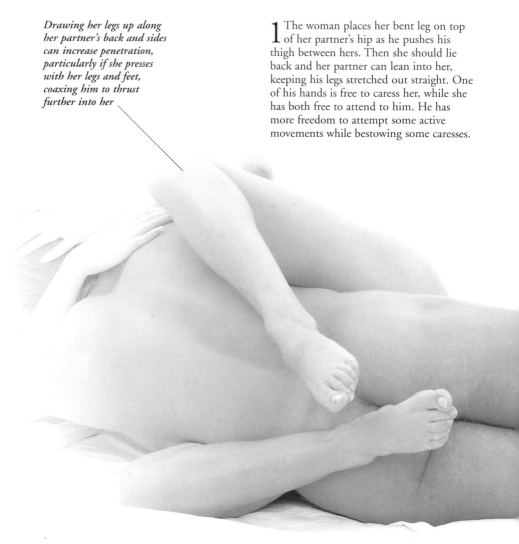

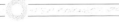

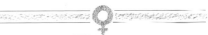

MAN

These positions provide plenty of body contact. The man has enough freedom to experiment with various movements to give new sensations. Movement is somewhat limited, but he is free to grasp his partner's buttocks and pull her on to his penis.

WOMAN

These positions can supply plenty of pressure to the vulva for increased stimulation. They also are good in late pregnancy because they allow a woman plenty of space from her partner, and his penetrating and thrusting can be restricted.

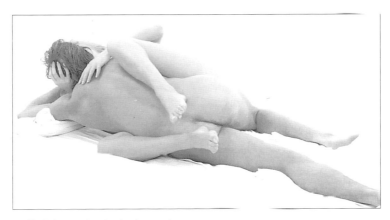

2 By bringing his leg back up, the man can now make strong pushing movements. He can increase the pressure by using his hands to press his partner's buttocks next to his hips.

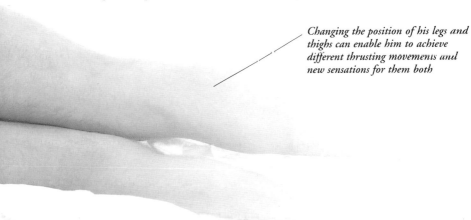

Changing the position of his legs and thighs can enable him to achieve different thrusting movements and new sensations for them both

REAR-ENTRY POSITIONS

Although not as popular or as romantic as face-to-face positions, couples who have frequent intercourse enjoy the variety that a change to a rear-entry position can bring. Rear-entry positions provide the man with considerable freedom to thrust, and with them he can alter most easily the angle and amount of penile movements. For those women who are fortunate enough to have sensitive "G" spots, these positions result in the greatest stimulation; for those who don't, the different sensations produced can still be extremely exciting.

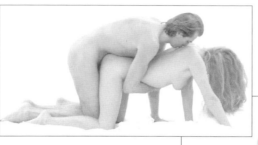

1 Probably the best known rear-entry position, this is known colloquially as the "doggie". The woman kneels on her hands and knees on the bed or floor, and her partner kneels behind.

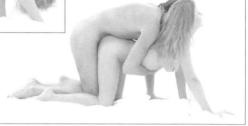

2 The vagina is turned straight back to the man pressed against her, and she can move the angle of her pelvis to give various sensations to both. She can also sway back and forth on her hands and knees.

This position can be very exciting for a woman, if lithe enough, as excitement mounts from her partner's penis rubbing against new areas of her vagina not normally stimulated

Attempting rear entry is highly stimulating for him as the sensation of dominance is very high

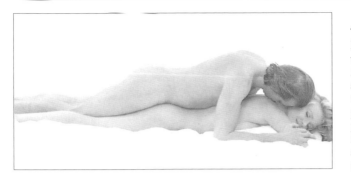

4 If she lies flat and presses her legs together, the woman's clitoris and inner lips will be stimulated indirectly, maintaining her pleasure, and her partner can remain inside, moving how and when he pleases to rekindle desire.

3 The woman will find it more restful to slide down gently on to her stomach and chest while the man takes most of his weight on his hands. (The position can also be initiated in this way.) Deeper penetration will be achieved if she raises her bottom off the bed.

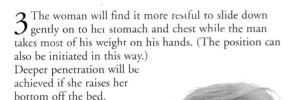

MAN

The sight of a woman's bottom is very exciting to most men. Here, he can caress much of her body and benefit from the greatest depth of penetration combined with a sense of mastery.

WOMAN

Rear-entry is a turn-on for many women who like feeling vulnerable. It also enables them to fantasize, their partners not being visible, and provides good access to the front vaginal wall.

AFTERPLAY

On all levels – physical, emotional and mental – men and women experience the period of resolution in different ways. While both feel relaxed, calm and satisfied, having experienced a type of communion that is ecstatic and timeless, a man returns to the normal world and becomes aware of his surroundings much more quickly than a woman does. Detumescence is very fast; the penis becomes flaccid within a minute. A woman takes much longer to surface from the depths of her orgasm, especially if her experience was intense. The engorgement of her genital organs resolves much more slowly, and so do her emotions.

Most women wish to stay in an embrace while their partners wish to get up or simply drift off to sleep. This is a classic instance of why it is important for partners to talk about their desires and to reach a happy solution. If they don't, in time the situation could well lead to unhappiness, frustration and resentment.

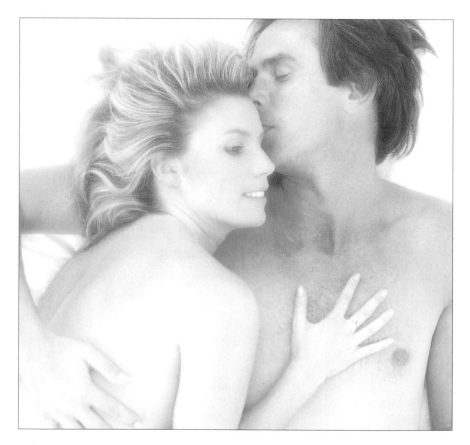

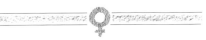

MAN'S EXPERIENCE

Once a man has ejaculated, his interest in sex, and possibly his partner, declines rapidly. His penis will shrink and his sex drive diminishes. For a period of time, depending mainly on his age and health, he can't achieve another erection and so his interest in sex is reduced.

For many men, the penis becomes exquisitely sensitive immediately after orgasm, necessitating instant withdrawal from the vagina. Such men will often withdraw physically from their partners, moving and turning away from them.

In addition, many men are frequently overcome by post-coital somnolence. During the arousal period, a substantial amount of blood flows into the man's pelvic area, and his muscles contract and tighten. This blood is rapidly diverted away from the area after sex, and his muscles relax so that the excitement is replaced by drowsiness and a general feeling of lethargy – something not experienced by the majority of women. A man will often roll over to his side of the bed and go to sleep, leaving his partner in the "damp spot".

Accommodating a partner Most men are totally unaware of how a woman interprets these movements, since she experiences very different feelings after orgasm (see right).

Even if a man is not able to combat his physiological reactions to orgasm, he can and should be sensitive to his partner's emotional needs. A last cuddle and goodnight kiss can be bestowed before he drifts off without too much effort, and it will make all the difference to the woman. A change to lovemaking during the morning, when both partners are fresher, or during the day, may help to stave off sleep.

WOMAN'S EXPERIENCE

During the slow phase of detumescence, while still savouring the effects of an orgasm, most women feel a strong desire to remain entwined in their partners' arms, and to lie quietly close to them enjoying non-passionate embraces and caresses. Some even will wish to lie with their partners' penises still inside them, flaccid though they may be.

There is a theory that a woman's instinct for sexual pleasure is so deeply ingrained in her nature that she has an overwhelming need to maintain body contact with her partner after orgasm, and thereby extend the period of enchantment for as long as possible.

But if her partner gets up, has a cigarette or simply rolls over and goes to sleep, a woman usually feels neglected and bereft, and this kind of turning off without explanation after sexual union usually leaves her feeling lonely. A sudden withdrawal of this kind seems uncaring, if not brutal, to her.

Prolonging a man's interest A man's usual physiological response to orgasm is one of drowsiness and lethargy, and this is enhanced if lovemaking is left to times when he is already feeling tired and ready for sleep. Therefore, a change to morning lovemaking may bring about a more affectionate afterplay.

To encourage your man to stay awake, keep conversation light and romantic; tell him how much you love him and how wonderful he is. It is a good idea to avoid discussing household problems, as this is certain to send him off to sleep. Make sure, too, that after having sex it is not you who rushes off immediately to the bathroom to get washed. If you must have a wash, suggest you have a bath together.

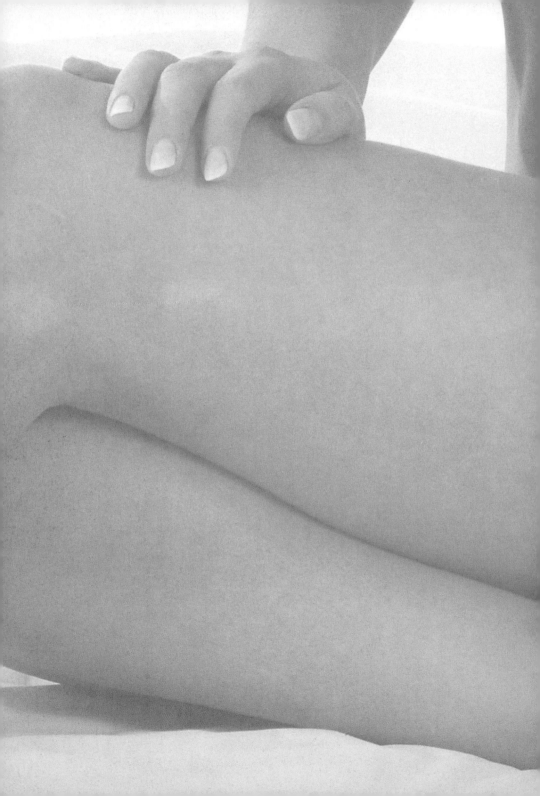

3

MENOPAUSE

INTRODUCTION

FOR MANY WOMEN, the menopause can be a psychological, emotional and intellectual turning point in their lives as well as a physical one, but it does not have to mean a decline. As your children leave home and you look forward to reducing your workload, you will have more time to yourself than you have ever had before. This can be liberating, and you can take the opportunity to reassess your lifestyle and decide what you want from the future.

As the menopause approaches, the ovaries begin to fail, and there is a sudden dip in our female sex hormones, oestrogen and progesterone, which causes the cessation of menstruation. About three-quarters of all women experience some menopausal symptoms, all of which can be treated.

Temporary symptoms of the menopause include hot flushes, night sweats and loss of libido and they may last for several years; long-term ones include the thinning and drying out of vaginal and genital skin and urinary troubles – all of which may become permanent. Fortunately, these complaints are not dangerous and can be remedied by many therapies. However, some of the other consequences of the menopause *are* dangerous. These include osteoporosis or brittle bones, and one in four postmenopausal women who is admitted to hospital with a fractured thigh bone never leaves, so it is important that we protect ourselves from this disease.

The menopause affects every organ of a woman's body, and any treatment, therefore, must be viewed in the context of what is good for the whole: this involves a healthy diet, lots of regular exercise, relaxation, yoga, minerals and whatever change in your lifestyle you think would help. Each of the complementary therapies, from aromatherapy to yoga, has its own champions.

1

What happens at the menopause

As the supply of eggs in the ovaries dwindles, oestrogen and progesterone levels fluctuate and begin to decline. This produces the end of menstruation and also has other effects on the body. Menopausal symptoms are felt largely because of the suddenness of oestrogen withdrawal. Many women experience few or no symptoms while others may be incapacitated. This chapter describes the classic symptoms associated with the menopause and gives self-help advice plus the most appropriate natural therapy available.

PLANNING YOUR FUTURE

The menopause is an important crossroads in our lives and, if viewed positively, can be rewarding and revealing. Life is a series of milestones and, whereas in our younger days we rushed past the markers, as we grow older, we tend to reflect more. The menopause gives us a perfect opportunity to look back at what we have done in the past, and decide what we might want to do in the future.

A woman who may have devoted half of her life to raising a family still has time to go back to college, start a new career and take care of her body so that she is fitter than she has ever been. The end of fertile life doesn't have to imply new restrictions and physical decline; our options can increase rather than decrease.

THE MENOPAUSE TIMETABLE

Most of the time we use the word menopause incorrectly. Strictly speaking, it means the end of menstruation and could, hypothetically, be a moment in time. The word climacteric more accurately describes the ongoing changes and symptoms, as it refers to a transition period that may last 15–20 years. During this phase, both ovarian function and hormonal production decline, and the body adjusts itself to these changes.

It may help to think of the menopause as being the counterpart of the menarche, when periods commence. The climacteric can then be compared with the years of adolescence or puberty when the ovaries begin to function and mature.

THE CLIMACTERIC

There are three stages in the climacteric: pre-, peri- and postmenopause. The menopause signals the end of the premenopause and the beginning of the postmenopause.

Premenopause This period of time refers to the early years of the climacteric, after the age of 40, when menstrual periods may become irregular and sometimes heavy, and the symptoms of the menopause start to emerge. You find yourself saying, "Is it hot in here or just me?" If your doctor tells you that you are premenopausal, ask for a precise definition of what he or she means.

Perimenopause This is the stage lasting several years on either side of your last menstrual period. Perimenopause is, in part, a retrospective diagnosis, since it's only when your periods cease that you can measure backwards two years in time to when it began. It's during this time that you notice most physical changes, when your periods may become irregular and when hot flushes may start.

Menopause This has a precise meaning – the menopause is your final menstrual period. This is another date that can only be identified retrospectively, when you have not had a menstrual bleed for 12 months. In other words, it is impossible for a woman to know the exact moment that she is experiencing the menopause.

Postmenopause This period overlaps with the end of the perimenopausal stage and will extend into the years that follow your last menstrual period. It lasts until the end of your life.

CAN I PREDICT MY LAST PERIOD?

The average age when women experience the menopause in this country is 51, an age that has remained fairly constant over the centuries, even though the average age for the onset of menstruation has become earlier. About half of all women will stop menstruating before they turn 51, and half will stop menstruating afterwards. There is no need to be alarmed if you stop menstruating before your 45th birthday; this happens to about a third of all women. At the other end of the scale, many women carry on menstruating into their early 50s, and a few into their mid-50s.

Although there is no way in which you can predict exactly when your menopause will occur, there are factors that may influence its timing. The age you begin to menstruate may affect the age that you experience the menopause, although no studies have yet proved this. And it is possible that the age at which your mother experienced the menopause will have some bearing on when you stop menstruating, but again this relationship has not been scientifically proven. Two factors that do *not* influence the time of your menopause are whether or not you took the oral contraceptive pill, or your age when you had your first and last child.

THE RANGE OF SYMPTOMS

The list of symptoms associated with the menopause is long, and at first glance may be daunting. Fortunately, no woman experiences the whole range – you will probably only have a few and many women have none. The list described here is long simply because it's helpful to know the array of disparate symptoms, especially if you need to discuss your treatment with a doctor. The physical effects of the menopause are so diverse, it is sometimes hard to connect them to a single cause. There are some classic symptoms, such as hot flushes and mood swings, that women may readily associate with the menopause, but others, such as poor bladder control or back pain, often appear to be just incidental. All the symptoms listed here are directly or indirectly related to a drop in oestrogen levels.

Back pain
Breast soreness
Chest pain
Itchy skin
Night sweats
Palpitations

Anxiety and low self-esteem
Depressed mood
Dry hair, eyes and mouth,
and dry, wrinkled skin
Feelings of pessimism
Forgetfulness
Headaches
Hot flushes
Inability to concentrate or
make decisions
Increase in facial hair
Insomnia
Irritability and tearfulness
Lowering of the voice
Mood swings and PMS
Thin hair
Tiredness and lethargy

Aches and pains
Brittle nails
Muscle soreness
Pins and needles
Swollen or stiff joints

Bloated abdomen
Constipation
Dry vagina
Heavy/irregular periods
Itchy vulva
Loss of bladder control
Loss of libido
Slower sexual arousal
and lubrication
Urgent urination

Signs of the menopause

The early symptoms associated with the menopause, such as mood swings, are different from later symptoms, which include dry skin and slower sexual arousal. This reflects the body's response to fluctuating oestrogen levels, and then to permanently lowered oestrogen levels.

HOT FLUSHES

Hot flushes are experienced by more than 85 percent of menopausal women, although both their frequency and severity can vary greatly from person to person. During a hot flush, a woman can perspire so profusely that perspiration runs down her face, neck and back; her skin will rise in temperature, her heart will beat faster and she may well also experience palpitations. From time to time a woman may actually faint during a hot flush, although this is rare.

Hot flushes occur because the brain decides that the body is overheated. We now know that this is because the natural temperature set-point (the temperature above which the brain considers the body too hot, and below which it considers it too cold) becomes lowered. This means that even under normal conditions the brain may think that the body's temperature is too high, and responds by increasing the blood flow through the skin to reduce it. The skin then reddens and begins to perspire, and when the sweat starts to evaporate, the body temperature cools down again. Even though a hot flush may feel most severe in the head, face and neck, the rise in temperature actually occurs throughout the body. Even finger and toe temperatures rise sharply at the beginning of a hot flush.

In a Danish study of menopausal women, one third of those interviewed continued to have hot flushes for ten years after their last period and in the most severe cases, women had hot flushes six or seven times every hour. Two out of three women suffered hot flushes well before their last menstrual period, but for most the frequency increased dramatically at the menopause and continued for about the next five or six years.

The discomfort experienced during a hot flush is unique – it is not the same as being overheated. In one study, investigators tried to induce hot flushes by using hot-water bottles and blankets but discovered that applying direct external heat does not produce the same dramatic changes in heart rate and blood pressure as a menopausal flush does.

HOT FLUSHES SELF-HELP

The following simple measures can relieve symptoms.

• *Record your flushes; try to avoid recurrence of situations that act as a trigger.*

• *Don't wear synthetic fabrics, and avoid clothes with high necks and long sleeves.*

• *Discover ways of cooling down: keep a thermos flask of iced water near you, take a cold shower, or use a fan.*

• *Give up smoking.*

• *Try taking vitamin E. One thousand international units a day is recommended. Avoid vitamin E if you suffer from diabetes or heart problems.*

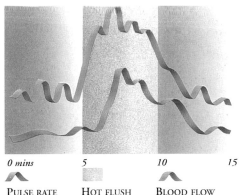

| 0 mins | 5 | 10 | 15 |

PULSE RATE   HOT FLUSH   BLOOD FLOW

Hot flush sensation
Before you experience a flush, your blood flow (see above) increases dramatically and your pulse rate becomes faster. Flushes usually last for about three to five minutes.

277

The following simple measures can relieve symptoms.

• *Keep your bedroom temperature fairly cool, and leave a window open if possible.*

• *Avoid nightclothes and bed linen made of nylon or polyester; cotton fabrics will be more comfortable.*

• *Keep a bowl of tepid water and a sponge by your bed so that you can cool yourself down easily. Never use cold water, as it can cause you to overheat. Allow the water to evaporate on your skin – as it does so it will take the heat from it and make you feel cooler.*

COMPLEMENTARY THERAPY

The products that are most frequently suggested by herbalists and homeopaths for hot flushes are lachesis, fo-ti-tieng, pulsatilla, white willow, wild yam root, dong quai, soya beans, black cohosh and sage. You can find all of them in most healthfood shops and at pharmacies that stock natural products. Alternatively, you can consult a qualified homeopath or herbalist.

Sage, dong quai and black cohosh contain oestrogen-like substances. It is the mild oestrogenic effect that they exert on the body that may help to compensate for declining levels of natural hormone.

Acupuncture can relieve hot flushes. Both electro-stimulated acupuncture (ESA) and superficial needles position acupuncture (SNPA) decreased the number of flushes by almost half in a sample of menopausal women in Stockholm. This change persisted for three months after the treatment.

DIET AND EXERCISE

Limiting your intake of foods and drinks that trigger hot flushes can help reduce their intensity. These include sugary, salty, spicy or hot dishes, chocolate, alcohol, coffee, tea and cola drinks. Avoid large meals (small, regular ones are better) and include soya-based products, such as soya sauce and tofu, and citrus fruits – all of which have oestrogenic properties – in your diet. Taking regular exercise helps too; women who exercise regularly have fewer hot flushes than those who do not.

NIGHT SWEATS

The night-time equivalent of the hot flush is the night sweat, in which you wake up hot and drenched in perspiration. Most women who experience night sweats also have hot flushes during the daytime but the reverse isn't always so. Night sweats can very occasionally be a symptom of stress, or a disease that is unrelated to the menopause – if you consult your doctor, he or she will be able to make a diagnosis.

Sleeplessness in menopausal women is nearly always linked to night sweats. Sufferers describe waking up, so drenched in perspiration that they have to get up to change their nightclothes and bed linen.

We know from research that a night sweat is a physiological process involving a fever that lasts a minute or two and then disappears. The heart rhythm goes wild, the body temperature rises and the woman is left with a sweaty face and chest, followed by a feeling of being chilled. Some women with severe and frequent night sweats become very depressed. Furthermore, their depression doesn't go away until the night sweats are brought under control.

COMPLEMENTARY THERAPY

There are several herbal remedies that may alleviate insomnia. Scullcap, for instance, is generally regarded as a good sedative herb, and can be combined with lemon balm to treat anxiety that leads to insomnia. Camomile also has soothing properties and makes a refreshing and effective herbal tea, as does sage. Sage tea has a particularly strong taste but if it is not to your liking, you can buy sage in tablet form from any good herbalist. Agnus castus is an excellent general herb for many menopausal symptoms including both hot flushes and night sweats; since it may help to normalize female hormone levels, it acts as a natural type of HRT.

Relaxation can be particularly therapeutic because it calms the mind and body, which in turn normalizes body chemistry and makes the skin sweat less. Meditation can be useful too. It slows down your metabolism, and it can slow down your brain waves from the fast beta waves that are characteristic of the normal working day to a slower alpha or theta wave, the wave pattern that occurs just before sleeping – if you can achieve this state it can be as restful as sleep. See pages 308–309 for a selection of simple but effective relaxation and meditation techniques. Or try yoga, which can have a calming effect. See page 346 for some easy-to-practise techniques.

DIET AND EXERCISE

Avoiding the types of food and drink listed on page 278 can help alleviate the frequency and intensity of night sweats as well as hot flushes. In addition, try to avoid eating large meals late in the evening if you suffer from night sweats; if possible, eat your main meal during the day at lunchtime and have only a light supper during the early part of the evening.

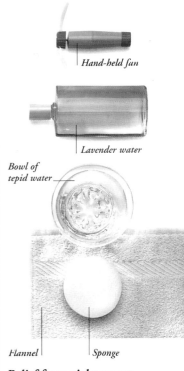

Hand-held fan

Lavender water

Bowl of tepid water

Flannel *Sponge*

Relief from night sweats
Cooling yourself with tepid water will help ease the discomfort of a night sweat. A battery-operated fan and scented lavender water can also be efficient cooling aids.

VAGINAL AND URINARY SYMPTOMS

Urogenital problems are very common during the menopause, yet only four in ten women consult their doctor about them. Anatomically, the vagina and the lower urinary tract lie very close together, separated by just a few layers of cells. They both decline when there is lack of oestrogen by becoming thin and dry.

Urinary symptoms include discomfort in passing urine, and frequent and urgent urination, even when there is very little liquid in the bladder. There may also be some dribbling because the sphincter muscle guarding the exit from the bladder becomes weak due to low oestrogen levels. From time to time, urine escapes from the bladder on laughing, coughing or carrying a heavy weight. This is called stress incontinence and is due to increased pressure inside the abdomen squeezing urine from the bladder. With many of these symptoms you could also have genital dryness and itching. Vaginal soreness, particularly during or after intercourse because the vagina fails to lubricate, is also very common among menopausal and postmenopausal women.

COMPLEMENTARY THERAPY

Herbs that may relieve urinary symptoms include buchu, cornsilk, and uva-ursi, which has some antiseptic properties. Goldenseal is believed to have some anti-infective properties.

DIET AND EXERCISE

Keep your bladder flushed out by drinking at least two litres (about four pints) of fluid a day – water is best. Try cranberry juice too; this is especially effective if you are prone to cystitis. Exercise can also help to keep your vaginal area supple. Swimming is a particularly good exercise – but so is regular sex or masturbation.

Kegel exercises strengthen pelvic muscles, combat urinary incontinence and make sex more pleasurable, and are simple to do. To find out which muscles to exercise, next time you go to the toilet stop urinating in midstream by contracting your muscles; these are your pelvic floor muscles. Using these muscles, draw them up, hold for a count of five, then relax. Repeat this five times and do at least ten times a day.

MUSCLE AND JOINT SYMPTOMS

Collagen is a protein that provides the scaffolding for every tissue in the body, and when it begins to disintegrate at the menopause, muscles lose their bulk, strength and coordination, and joints become stiff. Muscles become more prone to soreness and stiffness after exercise, and joints may swell so that their mobility becomes restricted. If you retain fluid, you may get pins and needles or numbness in the hands.

Osteoporosis (often called the brittle bones disease) causes aches and pains all over the body, especially in the upper back, due to the thinning of vertebral bones.

General fatigue at the menopause may be profound. Although underused muscles and joints can be a major factor, there are other causes of chronic fatigue that do not necessarily have any direct connection with the menopause, such as low blood sugar, anaemia and an underactive thyroid gland. Make sure that you get your doctor to check out all of these possibilities if you are experiencing disabling fatigue.

COMPLEMENTARY THERAPY

If you are suffering from stiff and swollen joints, a poultice made with cayenne pepper may be helpful. Other herbal remedies that could be effective include alfalfa, sarsaparilla, feverfew and white willow. Juniper, rosemary and lavender essential oils may relieve pain when they are diluted with a base oil and used in a local massage or compress, and basil diluted with a base oil may alleviate fatigue.

DIET AND EXERCISE

Diet can help protect your muscles, bones and joints, and in particular a diet containing increased amounts of calcium: dairy foods are high in calcium (cheeses such as Parmesan and cheddar are particularly good), as are oily fish, such as sardines and whitebait, and soya-based products, such as soya sauce and tofu. If you don't feel that you can increase your calcium-rich food intake easily, ask your doctor to recommend a good calcium supplement. In addition to a calcium-rich diet, weight-bearing exercises, such as skipping, brisk walking and dancing, are known to help strengthen bones.

MUSCLE AND JOINT SELF-HELP

Try to exercise regularly. If you keep your muscles strong with exercise you will be more agile and, if you do trip up, muscle strength and coordination will help you fall with less impact.

PREMENSTRUAL SYNDROME

If you have suffered from premenstrual syndrome (PMS) all your life, you are more likely to experience intensified symptoms, such as fatigue, anxiety, irritability, tearfulness, breast soreness, water retention, skin problems and insomnia as you become menopausal. If you suspect that your mood swings are PMS-related, you can confirm it by charting your symptoms daily for three months.

COMPLEMENTARY THERAPY

The standard remedy for PMS is evening primrose oil, which is widely available from healthfood shops and most chemists. Other herbs that may be useful include beth root, which can help alleviate very heavy or irregular periods, and black cohosh. Aromatherapists recommend the oils of ylang-ylang, lavender and lemon grass, which you can use in a warm bath.

DIET AND EXERCISE

Premenstrual symptoms should disappear along with your periods, but while you are still menstruating there is no instant cure. You can lessen the problem, however, if you try to avoid stressful situations and eat a regular,

CHANGES DUE TO COLLAGEN DEFICIENCY	
Skin	Dryness or oiliness, wrinkles, flaking, bruises easily, wounds heal slowly, patches of brown pigmentation, prominent veins
Nails	Brittleness, white spots, splinter haemorrhages
Eyes	Dryness, dark circles under eyes, small yellow lumps of fat on the white part of the eyes, night vision deteriorates, red blood vessels around the corners of the eyes
Gums	Bleeding and sponginess, recession leaving tooth roots exposed, infection and periodontal disease, which causes bad breath
Hair	Dullness, dryness, oiliness, split ends, poor growth, thin patches, dermatitis of the scalp, hair loss, dandruff
Mouth	Cracks on the corners of the lips, mouth ulcers that are slow to heal
Tongue	The sides may become scalloped and the tongue thinner and smoother

balanced diet throughout the month, avoiding sugar and salt (salt increases water retention and bloating). Avoiding alcohol before your period starts could also help. Exercise can alleviate premenstrual symptoms too: it's a great mood-lifter and can help work off tension and anxiety.

FACE AND SKIN SYMPTOMS

The lowered levels of oestrogen that occur at the menopause cause changes in the skin, hair, nails, eyes, mouth and gums. These changes are in part due to the disintegration of collagen fibres and the weakening of the protein elastin, which gives connective tissue its strength and suppleness. One of the most noticeable changes is the appearance of wrinkles in the facial skin. Deterioration of nerve endings in the ageing skin can lead to itchiness and a condition called formication, an intense tingling that some women describe as a feeling that insects are crawling across their skin. Formication is a classic symptom of menopausal distress. In a study of 5,000 women, one in five suffered from it within 12–24 months after their last menstrual period. About one in ten women continues to suffer from formication for more than 12 years after the menopause.

DIET AND EXERCISE

Make sure that you eat foods rich in vitamins A, B, C and E in addition to potassium, zinc, magnesium, bio-flavonoids, iron and calcium (for examples of vitamin- and mineral-rich foods, see page 316 and page 318). Drinking two litres (about four pints) of water a day will not only help keep your bladder healthy, it will have a noticeable effect on your skin and hair too. Regular exercise – even a daily brisk walk in the fresh air – can also benefit your skin.

SEXUAL SYTMPTOMS

A common myth about the menopause is that it marks the beginning of a woman's sexual decline. Nothing could be further from the truth. The majority of women can continue to experience sexual pleasure well into old age. Most menopausal women, however, notice some changes in the way their bodies respond during arousal and sex. This is often due to physical changes in the urogenital tract rather than a decreased emotional desire for sex. One of the most common sexual problems after

SEXUAL SELF-HELP

The following simple measures can help increase your sexual enjoyment.

• *Before sex, put sterile, water-soluble jelly on your vaginal entrance, and a small amount inside your vagina and on your partner's penis.*

• *Avoid douches, talcum powder, perfumed toilet papers and bath oils and foams; they can irritate the vagina.*

• *Avoid washing the inside of your labia with soap as it will dry the skin.*

• *Spend longer on foreplay to give your body more time to lubricate.*

The sexual woman
Ideally, the menopause should be a time when we become more open and uninhibited about our bodies.

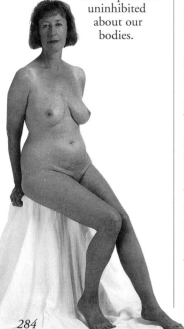

the menopause is lack of lubrication. The vaginal lining may actually crack and bleed and this can make penetration painful, and sometimes impossible.

In youth, blood flows quickly to the genitals during arousal, causing swelling and sensitivity to touch. After the menopause, however, there is less engorgement of the clitoris, the vagina and the vulva, leading to a more subdued arousal.

The breasts also increase in size during sexual arousal in young women – by as much as a quarter in some cases. The rush of blood to the tiny veins of the breasts that causes this does not occur so often after the level of oestrogen has declined and as a result the breasts may no longer be so sensitive to stroking. Another part of the sexual response that disappears is the "sex flush" – the rash that may appear on a woman's chest and body just before orgasm. This does not affect sexual enjoyment, but it does show that your body responds to sexual arousal differently from the way it used to.

In a young woman, the vagina expands during sexual arousal to allow easy penetration. After the menopause, the vagina does not expand so much, but it still remains large enough to accommodate an erect penis (as long as you allow time to achieve proper lubrication). Sexual desire can also be diminished by certain drugs, such as tranquillizers, muscle relaxants, antidepressants, amphetamines, diuretics, antihypertensives and hormones.

Women who have had a hysterectomy or surgical removal of the ovaries may also experience a diminished enjoyment of sex and a reduced ability to reach orgasm.

COMPLEMENTARY THERAPY

Herbs have always been used to treat low sex drive, although some, such as nutmeg, have been found to irritate the urogenital system and should be avoided. Many plants, such as ginseng and saffron crocus, are widely used for their aphrodisiac properties. The bark of an African tree, *yohimbine*, is the source of several drugs used to treat impotence.

DIET AND EXERCISE

Hypothyroidism becomes more common in the menopausal years, and may be a cause of low sexual desire. Since several minerals, most importantly zinc, can help activate the thyroid gland, adding zinc-rich foods such as wheatgerm and sardines to your diet can help symptoms, as can avoiding foods such as turnips, kale, cabbage and soya beans, which contain an anti-thyroid substance. Stress, such as bereavement, moving house and family problems can also adversely affect sex drive, and too much sugar, fat, coffee or alcohol place a strain on the body. Practising Kegel exercises regularly will give you better toned pelvic muscles, which will enable you to grip your partner's penis more tightly and increase your sexual enjoyment.

INSOMNIA

If you are feeling depressed or anxious, or if you are suffering badly from night sweats, it can become very difficult to get to sleep and quite common to wake early in the morning. Eventually, a good night's rest can become something of a rarity.

Women who have normal levels of oestrogen fall asleep faster than women who don't and spend more time in the deepest (dream) stage of sleep; they also feel more refreshed when they wake up. Dreaming seems to be particularly important for the feeling of rest and renewal that comes from sleeping. Without oestrogen, we can sleep for a whole night but we can still feel very tired when we wake up.

COMPLEMENTARY THERAPY

Valerian root has been used for many centuries as a sleep-inducing herb and its sedative effect can be very therapeutic during the menopausal years. Insomnia can also be alleviated by night-time infusions of herbs such as passion flower, catnip, camomile and hops.

DIET AND EXERCISE

The traditional glass of warm milk at bedtime does actually work for many insomniacs (this could be due to the action of calcium on the nerves) and is always worth trying. If you can, avoid eating large, heavy meals in the evening and in particular, eat your evening meal early, preferably before seven, and try to avoid caffeinated coffees and teas. A long walk about an hour before bedtime, or some other form of aerobic exercise, can also improve the quality of your sleep.

The following simple measures can relieve symptoms.

• *Rid yourself of night sweats or bring them under control so that you can sleep undisturbed.*

• *Read a good book, or a chapter from a good book; getting you "out" of yourself, will help you relax, which should make it easier to go to sleep.*

STOMACH AND BOWEL SYMPTOMS

Bloating with abdominal distension may be a problem during the menopausal years. As we age, small pockets of tissue may balloon out from the bowel, giving rise to the condition called diverticulitis. Within these small pockets (*diverticula*) food may lodge, become stale, ferment and produce large amounts of gas. The intestine may end up coated with food remnants that form small centres of fermentation. It is quite common for the sufferer to wake in the morning with a flat stomach and for the abdomen to swell as the day progresses, so that by bedtime the swelling resembles a six-month pregnancy! During the night, lack of food and sugar in the intestine allows fermentation to abate. After a breakfast that contains sugars and yeasts, fermentation in the bowels flares up again.

Because the female hormones progesterone and oestrogen affect the speed at which food moves through the intestines – progesterone reduces movement so that bowel motions become infrequent, dry and pebble-like while oestrogen speeds them up, enabling the stools to revert to a normal consistency and frequency – constipation is another frequent menopause symptom.

COMPLEMENTARY THERAPY

There are several homeopathic and herbal remedies widely available that can relieve stomach and bowel symptoms, such as the Bach Flower Remedies. Gentle "scouring" herbs and foods, such as sunflower seeds, may help, and senna has a mild purgative action. Some people recommend colonic irrigation, in which the lower part of the intestine is flushed out with water.

DIET AND EXERCISE

The classic cures for improving stomach and bowel symptoms are nearly all diet-based. Following a high fibre diet and drinking plenty of fluids will help keep your bowels normal (see page 319 for examples of high fibre foods). Foods that cause fermentation, such as yeast-based products and sugar, should either be avoided or eaten only in the early part of the day. And if you suffer from constipation, the best cure is still a natural one – lots of figs and prunes!

BREAST SYMPTOMS

Most women experience breast discomfort in the week before they menstruate, due to fluid retention in the breast tissue and a consequent increase in breast tension. As women reach their early 40s, this discomfort may develop into a more severe pain called mastalgia. The breasts become hard, tender and extremely painful. An attack of mastalgia can last for up to ten days.

In severe cases, the breasts can be so painful that you cannot bear anything to touch them. Pain is especially intense in the nipples, and may keep you awake at night; even turning over in bed can be agony. It is estimated that 70 percent of women in this country suffer from breast pain at some time in their lives, but particularly in the pre- and perimenopausal years.

Mastalgia can often be cyclical, fluctuating with the menstrual cycle and usually becoming worse immediately before menstruation. But non-cyclical mastalgia can occur at any time of the month and is most common in women over 40 years of age. The causes are not completely understood, but mastalgia may stem from abnormal sensitivity of breast tissue to the fluctuation of the female hormones at the menopause.

If you are suffering from severe mastalgia, you may be frightened that the pain is due to breast cancer. In the majority of cases, mastalgia is a benign condition, but you should see your doctor or have a mammogram if you need reassurance.

COMPLEMENTARY THERAPY

One of the essential fatty acids, gamolenic acid, which is found in evening primrose oil, significantly reduces breast pain in up to 70 percent of women and has not been found to have any side effects.

DIET AND EXERCISE

A bad diet can make breast problems worse. Women who suffer from breast pain tend to have low levels of essential fatty acids and eat high levels of saturated fat; saturated fat seems to exaggerate the effects of female hormones on breast tissue. Cutting down the amount of saturated fat you eat can help relieve your symptoms – see pages 320–321 for more information on this.

BREAST SELF-HELP

One of the simplest things you can do to help maintain breast health is to examine yourself for lumps regularly, at least once a month, by following the steps below.

* *Stand naked in front of a mirror with your arms by your sides.*

* *Now raise them and put your hands behind your head; look for differences in the shape or texture of both the breasts and nipples.*

* *Now feel your breasts; lie on your back with your shoulders slightly raised.*

* *Hold your fingers flat and carefully examine each section of your breasts, using gentle circular movements (use your right hand to feel your left breast and vice versa).*

* *Move your hand in a clockwise circular direction on the left breast and anti-clockwise on the right; keep the arm you aren't using by your side.*

* *Complete your examination by extending the arm you are not using behind your head and checking for lumps along the collar bone and in your armpits.*

MONITORING YOUR WEIGHT

Following the simple steps below will tell you whether you need to lose weight.

• *Check your weight (see right, below).*

• *Check to see if you carry more weight around your stomach and waist than around your hips and thighs – the former carries a greater risk of heart disease.*

• *Find your waist-to-hip ratio by measuring your waist at its narrowest point and your hips at their widest. Ratios above 0.8 are linked to an increased risk of diabetes, heart disease, high blood pressure, osteoporosis and arthritis. If you are in this category, discuss it with your doctor.*

WEIGHT GAIN

Some postmenopausal women strive to maintain their premenopausal weight. Medically this is quite unsound: the weight that you may gain at the menopause is due to a slower metabolism – something that affects men and women as they grow older – and a decline in oestrogen levels, which affects the way that fat is distributed.

Middle-aged women who are 3.5–4.5 kg (8–12 lb) underweight live less long than those who are 3.5–4.5 kg (8–12 lb) overweight. I don't wish to encourage any woman to become obese, but I do wish to free her from the pressure to be thin.

DIET AND EXERCISE

Unless you are so overweight that your health is being affected, a little weight gain at the menopause requires no treatment. But if your weight is posing a threat to your health, and you have other risk factors for heart disease, such as high blood pressure and smoking, then it is a good idea to make changes to your diet. It is important, however, to be realistic and to be aware that changes in body shape happen to all postmenopausal women. Excessive dieting is unhealthy, and it may mean that you fail to meet your daily calcium requirements. By eating healthy foods and exercising regularly, you should remain fit and not gain weight. If you were not overweight before the menopause and are no more than 6–8 kg (13–18 lb) more after it, and if your waist-to-hip ratio is not in the high risk category, then there is no health advantage in reducing your weight.

LOWERING OF THE VOICE

There are two reasons for the voice deepening after the menopause. First, there is a relative increase in the male hormones, or androgens, circulating in the blood. Long after ovaries stop secreting oestrogen, they continue to secrete androgens. This relative excess of male hormones has a masculinizing effect on various organs of the body, causing a deepening of the voice.

The second cause is a hypothyroidism (underactive thyroid), where the voice becomes deep, gruff and slightly hoarse, and there are other symptoms, such as hair loss, a tendency to feel the cold, and fatigue. If you are suffering from hypothyroidism, your voice will return to normal when you start to take thyroid supplements. If you feel medical treatment is necessary, you should consult your doctor as soon as you notice that your voice is deepening.

HEART SYMPTOMS

After the menopause, heart disease becomes as common in women as it is in men. Heart problems are rare in pre-menopausal women because of the presence of oestrogen. Angina, a crushing pain in the middle of the chest brought on by effort and alleviated by rest, is the warning sign. Without rest, the pain can worsen and radiate up into the neck, teeth and down the arm. Eventually the pain will become so bad that you will be forced to stop what you are doing. Angina is the sign that insufficient oxygen is reaching your heart muscle. You should take chest pain seriously and go to your doctor for a cardiac check-up.

Other symptoms relating to heart health include palpitations and shortness of breath on exertion. You may find that normal exercise leaves you unusually breathless and climbing up several flights of stairs gives you a pumping, fluttery feeling in your chest.

If you are suffering from other symptoms, such as dizziness, headaches or blurred vision, have your blood pressure checked, as you may have hypertension.

DIET AND EXERCISE

Because obesity is a risk factor in heart disease, you should try to lose weight if you are more than a few kilograms over your ideal weight. Cut back on saturated fats, avoid sugar and other "empty calorie" foods and try to limit the amount of salt you eat. A diet that is high in fruit and vegetables, oily fish and pulses, and low in animal fats and rich dairy products, can help lower your cholesterol levels and reduce the risk of heart problems. Garlic can improve your cardiovascular health, too; use it in cooking or take garlic pearls, which are odourless. There is a very clear, direct link between smoking and increased risks of heart disease; stopping smoking – the earlier the better – is therefore one of the most effective measures any woman can take to protect her heart.

Regular aerobic exercise helps to strengthen a weak heart and will also help to reduce high blood pressure, which can lead to heart problems. Try swimming,

MEDICAL TREATMENT FOR HEART SYMPTOMS

There is a wide range of drugs to treat heart conditions, including hypotensives, betablockers, diuretics, cardiac stimulants and coronary vasodilators.

Angina, for instance, can be controlled by taking a coronary vasodilator drug whenever you have an attack – you can even take one of these tablets before exercising to prevent angina in the first place.

If you suffer from high cholesterol, your doctor will probably prescribe drugs to lower it to reduce the possibility of serious heart complications, and will recommend that you change your diet (see left).

If you develop heart disease, treatments available include an artificial pace-maker, a coronary bypass operation or balloon angioplasty, depending on the type of heart condition you have.

Body shape and heart disease

Before the menopause, the waist-to-hip ratio is less than 0.8 and there is a correspondingly low risk of heart disease. After the menopause, fat distribution changes and the risk of heart disease increases. You can assess your risk by dividing your waist measurement by your hip measurement. If the resulting figure is over 0.8 you fall into a higher risk group for heart disease.

For example:

74 ÷ 99cm = 0.74 (low risk)
81 ÷ 99cm = 0.81 (higher risk)

KEY

■ WAIST MEASUREMENT

■ HIP MEASUREMENT

PREMENOPAUSE   POSTMENOPAUSE

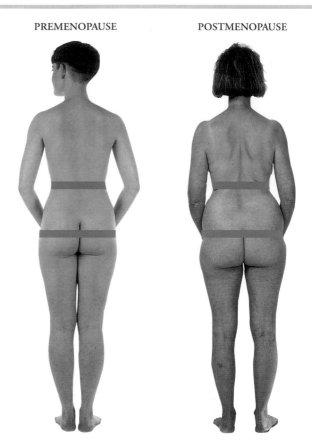

cycling and running, if you don't particularly like the idea of exercise classes. If you already have heart problems, consult your doctor before starting exercising.

EMOTIONAL SYMPTOMS

Feelings such as tension, anxiety, depression, listlessness, irritability and mood swings can occur at any age, but they rarely occur together, or as frequently, as they do during the menopause. This is because the centres in the brain that control your sense of well-being, a positive state of mind and a feeling of control and tranquillity are all affected by the absence of the oestrogen hormone, so for many women, menopausal mood changes resemble a roller-coaster ride. They describe subtle sensations such as trembling, fluttering, unease and discomfort. More severe feelings of anxiety or panic can arise with little or no provocation. Tasks that you used to be able to tackle easily can now leave you in total disarray. Mood swings from wild elation to deep despondency are quite common, and patience can be all too easily exhausted. The future may look bleak, your loss of self-esteem is precipitous and you may feel truly depressed.

A major depression, although rare, can descend upon you during your menopausal years, and this is distinct from any other emotional symptoms that you may experience, such as tearfulness and anxiety. The following are all possible predictors:
• A past or recent history of stressful events.
• A surgically induced menopause.
• Having negative expectations of the menopause.
• Severe hot flushes and night sweats.
• A family history of depressive illness.

Depression can be a debilitating illness that can last for weeks, months or even years if left untreated. As a woman, you're more likely to experience a depression than a man. Consult your doctor for professional help if you have experienced four of these symptoms for at least two weeks:
• Extreme eating patterns, such as bingeing.
• Unusual sleeping patterns.
• Being exceptionally lethargic or restless.
• An inability to enjoy a once pleasurable activity, including loss of sex drive.
• Debilitating fatigue or loss of energy.
• Feelings of worthlessness and self-reproach.
• Difficulty in concentrating and making even simple decisions.
• Thoughts of death or suicide, or suicide attempts (seek help straightaway).

COMPLEMENTARY THERAPY

Herbs that may have a calming effect are passion flower and valerian root. Passion flower helps insomnia and elevates the levels of serotonin in the blood, which creates a feeling of well-being. Adding an infusion of your favourite herbs to the bathwater can also be therapeutic.

Menopausal depression may be alleviated by ginger root, cayenne pepper, dandelion root and Siberian ginseng, all of which may work because they contain essential nutrients. Ginseng can have a tonic effect, and Siberian ginseng and liquorice root are also considered to be very effective in combatting lassitude and depression.

EMOTIONAL SELF-HELP

Emotional symptoms will be easier to cope with if you follow the guidelines below.

• *Share your feelings with your partner. Severe mood swings and irritability can distance you from your partner and can jeopardize a relationship.*

• *Think about joining a self-help group, or starting one yourself. Women who go to these groups may be better able to deal with depression.*

NATURAL PROGESTERONE

In the last few years there has been much media hype about the effectiveness of so-called "natural" progesterone for the treatment of menopausal symptoms. Lost in the hype, several important scientific facts have been ignored.

- *It is not natural to give progesterone for menopausal symptoms, nor is it scientifically or medically logical. Menopause symptoms are related to lack of oestrogen; progesterone in whatever form will not touch them.*

- *The original research work on progesterone for the menopause certainly does not show that it is useful for menopausal women.*

- *Advocates of natural progesterone claim it is beneficial for osteoporosis but the National Osteoporosis Society (NOS) opposes this view.*

- *It is claimed we are bombarded by xeno-oestrogens in packaging, plastics, foods and pesticides and so we need progesterone to restore the balance, an idea that is at best no more than conjecture.*

DIET AND EXERCISE

Exercise can help hot flushes and night sweats, which can often be a contributing factor to menopausal emotional problems and depression. Exercise can lift the mood and produce an "exercise high" that can last up to eight hours; try to have 20–30 minutes of short and sustained bouts of vigorous activity every morning to help you through the day. Relaxation techniques and meditation can promote tranquillity and combat anxiety and tension as well as improve suppleness, and are also worth trying on a regular basis). Yoga, with its unique combination of exercise and relaxation techniques, could also work well).

INTELLECTUAL SYMPTOMS

Forgetfulness is one of the most common symptoms that menopausal women complain of, and they may experience it long before they stop menstruating. You may forget where you put something, you may miss appointments and things that used to be simple to remember can suddenly require enormous effort. The ability to concentrate can also become difficult. These problems combined can make it hard to carry out work that involves complex assessments and major decision-making. Even minor decisions can sometimes be paralysing.

DIET AND EXERCISE

Relatively little research has been conducted on the effects that nutrients have on intellectual processes, but there is some evidence that vitamins such as B[1] and B[12] and minerals like calcium and potassium may all contribute to brain health. All of these are easy to incorporate into a normal healthy diet (see page 316 and page 318 for vitamin and mineral-rich foods). Bear in mind, however, that most vitamins need to be taken in conjunction with other vitamins and minerals in order to be absorbed by the body. A shortage of one vital element can cause the others to be less effective (see pages 315–321, for further information).

Regular exercise also helps you feel more alert and less sluggish, and can improve concentration too. A brisk walk in the fresh air every day for at least 20 minutes will tone you up mentally as well as physically.

2

MENOPAUSAL MEDICAL COMPLAINTS

The falling levels of oestrogen during the
menopause, combined with the natural ageing
process in the postmenopausal years, means
that women can become increasingly susceptible
to illness. One of the most painful conditions
is osteoporosis, but there are also other serious
conditions, all of which can be overcome or
controlled with a combination of medical
and self-help measures.

OSTEOPOROSIS

A painful, crippling and life-threatening condition, osteoporosis is the single most important health hazard for women past the menopause – it is more common than heart disease, stroke, diabetes or breast cancer. In its early stages, it has no obvious symptoms, so many women may be unaware that they have it. Because of its life-threatening nature, it is vital that every woman be told the facts about this disease; women must become vigilant and take measures to prevent osteoporosis from destroying their lives.

The clinical definition of osteoporosis is "a condition where there is less normal bone than expected for a woman's age, with an increased risk of fracture." However, some experts use the term "osteoporosis" to describe low bone density where fractures have already occurred.

WHY IT HAPPENS

As oestrogen and progesterone levels fall, bones begin to lose mass by 0.5–3 percent a year. By the time a woman is 80, she can easily have lost 40 percent of the bone mass in her body.

Oestrogen facilitates the uptake of calcium from the blood into the bone and inhibits its loss. A fall in oestrogen levels, therefore, leads to bone disintegration.

For a woman with severe osteoporosis of the spine, even minor knocks, jolts or falls can cause the spinal bones to fracture.

BONE DENSITY TESTS

There are several different ways of assessing bone density, and a scan is considered the best predictor of fracture. Bone density tests measure the density of the spine, wrist and other high-risk areas. A decrease in bone mineral density (BMD) measured in the spine or the hip may indicate a 200 percent increase in the chance of any fracture, and a staggering 300 percent increase in the chance of a hip fracture.

PHYSIOTHERAPY

Physiotherapy is often overlooked, but it should be an important part of your treatment for osteoporosis. A home exercise programme can be established to continue the treatment. Increased muscle strength, improved spinal power and posture, maintenance of bone strength, relief of pain, and toning of pelvic floor muscles to cope with stress incontinence are all benefits of physiotherapy.

Physiotherapists may also use various forms of electrotherapy or ultrasound to help relieve pain. Some now also use complementary techniques such as acupuncture, and recommend the use of heat pads, hot-water bottles or ice packs at home. TENS (Transcutaneous Electrical Nerve Stimulation) machines are available in most treatment centres for pain relief.

PREVENTING OSTEOPOROSIS

Since all of us are at risk of developing osteoporosis, it is important that we adopt self-help measures to build up our natural resistance. Fortunately, there are a number of ways we can change our lifestyles to help maintain healthy bones.

Regular exercise, a balanced diet and mental alertness can help to maintain overall fitness, and you should also have regular health checks with your doctor.

Where possible, reduce the hazards in your home by removing any trailing electrical flexes and loose carpets. Make sure that there is always a firm handrail on stairs and be particularly on guard when walking on slippery or uneven surfaces.

Women who take exercise twice a week have denser bones than those who take exercise once a week, who, in turn, have denser bones than those who never take exercise at all. It is never too late to improve your body. Bones can be strengthened to resist the effect of oestrogen depletion during the postmenopausal years.

Eat a calcium-rich diet The most important dietary advice for the early prevention of osteoporosis is to eat calcium-rich foods (see page 318 for examples of calcium-rich foods). In brief, to prevent your bones from becoming brittle, you need calcium for bone mass, vitamin D to absorb the calcium into your body and oestrogen to maintain the calcium inside your bones.

Common fracture sites
Women with osteoporosis characteristically suffer from fractures of the wrists, hip bones, vertebrae, pelvis and shoulder bones.

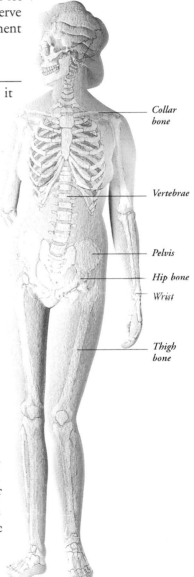

Collar bone

Vertebrae

Pelvis

Hip bone

Wrist

Thigh bone

HEART ATTACKS AND STROKES

Heart attacks and strokes stem from a disease of the arteries that narrows the artery channels, reduces blood flow and increases blood pressure (see below). Arteries become furred up by fat and prone to blockage.

RISK FACTORS

Your chances of suffering from disease of the arteries are increased by obesity, smoking, lack of exercise, high blood pressure and being menopausal and postmenopausal. Women who develop heart disease after the menopause should pay particular attention to the risk factors under their control, such as smoking, diet and stress levels.

When blood flow becomes impeded – generally after a number of years – you may experience angina, which is pain in the chest on exertion, or intermittent claudication, which is leg pain brought on by walking and alleviated by rest. If blood flow is restricted in the arteries supplying the brain, you may experience temporary stroke symptoms, dizziness and fainting attacks. Kidney failure is also possible if the renal artery becomes narrowed.

PREVENTION

Lowering risk factors, especially in early adulthood and midlife, can help prevent disease of the arteries from developing. You should try to give up smoking, have your blood pressure checked regularly, and get high blood pressure treated. Keep your diet low in saturated fats, and if your cholesterol levels still remain high, you may need medication. Regular exercise is essential.

HIGH BLOOD PRESSURE

Measurements for blood pressure are expressed as two figures: 120/80. A blood pressure that is consistently above 160/95 is considered high.

An increase in blood pressure occurs when there is resistance in the blood vessels to the flow of blood. Resistance rises in the large blood vessels because of increased rigidity due to age, and occurs in the small blood vessels when they become constricted because of nerve or chemical control.

RISK FACTORS

Apart from being postmenopausal, other risk factors for essential hypertension (high blood pressure) include smoking, obesity, excessive alcohol consumption, a family history of high blood pressure, a sedentary lifestyle, stress and old age.

SELF-HELP

High blood pressure can often be reduced by making changes to your lifestyle. If you smoke, you should give up or at the very least cut down. You should also assess your alcohol intake. If you are a heavy drinker you should cut down drastically or try and stop drinking altogether. If you are overweight, you should try to lose weight and exercise more. Dietary measures could include cutting down on salt intake and eating less fatty food (see Good Nutrition, pages 314–321).

Biofeedback training can be helpful to some patients in reducing their blood pressure. This involves learning breathing and relaxation techniques. During a biofeedback session your blood pressure is continuously monitored and you learn to respond immediately to any increase in blood pressure by practising breathing and relaxation techniques.

STROKE

This is a potentially fatal result of hypertension (high blood pressure). Sixty percent of strokes are caused by a cerebral thrombosis, when an artery in the brain becomes blocked by a clot (thrombus) that has built up in its wall.

About a third of major strokes are fatal. A third result in some disability with speech or movement and a third have no long-term ill effects. Strokes are rare before the age of 60, but thereafter the risk increases rapidly.

SELF-HELP

After hospital treatment, stroke patients spend most of their recovery period at home relearning how to use the parts of their body that may have been paralysed. There are many self-help aids available that can make life easier, such as easy-to-hold cutlery. Dressing in front of a mirror may speed up relearning.

UROGENITAL AGEING

When oestrogen is plentiful, the bladder, urethra and vagina keep healthy. When hormone levels fall during the menopause the urogenital system thins, atrophies and becomes susceptible to infection.

SYMPTOMS

Signs of genital atrophy include a dry, itchy vagina and vulva, which causes pain during sex. These symptoms are often combined with the frequent, urgent desire to urinate, and incontinence. This combination of symptoms, known as urogenital syndrome, is the most common reason for women over the age of 55 to visit a gynaecologist.

CYSTITIS

Oestrogen is so crucial to the health of the urinary tract that after the menopause the bladder is far more vulnerable to bacterial infection. Cystitis, inflammation of the inner lining of the bladder, is most commonly caused by the *E. coli* bacterium.

SELF-HELP

Drink lots of water or diluted fruit juice at the beginning of an attack. *E. coli* cannot multiply in alkaline urine, and you can make your urine alkaline by taking a teaspoon of bicarbonate of soda in a glass of water. Drink this three times within five hours of the first twinge. Soluble aspirin and a hot-water bottle can help to relieve pain.

Each time you pass urine, wash your hands carefully. You should also wipe your perineum from front to back once with damp cotton wool. Soap and water can dry out the perineum and vagina and make you more prone to infection. When you dry yourself, pat gently.

If your cystitis is provoked by intercourse, it is probably best to refrain from sex until you are more comfortable. Otherwise, reduce friction with a lubricating jelly and experiment to find the most comfortable sexual position. You should also wash carefully and pass urine after sex.

PRURITIS VULVAE

Itching is a sign of oestrogen deficiency, and pruritis vulvae, chronic, uncontrollable itching of the vaginal area, is usually worst in hot weather or during the night.

Diabetes, vaginal yeast infections, such as thrush, and urinary tract infections, can all cause pruritis vulvae. However, it can be pyschogenic in origin. Repeated scratching can become more and more pleasurable, even to the point of orgasm. Eventually the sufferer will develop profound soreness and thickening of the skin in the vaginal area.

SELF-HELP

You can prevent pruritis vulvae from getting worse by trying not to scratch the vaginal area. Consult your doctor if it persists for more than two days – if you don't, you may find yourself in an unbreakable itch-scratch-itch cycle. Pay particular attention to normal hygiene but, if possible, avoid the use of soap and detergents as they will strip the skin of oils and make it more sensitive. Use only warm or cool water, and try applying a silicone-based hand cream to the itchy area after each wash. Ice packs may also help to numb the itch. Don't use local anaesthetic creams and sprays as these may cause allergic reactions.

INCONTINENCE

This occurs when the sphincter muscle at the base of your bladder becomes so weak (or the bladder muscle becomes overactive) that you have little or no control over the flow of urine. There are several types of incontinence – see right for the most common.

SELF-HELP

Mild incontinence is often due to weakened pelvic floor muscles, and you can improve your bladder control by doing Kegel exercises. These involve repeatedly contracting and relaxing the muscles of the urogenital tract. If you are suffering from urge incontinence, self-help measures include emptying your bladder every two hours, and avoiding diuretic drinks, such as tea and coffee. There are a number of aids available for incontinence sufferers. These include waterproof bed sheets, incontinence pads, female urinals and waterproof pants. However, you should consult your doctor long before these become necessary. If you suffer from stress incontinence when you exercise, try emptying your bladder beforehand. Wearing a tampon during exercise can act as a splint to the urethra.

TYPES OF INCONTINENCE

The following are the three most common types of incontinence.

Stress incontinence This is the leakage of a small amount of urine caused by an increase in pressure inside the abdomen when you sneeze, cough, laugh or lift a heavy object.

Urge incontinence This occurs if you wait until you need to urinate urgently. The bladder starts to contract involuntarily and empties itself. This type of incontinence is often triggered by a sudden change in position, such as standing up.

Mixed pattern incontinence This is a combination of both urge and stress incontinence, and may be the result of two faults in the bladder function.

MEDIUM TO HIGH RISK FACTORS

The following conditions can make you more prone to breast cancer.

- *Having a family history of breast cancer (especially close female relatives).*

- *Early onset of menstruation and a late menopause.*

- *Being over the age of 40.*

- *Having children later than average.*

- *Being Caucasian.*

- *Obesity or a diet high in animal or dairy fat.*

LOW RISK FACTORS

The following conditions will make you less prone to breast cancer.

- *Having several children.*

- *Breastfeeding.*

- *Being short and thin.*

- *Late onset of menstruation and an early menopause.*

BREAST CANCER

This is the most common type of cancer in women, and is the leading cause of death in women aged between 35 and 50. In the UK, women have a one in 12 lifetime chance of developing breast cancer.

MEDICAL TREATMENT

Most doctors will refer a woman with a breast lump to a hospital so that further tests can be made. If you have a cyst, the fluid can be removed and examined, and a clear-cut diagnosis made.

If the lump is small and shallow it is possible to have an outpatient lumpectomy. The lump is removed with some surrounding tissue and then examined in the laboratory. If cancer is discovered, blood tests, X-rays and bone scans will be carried out to help decide upon the right treatment.

Radical treatments, such as mastectomy, do not necessarily improve survival rates. Many surgeons now recommend lumpectomy combined with radiotherapy or anti-cancer drugs (chemotherapy).

OUTLOOK

If a very small tumour is treated early, a complete cure is likely. All women who have had breast cancer will be asked to attend regular check-ups to detect any recurrence or spread of the cancer to the rest of the body. It is very important that regular breast self-examinations and early mammograms are carried out. Even if the cancer recurs, it can be controlled for many years with surgery, drugs and radiotherapy.

TYPES OF COMMON BREAST SURGERY

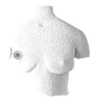

Lumpectomy
The whole lump and a small area of surrounding tissue is removed.

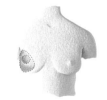

Partial Mastectomy
Removal of a substantial area of the breast tissue and the nipple.

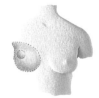

Extended Mastectomy
All of the breast is removed plus some lymph nodes from the armpit.

3

POSITIVE ATTITUDES

The menopause is sometimes incorrectly stereotyped as the start of a gradual decline into old age, when your body loses its feminine qualities and becomes sexually redundant. Women know from experience that this is far from the truth. With care your body remains one to be proud of, your mental resilience continues to be great and you still have a valuable role to play in society. By adopting a positive attitude to life in general, and to your changing lifestyle and body in particular, you can improve the quality of your life and be living proof that this is only the end of the beginning, not the beginning of the end.

STAYING POSITIVE

Try to act on the following positive statements.

• *Being well-informed helps me to deal effectively with any menopausal symptoms that arise.*

• *The speed of ageing does not accelerate after the menopause.*

• *Femininity does not have to equal fertility.*

• *I deserve understanding from my partner and family.*

• *If I experience menopausal symptoms, talk about them. The more open I am, the more I will help to break down taboos.*

• *I have the right to take control of my life. If I don't want to rely on doctors or medicines, I won't. There are good relaxation techniques as well as complementary and dietary approaches that can help deal successfully with any symptoms.*

• *I can take steps to maintain and even improve the quality of my sex life. There is no reason why the menopause should be the beginning of a sexual decline.*

• *There's no time like the present for developing a new skill, hobby or project. I can even begin a second career.*

• *I will embark on financial planning for retirement as early as possible, to take advantage of what could be my most creative years.*

THINKING POSITIVELY

Referring to the menopause as the change of life is both misleading and counterproductive. The menopause isn't the only change that will occur during your life and it is unlikely to be the most significant one. Life is a series of gradual changes – we don't suddenly reach a turning point and start growing old when we reach midlife. Ageing is a continuous process that begins the moment we are born and continues until we die. I believe that a healthy attitude to the menopause is to see it as a time in which to rediscover yourself, to assess (or reassess) your life and its purpose, and to establish new aims and goals.

By the time we reach middle age most of us carry around the received wisdom of society, leftovers from old traditions, fears that are often obsolete, and beliefs that may be borrowed. Without clearing out all these redundant feelings, we can lose touch with our inner selves.

RESISTING NEGATIVE STEREOTYPES

It is important to resist negative stereotypes associated with the menopause. These are very often culturally created and do not reflect the reality of our individual experiences. In countries where age is venerated and older women are respected for their experience and wisdom, fewer physical and psychological symptoms of the menopause are reported. In countries that lack a tradition of myths and misconceptions about the menopause, ageing seems to be regarded as a more natural process; women aren't adversely affected by negative images and may feel less confused by what is happening to them.

If you believe that in order to be beautiful and successful you must be young, then you may not enjoy your middle age to the full. If you are convinced that the quality of life deteriorates from the age of 50 onwards, this can become a self-fulfilling prophecy. Because you believe it is going to happen, you may inadvertently make it happen by not taking care of yourself and by adopting resigned, negative attitudes.

TAKING CONTROL OF YOUR BODY

The first step towards taking charge of your life and managing your menopause is to take charge of your body. You need to play an active role with all of your medical and health providers. Be aware of all your options and exercise them in order to eliminate as many health problems as you can. The strategy you choose to deal with any menopausal symptoms you may suffer from is up to you. You could decide to try self-help measures, for instance, or complementary medicine. Alternatively, you may feel that your symptoms warrant conventional medical help.

To achieve these goals, you need to have a firm sense of your own self-worth and optimism about the future, and you must be prepared to make an effort. As soon as you start to take control of your menopausal symptoms, your health and sense of well-being will benefit enormously.

TAKING CONTROL OF YOUR MIND

The second step towards taking charge of your life and managing your menopause is to take charge of your mind. As with your body, you need to be positive in your attitude and prepared to make a real effort to get what you want from both your family and friends, and from medical and other professionals with whom you come into contact. Try to keep in mind the positive statements listed on the left – and remember that the menopause is not the beginning of the end; it's the beginning of the rest of your life.

THE POWER OF POSITIVE THINKING

While health and vigour during the menopausal years depend a great deal on following a good diet and taking plenty of exercise, these are by no means the only resources you have to draw upon. Rest, relaxation and a variety of leisure activities will help you keep active and mentally alert. You also need self-affirming thoughts to maintain your self-confidence and prevent self-criticism. Never allow yourself to think that you are unattractive, lacklustre or out-of-touch. The strong interaction between your mind and your body means that you can make your menopause more difficult with negative thoughts. In other words, if you believe you're sick, you can start to behave like a sick person.

If you try to repeat some of the statements on the right like a mantra each day, you will gradually become more and more convinced of their truth.

A PERSONAL MANTRA

Positive thoughts and attitudes will maintain your self-esteem.

• *My body is strong and healthy and can become healthier each day.*

• *My female organs are in good shape.*

• *My body chemistry is effective and balanced.*

• *I eat healthy, nourishing food.*

• *I'm learning to handle stress.*

• *I'm calm and relaxed.*

• *I work efficiently and competently.*

• *I have the freedom and confidence to enjoy life.*

• *I can be happy and optimistic at this time of my life.*

• *My life belongs to me and it brings me pleasure.*

• *I devote time to myself each day.*

• *My friends and family are more enjoyable than they have ever been.*

• *I'm going through the menopause more easily and more comfortably with each passing day.*

CHANGING FAMILY ROLES

The structure of the family is constantly changing. For many of us, the time when we really need stability and continuity may be the very time when we may have to cope with a major upheaval in the family, such as a divorce, remarriage and new relations with various children and children-in-law. And as we get older, we may have to decide with whom or near whom we are going to live.

The extended families that can arise from divorce and remarriage may include young adults who have grown up with the idea that their parents are fixed points in the universe. Suddenly they may acquire new grandparents. Similarly, grandparents may find themselves with new grandchildren. At first, this may be hard to deal with, but people often overcome these difficulties through love and generosity. Newly formed family ties can be just as strong as old ones.

CARING FOR ELDERLY PARENTS

Although family relationships have changed radically in the last century, one thing that has remained fairly consistent is the way in which younger members of a family assume responsibility for older ones. There is no doubt that this can place severe emotional, physical and economic stress on us. The mobility of today's society means that the family is not always gathered in one place. Even a few minutes' travelling time can make support difficult, especially if we have other commitments, such as work.

Sometimes the responsibilities of looking after home, husband and aged parents, as well as dealing with postmenopausal symptoms, can be overwhelming. Try to delegate as much as you can. Enlist the help of your partner, children and siblings. If you have a very old or infirm parent, you may have to take the decision to house him or her in sheltered accommodation. No family should feel guilty about this – it's a responsible option, ensuring that your parent is well cared for.

BECOMING A GRANDPARENT

One of the joys that many people have in store for them in midlife is becoming a grandparent. Once past childbearing age, many women begin to look forward to their second chance at mothering and find that few experiences compare with spending time learning from and teaching their grandchildren. In my opinion, grandparents are an important part of the family in that they can teach a child how to relate to older people. Grandparents, by virtue of their age, may be more philosophical, tolerant and sympathetic than parents. Long practice means they have learned the knack of handling children with ease. These qualities enable children to develop in a relaxed, familiar environment.

It's sometimes said that grandparents spoil their grandchildren. This must be a misuse of the word "spoil". If spoiling a child means giving him explanations instead of dismissals, suggesting alternatives instead of negatives, and helping him instead of ignoring him, then grandparents do indeed spoil children. As a grandparent you are in a position to share your passions with your grandchildren, whether they be gardening, sewing, sketching or swimming. As grandchildren grow up, you can be a valuable confidante to them. You, of all people, are best equipped to teach them how they can cope with change, having lived through some of the most dramatic upheavals the world has known. You have a valuable historical perspective on employment, politics and social change. Recount your past experiences and encourage them to ask you questions.

You can provide a positive role model of middle and old age for your family. You can be independent. You can also listen. Parents don't always have a lot of time for this, but you are in a position to listen to family members without giving advice. You can tell your family about your own experience and what it has led you to believe.

You may find that you have much more in common with teenage grandchildren than you had ever imagined. At opposite ends of life, you are both likely to be experiencing changing identities and asking the same questions: Who am I? What do I really want? How do I get it? Very frequently adolescents can have more in common with grandparents than with parents, who are too busy to be self-aware and introspective. Grandparents can give a unique kind of loving and caring, and grandchildren relish knowing that they hold a special place in their grandparents' lives.

ROLE OF GRANDMOTHERS

You can maximize your enjoyment of your grandchildren by acting on the following advice.

• *Find free time to spend talking and listening to grandchildren.*

• *Find time to spend on activities that are fun, rather than routine.*

• *Live apart from grandchildren, allowing the children to feel they have a second home.*

• *Provide personal information to daughters or daughters-in-law from their own experience.*

• *Have an overview about general child care.*

• *Create more time for mothers by taking care of children.*

MENTAL AGILITY

Most of us are concerned about our physical fitness, but fewer of us stop to consider our mental fitness. Women, regardless of their marital status, suffer more from mental illness than men, and can become even more vulnerable around the time of their menopause. During middle age, some women feel that their freedom of choice becomes more restricted, and this can lead to frustration, conflict, unhappiness and mental trauma.

Mental fitness can be as easy to develop as physical fitness. We must strive to maintain a basic level of mental health so that we can rise to cope with any challenges that present themselves, deal with emergencies and generally have the resilience to survive stressful situations in the long-term. As we get older, we have to deal with emotional trauma, such as the loss of parents and possibly our partner.

Self-knowledge requires supreme realism: we have to learn that we are not unique in suffering, that difficult times come and go, that adversity is normal and that some failures are inevitable. As we grow older, we should leave behind preconceptions and prejudices, and be constantly prepared to change our attitudes. We need to work with our emotions in a constructive way, and yet still be affectionate and tender with ourselves.

STAYING MENTALLY FIT

We can learn a lot by observing the qualities of people whose mental and emotional resilience we admire. The following qualities come from emotional openness, flexibility and self-reliance.

• Independence and recognition of others' independence, privacy and peace.

• Lack of self-pity, so that when a problem arises it is looked at objectively.

• The attitude that nothing is hopeless and problems are there to be solved.

• A sense of inner security rather than security gained from controlling others.

• Being prepared to take responsibility for our own mistakes.

• A few close and loving relationships rather than many superficial ones.

- A sense of realism about the goals we set ourselves.
- Being in touch with our emotions and feeling free to express them.

Just as a muscle becomes weak if it's not exercised regularly, so your brain will slow and become feeble if it is not stimulated. The best mental exercise is work. A recent experiment performed on Japanese octogenarians showed that those who kept going into their offices, even for one hour a day, had greater mental powers than those who had retired at 60 and given up disciplined thinking.

The first tip to maintain mental fitness is daily intellectual work. It helps if your efforts are judged by your peers, but work of any kind provides mental stimulation. Interaction with other people forces you to assess what they are saying and respond with questions and comments. Your brain has to assimilate information and your cognitive processes remain active.

As we get older, we lose the ability to form new brain connections, so we have to make certain that old and well-established connections are continually used. The only way to do this is through thinking. Don't make the mistake of believing that thinking is a passive process – it means engaging in, questioning and absorbing what is happening all around us. For example, arithmetical "exercises" are often encountered in daily life and you can engage in them more actively. Anticipate your supermarket bill by adding up the cost of your shopping or estimate how much change you'll receive. Try to judge the size and quantity of objects and then measure them to check on your judgement.

Try to add to your vocabulary daily by noting down each new word you see or hear. Keep a dictionary handy to check on meanings and use the word in subsequent conversations. Read a daily newspaper article or watch the television news and discuss the main events of the day with a friend.

If you have the opportunity, think about taking an evening class. The range of courses available to adults is huge – there are crafts courses that take up a couple of hours a week, or you can take full-time courses in academic subjects such as history or English literature. Your local library is the best source of information on continuing education.

MEMORY MAINTENANCE

Follow the simple measures below to improve your memory.

- *When you read a book or magazine article, summarize the plot or the points made in it to a friend.*

- *When you're going shopping, try to collect as many items as possible without referring to your shopping list.*

- *If you want to remember several things, do it with a mnemonic. For example, you can abbreviate tasks such as ironing, making a phone call and typing a letter into the single word PIT (Phone/Iron/Type), which will act as a memory aid.*

- *If you walk into a room and forget why you're there, go back to where you came from and don't leave until you have remembered.*

- *If you have lost something, track it down. Write down the last six things you did prior to losing it and where you were for each activity. Draw a grid with what you were doing along one side and where you were along the bottom. The item you've lost lies in one of those squares; check each one out until you come across it.*

DEEP MUSCLE RELAXATION

Follow the steps below to relax your body.

1 Find a peaceful place, lie on your back, or sit in a comfortable chair and close your eyes.

2 Tense your right hand (or left, if you are left-handed), then let it go loose. Imagine it feels heavy and warm. Repeat with your right forearm, upper arm, and shoulder, then move on to the right foot, lower leg, upper leg. Now do exactly the same thing with the left side of your body. By the time you have finished, your hands, arms and legs should feel heavy, relaxed and warm. Allow a few seconds for these feelings to develop and to get used to the sensation.

3 Now relax the muscles around your hips and waist. Let the relaxation flow up the abdomen into the chest. You will find that your breathing starts to slow down.

4 Let the relaxation go into your shoulders, facial and jaw muscles. Pay special attention to the muscles around your eyes and forehead – tense them, then let the frown melt away. Finish by imagining that your forehead feels cool and smooth.

RELAXATION

If you are relaxed, you will be better able to deal with problems and conflicts at home and work, and you will find personal relationships easier to manage. Irritability and aggressiveness will dissipate and you will find you have energy to spare. Relaxation can often help you to deal with menopausal symptoms such as hot flushes.

DEEP MUSCLE RELAXATION

The deep muscle technique described on the left has been taken up by most relaxation experts around the world. It may take time to learn, but it will help you cope with stress, lower your blood pressure, decrease your chance of getting headaches and make you sleep better.

If you can, practise this technique twice a day for 15–20 minutes each time. However, even as little as three minutes will be sufficient time to give you a sense of well-being. The best time to practise is just before mealtimes or an hour afterwards.

DEEP MENTAL RELAXATION

Once you've mastered deep muscle relaxation, you're ready to go on to deep mental relaxation (see opposite). This technique is designed to clear your mind of stressful thoughts and tension. It is a form of meditation in which you attempt to separate your body from your thoughts in order to create a personal space that is free from worry and negative thoughts. You can retreat or escape to this whenever you want to. Find a place where you know you will not be disturbed and lie down or make yourself comfortable in a chair. Before you start the steps themselves, close your eyes and begin by breathing deeply several times.

When you've mastered both deep muscle and deep mental relaxation, they can be done together. They're fairly easy to combine, and you should practise them twice a day until you become competent.

INSTANT RELAXATION

Once you have trained your body to achieve deep muscle and mental relaxation, you should be able to achieve partial relaxation within about 30 seconds. If you are feeling stressed, try the following exercise.

Sit, lie or stand comfortably. Take a deep breath to the count of five, then breathe out slowly and tell your muscles to relax. Repeat three times until you're feeling relaxed. Imagine yourself in a pleasant situation, such as walking along a beach. If a situation panics you, regain control by breathing deeply. This should calm you and lessen the stress.

MENTAL IMAGERY

Use your imagination to get in touch with your body. For example, focus on your left hand and make it feel warm. Now concentrate on your right thigh and make it feel warm and heavy. Try to imagine that one leg is heavier than the other. Once you've mastered this, you can apply it in any situation by imagining that your body has the inner resources to overcome the symptoms you are experiencing. As part of cancer therapy, patients are trained to imagine their body's defences as warriors, physically killing their cancer cells. You can use this technique to combat menopausal symptoms.

BREATHING TECHNIQUES

Almost all muscle relaxation programmes involve proper breathing as the key to controlling stress and anxiety. This may be simple deep breathing, yoga breathing or deep abdominal breathing.

Most people breathe incorrectly, using no more than a third of their lung capacity, and hardly using the abdomen at all. Most of us only use the upper part of the chest, so we are depriving the body of oxygen. Try to change your shallow breathing to deep, slow breathing. Besides improving the function of your lungs and the muscles of your abdomen, it will relax your whole body.

To do deep abdominal breathing, place one hand on your stomach and breathe in slowly through your nose to a count of five. As you inhale, let it balloon out. The further out it goes, the more lung capacity you use, and the more oxygen you are getting to your tissues. When you think your lungs are absolutely full, try to take a little more air in to the very bottom of your lungs. Then breathe out deeply, through your nose if you can, but through your mouth if it allows your stomach and chest to collapse completely. This "oxygen fix" is wonderfully refreshing and you can do it as often as you like.

DEEP MENTAL RELAXATION

Follow the steps below to relax your mind.

1 Allow thoughts to associate freely in your head.

2 Stop any recurring thoughts by saying "no" to them under your breath, and repeating "no" until they go away.

3 With your eyes closed, imagine a tranquil scene such as a calm blue sea. Whatever you imagine, try to see the colour blue, because this is very therapeutic.

4 Concentrate on your breathing – and make sure it is slow and natural. Follow each breath as you inhale and exhale.

5 By now, you should feel calm and rested. You may find it helpful to repeat a soothing mantra, such as "love", "peace" or "calm".

6 Remind yourself to keep the muscles of your face, eyes and forehead relaxed, and imagine that your forehead is cool and smooth.

YOUR APPEARANCE

Many women first become really conscious of the signs of ageing on their faces and bodies during the menopause. It is very important to feel comfortable with the way you look – not only will your confidence improve, but your whole outlook will benefit. A feeling of self-esteem is particularly important as you get older, and looking after your appearance is a good way of promoting self-worth.

Your body will look better if you eat a healthy diet containing the right vitamins and minerals and exercise regularly; you can make the most of your skin and hair if you take proper care of them. Paying attention to your figure will mean not only that your clothes fit more comfortably but that they will look more flattering too.

There's no secret formula for looking good. You have to think carefully and logically about how to make the most of your good points and how to conceal your bad ones successfully. There's no need to buy expensive cosmetics or clothes; it's much more important to look natural and feel comfortable. The truly wonderful thing about reaching the menopause is that there are no prescribed roles for you to play, and no set of rules that you have to follow.

POSTURE

Shapelessness and poor posture can give the impression of age, and a relaxed, upright posture and a supple figure can make you look much younger. Bad posture can also make you look fat (or at least fatter), while good posture can take pounds off as well as years. Make sure that you stand with your feet parallel, your pelvis straight and your spine vertical. Your shoulders should be relaxed rather than hunched. You will not only improve your appearance by paying attention to your posture and gait, but you will help maintain the health of your spine, and back muscles.

CLOTHES

If you remain in good shape, there's nothing to prevent you from continuing to wear the kind of clothes you have always worn. However, ageing inevitably brings changes to body shape, and you may want to accommodate these. Comfortable good-quality garments with flattering lines suit mature women, but you should avoid viewing your age as a constraint upon what you should and shouldn't wear.

If you suffer from hot flushes or night sweats, avoid synthetic fabrics such as polyester or nylon and wear cooling, natural ones such as cotton. It may also be wiser to avoid wearing wool next to your skin, although it is a natural fabric. And don't wear tightly fitting garments whatever the material – they'll make you sweat even more.

Choose your shoes very carefully too. High heels can throw your body out of alignment and increase the likelihood of falling. Shoes that are too narrow will cramp your toes and cause corns and ingrowing toenails. When you are at home, make a point of taking your shoes and tights off and allowing your feet to spread and relax.

UNDERWEAR

Even if your waistline and hips start to spread, you shouldn't be tempted to wear rigid corsets. If you feel you must wear foundation garments, then choose light ones that allow you to move and breathe freely. Lightweight undergarments make hot flushes easier to cope with. If possible, wear underwear that is made of natural fibres such as cotton and silk, since these are the most comfortable fabrics to have next to your skin, particularly in hot weather. Avoid wearing harsh, coarse fabrics next to the skin, and look for fastenings that are easy to reach and operate.

Your underwear should always be chosen on the basis of comfort and fit. Make sure you choose a bra with wide straps that don't cut into your skin, and try wearing an underwired bra for extra support, particularly if you have large breasts. Two tips to remember when you are buying a bra: if it rides up and sits high on your back, this means that it is too big; if you cannot comfortably slide a finger underneath the straps at the front, then it is too small. You should also check carefully that there are no bulges of flesh around your cleavage; this is a good indication that the cup size is too small.

CHOOSING A BRA

Underwired bras give support and can prevent the appearance of sagging breasts. Make sure the wired part lies flat against your skin and extends underneath your arms. Choose a bra with wide, soft straps and no lace – lace digs into the skin and makes it sore.

HAIR SELF-HELP

Follow the steps below to perfect hair.

• *Do not scrub your scalp when you wash your hair. You will loosen hairs from the soft wet hair follicles.*

• *Do not tug or pull at wet hair as you comb it; this will remove or tear it. Use a wide-toothed brush or comb.*

• *Do not brush or comb your hair too frequently, as this may make it look lank and dull.*

• *Do not use anti-dandruff shampoos more than once every two weeks, because they contain ingredients that can irritate the scalp.*

YOUR HAIR

As you get older, new hair grows in with no pigment. Grey hair is just as healthy as pigmented hair and needs no special treatment. As far as general hair care is concerned, use the mildest shampoo you can find, and only shampoo your hair once – shampoos are now so efficient that shampooing twice is unnecessary. Mix two teaspoonfuls of shampoo in a glass of warm water and pour it over your already wet hair. Then massage the shampoo very gently into your hair. It's not necessary to scrub hard to work up a lather, just leave the shampoo on for about a minute, and then rinse until the hair is clean. If your hair is slightly dry, you will need a conditioner; these work by coating, or softening and swelling, the hair fibre. After you have washed your hair, dab it dry with a towel rather than rubbing it vigorously.

Grey hair can be hidden with temporary or permanent colouring but, to avoid a harsh contrast with your skin, it's probably better to use a shade that is lighter than the original colour of your hair. The way your hair responds to artificial colourants depends on how porous your hair shafts are. There are several types of colouring.
• Restorers can be combed through or sprayed on. They work by coating the hair and eventually may make it brittle and easily damaged.
• Temporary colour, dry or liquid, gives highlights to grey hair, but it doesn't last beyond one shampoo.
• Semi-permanent colour blends grey hairs into your natural colour and completely covers them. It fades over a period of time, especially in the sun, so reapplication is necessary every few weeks.
• Permanent hair colour penetrates the hair shaft itself and cannot be shampooed away. It has a chemical base that can dry out the hair. It also leaves a regrowth when new hair grows in, and has to be reapplied every four to six weeks depending on the rate of growth. Try to avoid bleach, since this strips the hair of natural oils. Make sure your hair is regularly looked after, and pay as much as you can afford for a style that really suits you. Don't let yourself be pressured into expensive perms and colours. Grey hair can be very attractive and you may not want to go to the trouble of regular colouring.

PHYSICAL HEALTH

Monitoring and maintaining your health is the key to continuing a healthy, happy and active life. Observing and reading the messages your body sends, and responding sensitively to them, bring a real sense of achievement as well as well-being. And there is simply no doubt about it: it is not difficult to enjoy natural good health. Eating healthy food *does* make you feel better; controlling your weight *does* make you look better; and keeping fit *does* make you more energetic. What's more, any efforts you make quickly become apparent, giving you the incentive to continue the good work.

GOOD NUTRITION

As you get older, your digestive tract becomes less efficient and digestion can take longer; your body no longer finds it as easy to cope with foods that contain a lot of calories but little nourishment. Although you need fewer calories than you did when you were younger, you still require the same amount of vitamins and minerals. The healthiest diet during the menopause, therefore, is one that consists of unprocessed fresh foods, such as wholegrains, vegetables, fruits, fish, seafood, some oils and eggs. A whole range of healthy foods is now widely available in every high street, so it has never been easier to experiment. Concentrate on building up a regular diet of unprocessed, high-grade carbohydrates to which protein can be added as a "condiment".

As your body's metabolism and chemical reactions slow down, an adequate intake of vitamins and minerals is essential; eating the right diet can have a powerful and beneficial effect on menopausal symptoms, making you independent of doctors and drugs.

Some protein is essential for health, but too much, especially in the form of fatty meats, can lead to deficient calcium absorption. If you've been a heavy meat-eater in the past, this could increase your risk of developing the bone disease, osteoporosis. Start to cut down on the amount of meat in your diet as soon as possible, and try to replace it with foods such as fish, rice, beans, vegetables and pasta.

A certain amount of fat is needed for functions that cannot be performed by any other nutrient, however; essential fatty acids are necessary for the metabolism of calcium, for instance, and they cannot be manufactured by the body. The best forms of fat are those found in whole natural foods, such as vegetable oils and fish oils. Fats to avoid are saturated fats, that is, fats that are solid at room temperature; these include butter and lard, and certain vegetable oils, such as coconut or palm oil found in processed foods.

Fermented milk products, such as yoghurt, can be particularly effective at encouraging calcium absorption. Even those who have problems digesting whole-milk products can usually tolerate fermented ones because they are partially predigested.

BASIC ESSENTIALS

Vitamins, minerals, fibre and water are some of the basic essentials of any diet. Making sure your diet contains adequate amounts of all of them should be one of your most important priorities. In addition to the general information listed below, see the charts on page 316 and page 318 for specific guidance on vitamin- and mineral-rich foods, and how they can help you become healthier.

VITAMIN A

This is necessary for the health and growth of the skin, eyes and mucous membranes. A vitamin A deficiency can cause night blindness and an increased susceptibility to infections. The lack of vitamin A may also contribute to heavy menstrual bleeding and to skin conditions related to the ageing process.

VITAMIN B COMPLEX

Several B vitamins are useful during the menopause. Their effects include helping us to handle sugar, keeping the liver healthy and stabilizing brain function. Low levels can lead to emotional distress, fatigue and irritability. Folic acid (another B vitamin) may help to prevent precancerous changes in the cervix. If you're taking hormone replacement therapy (HRT), you may want to take a vitamin B6 supplement because HRT can lead to a deficiency that may make you prone to depression.

VITAMIN C

This is often dubbed the "healing" vitamin; it helps to mend wounds and burns, and it maintains collagen, which helps lubricate the skin so, to a degree, it could be called an anti-wrinkle vitamin. Since the need for collagen regeneration increases with age, we require greater amounts of vitamin C as we grow older. Vitamin C also helps the adrenal glands and the body's immune system to fight infections and allergies.

VITAMIN D

Along with calcium and oestrogen, vitamin D is essential to maintain bone mass and prevent the onset of osteoporosis after the menopause. Vitamin D promotes the absorption of calcium and phosphorus from the intestine. All menopausal women should include adequate quantities of this vitamin in their diet to maintain strong, straight bones in later life.

VITAMIN E

Vitamin E has been used with some success as an oestrogen substitute. It is possible that vitamin E may relieve hot flushes and the psychological symptoms of

VITAMINS THAT WILL BENEFIT MENOPAUSAL COMPLAINTS

VITAMIN	SOURCE	COMPLAINT
Vitamin A *(Retinol and carotene)*	Carrots, spinach, turnips, apricots, liver, cantaloupe melon, sweet potatoes	Excessive menstrual bleeding, Cervical abnormalities, Fibrocystic disease and cancer of the breast, Leukoplakia and other skin conditions
Folic Acid *(Vitamin B complex)*	Green leafy vegetables, nuts, peas, beans, liver and kidney	Cervical abnormalities and cancer, Osteoporosis, Diabetes mellitus
Vitamin B^3 *(Niacin)*	Meat and poultry, fish, pulses, whole wheat, bran	Hyperlipidaemia (high concentration of blood fat), Hypoglycaemia (low blood sugar)
Vitamin B^6 *(Pyriodoxine)*	Meat and poultry, fish, bananas, wholegrain cereals, dairy products	Cervical abnormalities and cancer, Diabetes mellitus
Vitamin B^{12} *(Cyanocobalamin)*	Fish, poultry, eggs and milk, B^{12} enriched soya produce (no vegetable contains B^{12})	Anxiety, Depression, Mood swings, Fatigue
Vitamin C *(Ascorbic acid)*	Citrus fruits, strawberries, broccoli, green peppers	Excessive menstrual bleeding, Cervical abnormalities and cancer, Chloasma
Vitamin D *(Calciferol)*	Sunlight, oily fish, fortified cereals and bread, fortified margarine	Poor calcium absorption, leading to an increase in the risk of osteoporosis
Vitamin E *(Tocopherol)*	Vegetable oils, green leafy vegetables, cereals, dried beans, wholegrains, bread	Hot flushes, Anxiety, Vaginal problems (e.g. dryness), Hypo-thyroidism, Chloasma, Atherosclerosis, Osteoarthritis, Fibrocystic disease of the breast

the menopause, but this has not been medically verified. It may also relieve vaginal dryness when applied as an oil directly to the vagina, as well as when it is taken in the diet.

CALCIUM

Experts recommend that women over 40 should take the equivalent of 1,500 mg of calcium a day (1,000 mg if they are on HRT) and women over 60 should take 1,200 mg. Calcium is essential for long-term bone health to protect you against osteoporosis; it will also protect your heart and lower blood fats.

Calcium absorption There is a misconception that in order to increase your daily calcium intake you can simply take calcium tablets. Unfortunately, taken on their own, these are difficult to absorb, and the calcium that is absorbed cannot be utilized by the bones and is excreted in the urine. To maximize the effect of calcium supplements, it is essential that both oestrogen and small amounts of vitamin D are present.

Calcium supplements If you think you need a calcium supplement, seek medical advice. There are many types on the market, and deciding which one to use is a decision you should reach with your doctor. Different tablets are derived from different sources, and some are combined with other nutrients for better absorption or because the nutrients work as a unit within the body.

Calcium and phosphorus Taken correctly, phosphorus will enhance the amount of calcium absorbed by the bones. The diet of most people is too high in phosphorus, adversely affecting retention of calcium. To re-establish the correct ratio, reduce your intake of high-phosphorus foods drastically. This means eliminating processed foods, such as canned meats, instant soups and soft drinks, which offer little nutrition. Check food labels and avoid those that contain sodium phosphate, potassium phosphate, phosphoric acid, pyrophosphate or polyphosphate.

OTHER BENEFICIAL MINERALS

Magnesium is instrumental in keeping calcium soluble in the bloodstream and may also help if you have low energy and a lack of vitality. A magnesium deficiency disturbs the

ACHIEVING A HEALTHIER DIET

The following simple guidelines may make it easier to change your eating patterns.

● *Keep your meals simple and easy. Cut down preparation time.*

● *Eat the largest meal of the day early; have a hearty breakfast, a light lunch and an even lighter dinner.*

● *Eat a variety of foods so that you get a range of nutrients; don't eat the same foods every day out of habit.*

● *Make the transition to raw, high fibre food slowly; don't worry if it takes a few months to change your dietary habits.*

● *Identify any "high stress" foods and start substituting these with low stress ones.*

calcification of bone, impairs bone growth and reduces calcium levels; diets deficient in magnesium may lead to skeletal abnormalities, including osteoporosis. Potassium is essential for normal muscle contraction and heart function; zinc is needed for hormone and brain function, and for building new cells. Fortunately, many foods contain magnesium, potassium and zinc together.

MINERALS THAT WILL BENEFIT MENOPAUSAL COMPLAINTS

MINERAL	SOURCE	COMPLAINT
Calcium	Milk and milk products, dark-green leafy vegetables, citrus fruits, dried peas and beans	Osteoporosis, Hyperlipidaemia (high concentration of blood fat), Hypertension (high blood pressure)
Magnesium	Green leafy vegetables, nuts, soya beans, wholegrain cereals	Osteoporosis, Fatigue, Diabetes mellitus, Coronary artery disease, Anxiety, Depression
Potassium	Orange juice, bananas, dried fruits, peanut butter, meat	Fatigue, Heart disease, Hypertension (high blood pressure), Anxiety, Depression
Zinc	Meat, liver, eggs, poultry, seafood	Osteoporosis
Iron	Nuts, liver, red meats, egg yolk, green leafy vegetables, dried fruits	Anaemia due to excessive menstrual bleeding
Iodine	Seafood, fish, seaweed	Hypothyroidism, Fibrocystic disease of the breast
Chromium	Meat, cheese, wholegrains, breads	Hypoglycaemia (low blood sugar)
Selenium	Seafood, meat, wholegrain cereals	Fibrocystic disease of the breast, Breast cancer
Manganese	Nuts, fruits and vegetables, wholegrain cereals	Atherosclerosis
Bioflavonoids	All citrus fruits, especially the pulp and pith	Hot flushes, Excessive menstrual bleeding, Vaginal problems, Anxiety, Irritability and other emotional problems

You require magnesium for the efficient absorption of calcium, vitamin D and phosphorus, thus emphasizing the importance of nutrient inter-relationships; recent evidence suggests that the balance between calcium and magnesium is an especially important one. If the calcium level is raised, magnesium intake needs to be increased as well. The optimum calcium/magnesium ratio is two to one. So if you are taking 1,000 mg of calcium, you will need to take 500 mg of magnesium to maintain a balance.

FIBRE

Roughage is a particularly important part of any healthy diet. It keeps your gut healthy and promotes regular bowel movements, which helps to prevent the distension and bloating that many women experience during the menopause. It also helps bowel conditions such as irritable bowel syndrome and diverticulitis. Fibre can also give you a feeling of fullness and satisfaction that will help you to control your appetite, combat cravings and avoid binges. There is good evidence to show that a woman who eats a high-fibre diet is less likely to suffer from a variety of cancers, including cancer of the colon and cancer of the breast. It may also protect against heart disease. Foods that are rich in fibre include wholegrains (brown rice, wholemeal pasta), dark-green leafy vegetables (spring greens, spinach), pulses (peas, beans, lentils), cereals, and nuts such as peanuts and cashews. See right for easy ways to increase the fibre content of your diet.

WATER

Water is a much neglected dietary element that is particularly important during the menopause. Water performs a wide range of functions in the body: it acts as a solvent for nutrients, oxygen, hormones, antibodies and waste products; it helps to eliminate waste from the body as urine; it keeps both the skin and the mucous membranes plump and moist; and it lubricates the joints.

Water leaves the body in the form of urine and faeces; it is also expired as water vapour and perspired as sweat. It serves as the body's natural radiator, keeping the skin cool – when perspiration evaporates from the surface of the skin, it turns into water vapour, using the body's internal heat to do so.

INCREASING FIBRE

The following simple ways will help you increase your fibre intake.

- *Switch to high-fibre bread.*

- *Have high-fibre cereal for your breakfast.*

- *Eat high-fibre soups – such as bean, lentil or sweetcorn.*

- *Use different types of beans and peas in your green salads.*

- *Use dark-green salad leaves, such as spinach, rocket and endive, instead of pale iceberg lettuce.*

- *Eat bean dips with raw vegetables or wholewheat pitta bread.*

- *Use unprocessed flour, nuts and sesame seeds in your standard recipes, where appropriate.*

- *Snack on wholegrain crackers and dried fruits.*

- *Eat wholemeal muffins instead of cakes and biscuits.*

REDUCING SUGAR

Most people eat too much sugar – follow the guidelines below to cut down.

• *Reduce your intake of convenience foods, relishes, ketchup, cakes, biscuits, sweets and fizzy drinks, all of which have high levels of sugar.*

• *Avoid refined carbohydrate foods such as white flour, white bread, white sugar or white rice, which are low in fibre and can contribute to obesity.*

• *When cooking, try to cut the amount of sugar in a recipe by about one-third; this won't spoil the taste at all.*

• *Satisfy cravings for chocolate and other sweet foods with healthier sweet alternatives, such as fresh fruit and fruit juice.*

• *Eat more fibre. A high-fibre diet will fill you up so that you are less likely to want a snack.*

• *If you have a sweet tooth, substitute a healthier sweetener, such as honey, which also has a sweeter taste weight for weight. You can also substitute fruit for sugar in pastries, cakes and biscuits.*

• *Use artificial sweeteners to sweeten without adding calories.*

• *Replace chocolate and cocoa with carob. It tastes similar to chocolate but is better for you and can control a sugar craving. Unfortunately, it is high in fat and should only be eaten occasionally.*

On average, we need about two to three litres (about four to six pints) of fluid every day, simply to replace the amount we lose. Half of what we need comes from food, in the form of fruits and vegetables; the other half must come from drinking – approximately six to eight glasses a day. Any fluid is better than no fluid, but pure water is best, followed by fresh fruit juices and low-fat milk. Beverages containing caffeine or alcohol are not such good choices because they are diuretic and increase the amount of water we lose. Drinks containing lots of sugar are fattening and bad for the teeth.

BAD FOODS

There are two food groups that are detrimental to menopausal women: "non-foods", such as sugar, which are high in calories but low in nutrients; and highly processed prepared foods, which are nutritionally inferior and don't contain the mysterious micronutrients, enzymes and trace elements that are found in natural foods. Many prepared foods contain salt, and blood pressure, bloating and fluid retention are all adversely affected by salt. See page 321 for ways of reducing your salt intake.

There are also foods and substances that can be described as "nutrient depleters" because they diminish the effect of many healthy foods. Nutrient depleters include alcohol, cigarettes, caffeine and some drugs, such as barbiturates, antibiotics, cortisone (an antirheumatic drug), laxatives and diuretics. For instance, vitamin A is lost by coffee, alcohol and processed foods; vitamin E is depleted by smoking cigarettes and from polyunsaturated fats by freezing; vitamin B is depleted by sugar, processed foods, dieting, coffee and tea, and also by taking some drugs, such as cortisone and antacids; calcium by sugar, fat and spinach; and potassium by fasting, salt and coffee. Try to keep your intake of nutrient depleters low.

FAT

Most of us consume nearly half our calories in fat, and most of this comes in the form of saturated fat, that is, from dairy products such as cheese, butter and cream, and from meat such as beef and pork. It is also found in many processed and canned foods. Saturated fat can be particularly dangerous for menopausal women because a high intake is directly linked to heart disease, strokes, high blood pressure, cancers and obesity and, because of lowering levels of oestrogen, women are becoming more vulnerable to these diseases at this point in their lives. However, polyunsaturated fats, such as those found in certain vegetable and fish oils, can help remove cholesterol from the tissues and protect the heart against heart disease.

To obtain essential fats and oils, eat raw seeds and nuts sparingly. Cook with vegetable oils such as corn, olive, sunflower, soya-bean or safflower. Eat low-fat dairy products, such as skimmed milk, and substitute natural yoghurt for cream in desserts and main dishes. Be sparing with cheese when cooking – use it as a garnish rather than as a main ingredient; alternatively, replace cheese with tofu, which is high in calcium. You can also replace milk in recipes with soya milk.

HIGH-STRESS FOODS

These are substances, such as sugar, caffeine and alcohol, that contribute to various menopausal problems. High-stress foods contain few nutrients and, in some cases, they may be addictive. In addition, avoid black pepper, monosodium glutamate (MSG) and very hot spices (which worsen hot flushes), or cut the amount by half.

REDUCING SALT

Follow the guidelines below to cut back your salt consumption.

- *Cut down on prepared foods, such as hamburgers, salad dressings, hot dogs, pizzas and French fries. If you're buying these foods, always look for brands that have no added salt.*

- *Avoid adding salt to already-cooked food. Fruits, vegetables, meat and grains contain all the salt you will ever need.*

- *Enhance natural salt in foods by using flavourings such as garlic, herbs, spices and lemon.*

- *Substitute potassium-based salt for table salt – it's healthy and doesn't exacerbate high blood pressure or heart disease.*

SUBSTITUTES FOR HIGH-STRESS FOODS

HIGH-STRESS FOOD	SUBSTITUTES
135 g (4 oz) white flour	135g (4 oz) wholewheat flour
1 square chocolate	1 square of carob or 1 tablespoon powdered carob
1 tablespoon coffee	1 tablespoon decaffeinated coffee
½ teaspoon salt	½ teaspoon of one of the following: potassium salt substitute, yeast extract, basil, tarragon, oregano
125 ml (4 fl oz) wine	125 ml (4 fl oz) low-alcohol wine
250 ml (8 fl oz) beer	250 ml (8 fl oz) low-alcohol beer
250 ml (8 fl oz) milk	250 ml (8 fl oz) soya milk
150 g (5 oz) sugar	One of the following: ¼ cup molasses, ½ cup honey, ½ cup maple syrup, ½ cup barley malt, 2 cups apple juice

CHANGING SHAPE

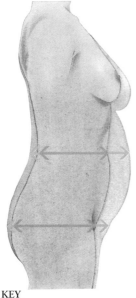

KEY

↔ Premenopausal figure: waist smaller than hips, healthy pattern.

↔ Postmenopausal figure: waist larger than hips, high-risk pattern.

Obesity and risk
The pattern of obesity is important in determining risk, with deposits of fat on the waist and stomach conferring a higher risk than fat on the hips and thighs. This pattern is characteristic of postmenopausal women and is also related to an increased risk of heart disease.

WEIGHT CONTROL

Being too thin at any time of life means that a woman is unhealthy. Some fat is essential for good health and this is never more true than at the menopause. We now know that women are healthier after the menopause if they are 6–8 kg (13–18 lb) heavier than they were before. If you were not overweight before the menopause, therefore, and providing your weight gain during and after stays within this bracket, your extra pounds should not affect your health. If you have gained more than this, however, and if your waist-to-hip ratio is higher than 0.8, you should take steps to control your weight. Obesity is potentially dangerous and can make you more susceptible to heart disease and high blood pressure, among other conditions.

Weight increase is gradual in both men and women as they age, but for women it may become especially noticeable during the menopausal and postmenopausal years. There are at least two factors involved here. First, lack of oestrogen leads to changes in body shape and fat distribution so that the waist thickens and fat is deposited on the front of the abdomen. Second, our metabolic rate slows down as we mature and, by about 55, we need fewer calories. Unless we have a regular and frequent exercise regime incorporated into our lives, continuing to eat at our usual rate will lead inexorably to weight gain.

POSITIVE EATING PATTERNS

Although you need fewer calories at this time of your life, your body's nutritional needs remain the same. Calorie-counting may be too time-consuming for anyone to maintain in the long term, so it's much better to concentrate on eating a diet that is well balanced and contains no "empty" high-calorie foods, such as sugar and fat. It's within your power to change not only what you eat, but how you eat. Eating five or even six small meals at regular intervals, for instance, is very effective in terms of weight control because each time you eat, you use energy for digestion and, if you eat very small quantities, the amount of energy expended in digestion can help compensate for the energy absorbed from the food. Small, frequent meals also prevent blood sugar levels from dropping, which can be accompanied by cravings for food.

Many studies have been carried out to show the differences between people who eat small, frequent meals and those who eat fewer, larger ones. The latter invariably have more body fat than the former. Some dieters find that a diet based on a nibbling pattern helps to prevent hunger pangs, and there is some evidence that this may speed up weight loss. Your digestive system will probably prefer a nibbling pattern diet, particularly if you suffer from indigestion or peptic ulcers.

Try not to go on crash diets or long-term diets that are little more than starvation. The initial weight loss may be impressive but less than half of this will be fat; most will be water, and it could include some of your precious body protein. A diet that restricts total calorie intake to under a thousand calories is only just adequate. Very strict diets, those around 500 calories, cannot provide all the required nutrients for an adult woman.

The attraction of a crash diet is that it offers severely obese people a chance to lose up to one to two kilograms (three to six pounds) per week. However, there is a great deal of research to show that towards the end of a long period of this kind of dieting, the rate of weight loss decelerates and the weight starts to go back on when normal eating patterns are resumed. In other words, the body adapts to starvation.

The fewer calories we give the body, the less it needs, until it can finally get by on less than 300 a day. A return to normal eating will cause an inevitable increase in weight as body stores of glycogen are replaced – extremely depressing if you have made a great effort to shed excess weight. It is common for a person coming off a starvation diet to go on eating binges and find herself on a treadmill of intermittent starving and bingeing that is extremely damaging to her health and self-image.

CHANGING MEAL PATTERNS

Rather than having a set menu for breakfast, lunch and dinner, think in terms of what type of food you would like to eat and how much time and energy you have to prepare it. For example, choose to cook a more elaborate meat meal at the weekend when you have plenty of time both to prepare and eat, and a nutritious but simple to-make soup or pasta meal during weekday evenings, when you have less energy to devote to either.

WATCHING YOUR WEIGHT

Try the following tips to help curb your appetite.

• *Drink half a pint of water before you start to eat. This will make you feel more satiated at the end of a meal.*

• *Put your food on a small plate. This controls the amount you can reasonably eat at one sitting.*

• *The more time you take eating food, the more satisfied you're likely to feel. People who over-eat usually eat quickly, and have to eat more in order to feel satisfied.*

• *Taking exercise an hour or so before a meal can help suppress your appetite.*

• *Eat your largest meal early in the day, when you have more time to burn up the calories you've eaten. Avoid eating large meals late in the evening – sleeping during the night does not burn off very many calories.*

OVER-TRAINING

Although many of us don't take enough exercise, a small percentage of women become psychologically addicted to exercise, experiencing the need to train every day, and feeling guilty if they miss a single session.

• *If you are addicted to exercise, don't be afraid that if you stop, even for a while, you will become unfit and overweight. This is quite untrue. Even competitive athletes have breaks in which they train lightly or not at all.*

• *If you feel your need to exercise is compulsive, or if it is accompanied by anxiety and depression, seek medical help.*

KEEPING FIT

Without doubt, exercise is the menopausal woman's best friend in that it allows you to control your body and emotions by using your internal resources. Each time that you take exercise, your adrenal glands are stimulated to convert the male hormone androstenedione into oestrogen. A minimum of four 30-minute exercise sessions each week will be enough to keep you topped up with oestrogen. As you become older, your cardio-respiratory fitness, your strength and your flexibility all begin to decline. For people who remain active, however, these things decrease at a lower rate (an average of five percent per decade after the age of about 20, as opposed to nine percent per decade).

Long-term exercise also means that you will have stronger bones and a lower risk of osteoporosis than non-exercisers. Although every woman is different, most of us lose 25–35 percent of our bone mass by the time we reach the age of 65. Bone loss begins around the age of 35, proceeds slowly up to the menopause, and then accelerates during the five to seven years after the menopause, when oestrogen levels are low.

Women who do weight-bearing exercises, such as low-impact aerobics, walking, running or weight training in their 20s and 30s can increase their bone density before loss sets in. Beginning exercise later in life can restore small amounts – about four percent. Unfortunately, you cannot "store" the benefits of exercise; it must be ongoing to confer its many benefits.

EXERCISE AS A MENTAL TONIC

Regular exercise may also have a significant effect on our mental agility by increasing the amount of oxygen supplied to the brain. In a recent comparison between sedentary older women and older women who exercised regularly, after four months the latter group processed information faster in tests.

Apart from increasing the oxygen supply to the brain, exercise may also slow down the loss of dopamine in the brain. Dopamine is a neurotransmitter that helps to prevent the shaking and stiffness that can come with old age (a severe shortage of it results in the exaggerated tremors of Parkinson's disease). Since exercise can slow down dopamine loss, it is therefore particularly beneficial as we grow older. Exercise can also prevent our reaction times from slowing down.

THE BENEFITS OF REGULAR EXERCISE

- A reduced risk of heart disease.
- A lower chance of developing diabetes.
- Maintenance of muscle strength.
- Higher levels of the healthy type of cholesterol in the blood.
- Healthier bones and less chance of developing osteoporosis later in life.
- A more efficient immune system.
- Reduced body fat.
- Better appetite control.
- Increased mental agility.
- Fewer headaches.
- Improved sleep quality.
- Flexible joints.

The type of exercise that you take obviously depends largely on resources, how much time is available and your own personal preference. Nowadays there is a wide range of opportunities available, and not only in sports centres and fitness classes. If you need or prefer to exercise in your own home, you will find on the pages that follow some basic effective exercises you can do at home to preserve muscle strength and tone. And there are also many excellent exercise videos and other publications on this subject on the market.

You may prefer a sport such as tennis, badminton or squash, all of which offer the added attraction of meeting and socializing with people. Likewise, joining any aerobics or exercise class can provide a social aspect that may encourage you to exercise regularly. Less rigorous and more traditional forms of exercise such as walking and swimming offer viable alternatives, and will keep the body fit and supple.

Recently, there has been a move away from aerobics towards strength training and weight-bearing exercise. Research suggests that any exercise involving weights can delay loss of bone and muscle tissue, a natural consequence of ageing. Weight-bearing exercise also helps the flow of sugar from the blood into muscle tissue, which may lower the risk of diabetes and heart disease.

Stretching exercises tone the body and maintain joint flexibility

Staying healthy
Exercise not only increases your physical fitness and resistance to disease, it also has an uplifting effect on your mood.

325

GENERAL EXERCISES

These exercises encourage mobility and preserve muscle strength and tone. Try to do each set at least 10 times a day.

UPPER BODY EXERCISES

These promote flexibility of the shoulders, neck and back, and alleviate problems such as headaches and painfully knotted muscles in the neck and back. They also improve your posture.

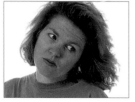

Head rolls
Starting with your chin on your chest, slowly roll your head around to your right shoulder. Hold this position and then slowly roll your head back, and around to your left shoulder.

Throwing off back and shoulder tension
Let your arms hang loosely by your sides, and let your head drop forward. Throw your right hand over your left shoulder as if you have a ball in your hand. Repeat this on the other side.

Lean back simultaneously with your weight evenly balanced

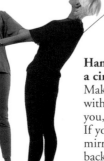

Hanging back in a circle
Make a circle, hold hands with the person next to you, and lean backwards. If you do this with a mirror behind you, bend back so you can see your face in it. You can do this with one other partner.

FEET AND LEG MOVEMENTS

Maintaining mobility and flexibility in your feet and weight-bearing joints is important as you get older, since it will help to prevent debilitating physical conditions such as arthritis.

Kicking your boots off
Kicks not only increase articulation in the knees and hips, they also relieve anger and tension. Support yourself by holding on to a door frame and kick forwards, as if you were kicking off shoes. Do this several times with each leg.

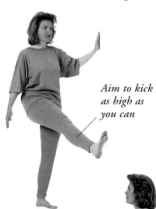

Aim to kick as high as you can

Bouncing
Stand with your feet parallel and slightly apart. Lift your arches and bounce gently up and down without bending your knees. This improves strength and flexibility in your feet and calves.

Knee moves

Lie on your back, raise your right knee and place your left palm on your right kneecap. Gently bend and stretch your leg. Now move your foot round and round in a circle, keeping your knee still. Repeat with the other knee.

Stepping up and down

Stand on a soft mat with your feet slightly apart and kneel down on your right knee, followed by the other knee. Now, leading with your right foot, and keeping your spine vertical, go back to a standing position. Repeat until your thigh muscle gets tired and then repeat with your left leg. This is the way that you should stand up after you have been sitting or working on the floor.

Move your leg slowly, drawing as big a circle as you can with your foot

Your back should be straight as you come up from the floor

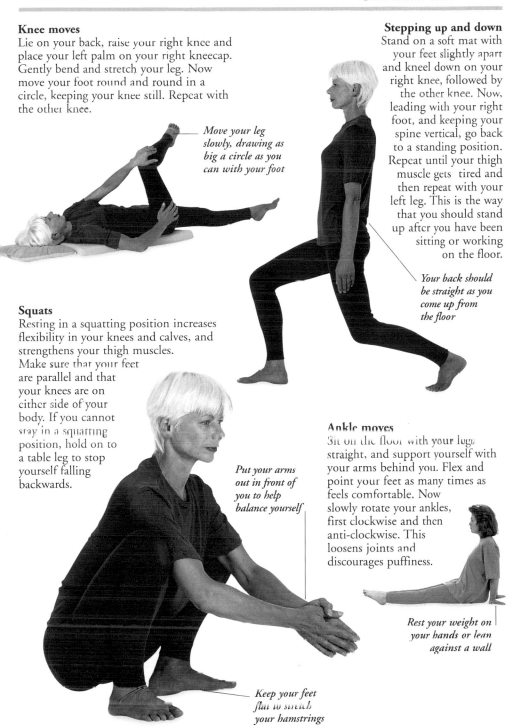

Squats

Resting in a squatting position increases flexibility in your knees and calves, and strengthens your thigh muscles. Make sure that your feet are parallel and that your knees are on either side of your body. If you cannot stay in a squatting position, hold on to a table leg to stop yourself falling backwards.

Put your arms out in front of you to help balance yourself

Ankle moves

Sit on the floor with your legs straight, and support yourself with your arms behind you. Flex and point your feet as many times as feels comfortable. Now slowly rotate your ankles, first clockwise and then anti-clockwise. This loosens joints and discourages puffiness.

Rest your weight on your hands or lean against a wall

Keep your feet flat to stretch your hamstrings

WAIST, HIPS, STOMACH AND BOTTOM EXERCISES

After the menopause, fat distribution changes so that more fat is laid down on the waist and abdomen. These movements help to keep your abdominal muscles toned and your hip joints loose and flexible.

Spinning top

Following the four steps on the right, kneel on the floor and shift your weight on to your bottom on the right-hand side of you. Bring your knees up and over on to the left side. Return to a kneeling position, then lift up your bottom and sit on your right-hand side again. If you repeat this movement, lifting your bottom over your feet, you should move around in a complete circle. You may need to use your hands to help you at first.

Move your knees slowly in an arc across your body to the left

Pull your stomach muscles in

Make your movements smooth and fluid

Rest your weight on your right thigh

Full hip circling

Following the three steps on the right, lie on your back on the floor and slowly bring your right knee over to touch the floor on the left side of your body. Bring your right knee up towards your chest and hug it with your arms. Lower your bended leg to the floor, keeping it at right angles to your hip. Now slide the leg back into the original resting position. Repeat with the left leg.

Your arms should be above your head

Keep your thigh at right angles to your body

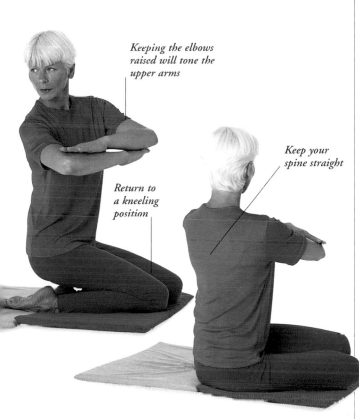

Keeping the elbows raised will tone the upper arms

Return to a kneeling position

Keep your spine straight

Bottom and thigh toner

This exercise is so simple it doesn't require an illustration. Lie on your front and cross your ankles. Keeping your knees straight, raise both your legs a short distance off the ground and hold them there for a count of ten. Now cross your legs in the other direction and repeat. (Avoid this exercise if you suffer from back pain.)

Bottom racing

Practising this simple exercise regularly will keep your buttocks toned. Sit with your legs straight out in front of you and move forwards on your buttocks as fast as you can. Keep your arms stretched out straight in front of you.

Standing spiral twists

This straightforward exercise will help keep your spine supple. Stand with your feet apart, your arms loosely by your sides, and twist at the waist as far as you can. Now twist in the other direction and increase your momentum. Let your arms swing under their own gravity.

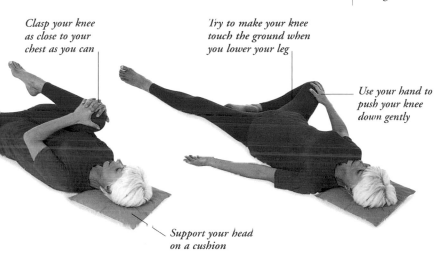

Clasp your knee as close to your chest as you can

Try to make your knee touch the ground when you lower your leg

Use your hand to push your knee down gently

Support your head on a cushion

329

*Try the following to reduce
nicotine intake.*

• *Smoke less than five
cigarettes a day.*

• *Always throw away
a long stub.*

• *Don't inhale.*

• *Always smoke low-tar
cigarettes.*

• *Always smoke filter-tip
cigarettes.*

• *Keep cigarettes as far away
from you as possible, so that
getting one involves the
maximum effort.*

ABANDONING BAD HABITS

Maintaining optimum health depends not only on adopting good habits but also on abandoning bad ones. For example, even if you eat the recommended daily amount of calcium and vitamin C, and you are a smoker, this amount will not be sufficient, since smoking depletes essential vitamins and minerals.

SMOKING

It has been proved that inhaling cigarette smoke causes lung cancer, bronchitis and heart disease. For women of any age, it is bad for your health, and it speeds up ageing of the skin. If you are still smoking, it is particularly important that you stop before the menopause. Smokers reach the menopause up to five years earlier than non-smokers (this includes passive smokers). Hot flushes tend to be more troublesome; smokers are more likely to get osteoporosis; and smokers are also more likely to have a heart attack.

Giving up smoking is difficult and some people only succeed when they have a dramatic health reason: the menopause, in my opinion, is a dramatic health reason. If you really find it impossible to give up completely, try to follow the controlling tips on the left.

ALCOHOL

Although drinking can have a relaxing effect, hot flushes can be triggered by alcohol and, for this reason alone, you should keep a careful eye on your intake.

A woman's response to alcohol differs according to the point she is at in her menstrual cycle: drink for drink, she will have higher alcohol levels during the pre-menstrual and ovulatory phases than at other times of the month. A woman's body contains 5–10 percent less water than a man's, so the same amount of alcohol will be more concentrated in her system and thus have a greater toxic effect on the body. Consequently, it takes less alcohol, consumed over fewer years, to cause liver damage in women than men.

Excessive drinking usually has a psychological origin, and menopausal women may be more vulnerable to alcoholism, especially if they feel that their former role is being eroded. We may also drink heavily if we are bored or unfulfilled. Understanding why we drink heavily is the first step to overcoming the problem.

Alcohol consumption is measured in units per week. Fourteen units per week is considered the healthy amount for a woman to drink. Half a pint of beer, a pub measure of spirits or a glass of wine is one unit. A light drinker would drink one to five units per week, and a moderate drinker 6–14 units. If you drink more than 14 units a week, you could be damaging your health, and if you drink more than 21, you may be on the verge of alcoholism. If the latter applies to you, or if you feel that your drinking is becoming a problem, you should seek medical help.

Menopausal women have acute reasons for limiting alcohol intake. Alcohol is an anti-nutrient, depleting the body of vitamins A, B and C, and it is a powerful oxidant and can lead to premature wrinkling of the skin.

CAFFEINE

Caffeine is a powerful drug that has a stimulating effect on the brain and a diuretic effect on the kidneys – it increases the amount of urine you pass. Although caffeine is present in the greatest quantity in coffee, it is also contained in some medications and in tea, chocolate and cola drinks. It can be a pick-me-up and, in small doses, may result in clearer thinking and sharper awareness. Larger doses, however, can give you "coffee nerves" – an anxious, fluttery feeling.

Caffeine can be particularly bad for menopausal women because it can actually trigger a hot flush. It also causes a temporary rise in blood pressure. If you have a weight problem, you should monitor your caffeine intake carefully, since too much can encourage the pancreas to release more insulin. This lowers your blood sugar, making you hungry and therefore inclined to binge.

Trying to cut out caffeine from your diet in one fell swoop may bring on withdrawal symptoms. Reduce your intake gradually, make sure your diet is rich in fibre, and drink plenty of water.

One way to reduce your consumption is to use a mixture of regular and decaffeinated coffee, gradually increasing the amount of the latter until the caffeine part is replaced. You can also substitute herbal teas, but check out the ingredients, since some herbal teas contain caffeine.

CONTROLLING YOUR ALCOHOL INTAKE

Try the following to reduce your alcohol intake.

- *Try to drink an equal quantity of water with alcohol.*

- *Eliminate drinks before and after meals, such as aperitifs and liqueurs.*

- *Always eat when you drink.*

- *Offer friends more non-alcoholic drinks, and drink more of these yourself.*

- *Skip the occasional round of drinks.*

- *If you have been drinking during the evening, have some water before you go to bed; put a full glass by your bedside in case you need a drink during the night.*

CARING FOR YOUR BODY

Keeping your body in good condition throughout the menopausal years requires the same combination of exercise, health-monitoring and hygiene that it always has. However, you need to pay more attention to certain parts of the body such as the teeth, eyes, ears and legs.

EYES

Visual defects that occur with age usually result from the changing shape of the eye, rather than the impaired functioning of its various parts.

Presbyopia becomes quite common in middle age, and develops because the lens is less able to change its shape to focus on what you are looking at. As a result, vision becomes blurred. Your optician will fit you with inwardly curved (convex) lenses to increase the power of your own lens, so that objects focus on the retina.

The cells of the retina also become less sensitive to light as you grow older, and it can become more difficult to read or see when brightness levels are low. On average, an 85-year-old woman needs approximately eight times as much light as a young person in order to see as well. The lens can also become yellowish, which makes it difficult to distinguish between different colours. Blue and green are filtered out, but warm colours, such as red and orange, are easier to see.

Even if you think your eyesight is perfectly all right, always have regular check-ups because a variety of disorders, such as glaucoma or cataracts, are more common in older people.

EARS

By the age of 50, some of us will be less able to hear higher-pitched sounds, but most of us should be able to look forward to normal hearing beyond the age of 60. Hearing loss is usually due to changes in the inner ear.

As we get older, we tend to lose the fine hair cells within the cochlea (inner ear) that activate the neurons in the auditory nerve. This is the most common cause of hearing loss, one that cannot be helped by a hearing aid. If impairment is not due to damage to the auditory nerve, or to the hair cells inside the cochlea, a hearing aid can make a big difference in your ability to cope.

The outer ear is rich in sebaceous glands that produce wax. Ear wax has several useful functions: it's an antiseptic and a lubricant, and it prevents foreign substances from reaching the eardrum and the middle ear. Daily washing is all that's needed to keep the outer ear clean. Wax should never be removed by a cotton swab – it will be driven down the ear canal where it will become impacted. It can then only be removed with warmed ear drops that dissolve the wax.

Even if you feel that both your ears and hearing are fine, always have regular check-ups to make sure that they both remain healthy.

MOUTH

The mouth is kept clean and healthy by the acts of talking, eating and drinking. Halitosis (bad breath) can be due to bad dental hygiene, mouth infection, dental decay or smoking. Regular tooth brushing is essential. Mouth washes and deodorant sprays do not compensate for bad hygiene and only cure bad breath temporarily.

By mid-adult life, most of us will have fillings, inlays and crowns, and we may also have a bridge or partial denture. At the menopause, the gums begin to recede due to lack of collagen, so the teeth become more exposed. Care of your mouth and teeth are as crucial now as they were when you were a child; follow the care tips on the right for optimum dental health.

Any sore patches on your tongue, gums or the inside of your cheeks that last two weeks or more should be seen by your doctor or dentist. A dry mouth can be relieved by sucking a sugarless sweet or having a drink of water. Always have the sharp edge of a tooth attended to by a dentist since it could cause an ulcer. Gum shrinkage that leads to loose dentures should also be attended to.

GENITALS

The vagina is a self-cleansing organ that does not benefit from excessive cleansing; in fact, over-zealous washing can upset the delicate bacterial balance necessary for vaginal health. It's far better to underclean than to overclean, and this applies to all parts of the body lined with delicate mucous membranes.

You should try to avoid using douches, antiseptics in the bath and vaginal deodorants. Overuse can kill off the bacteria that are the first line of defence against invaders

CARING FOR YOUR TEETH

Try the following simple guidelines to keep your teeth strong and healthy.

● *Keep plaque at bay by regular tooth brushing in the morning and at night, and after eating sweet foods. (Plaque causes calculus, which in turn can lead to pyorrhoea, the worst enemy of middle-aged teeth and gums.)*

● *Take care to clean in between your teeth (we develop spaces between our teeth as we get older). Dental floss or a tiny brush with a specially designed handle is suitable.*

● *Take a toothbrush with you if you're eating out so that you can brush your teeth after your meal.*

● *Visit your dental hygienist every three months for plaque removal, and visit your dentist every six months for general check-ups.*

such as *candida*, the fungus that causes thrush. The natural vaginal smell is preferable to an artificial perfume, and it plays an important part in sexual attraction; you may be less attractive to your partner if you take pains to camouflage it.

Under ordinary circumstances, bathing daily is sufficient to keep your genitals clean, although in hot weather you may feel comfortable washing more frequently. When you are washing, try not to use soap inside the outer lips of the vulva. You can wash the anal area as much as you like – it will not be harmful – but the vulval area is much more delicate and you should treat it gently. Unless you are sweating profusely or having sex a great deal, never use soap and water more than twice a day, and always use a gentle soap. At other times, it's quite sufficient to use water alone. You can wet a couple of cotton wool balls in water and wipe once from the front to the back of the perineal area, then throw them away. If you can't wash yourself during the course of the day, use baby wipes after you've been to the toilet, again from front to back, using them only once before disposing of them.

LEGS AND FEET

To maintain an active lifestyle, we should pay special attention to our legs and feet. Hardening of the arteries and increasingly poor circulation take their toll, especially on lower limbs and feet.

You'll avoid blisters and sore heels and toes if you wear comfortable, supple, low-heeled shoes most of the time. A shoe that fits well should grip your heel and instep, and not press on your toes. Whenever you can, sit with your feet up so that any fluid can drain away and the blood can flow more easily. This will also speed healing if you get any kind of cut, abrasion or sore. As you get older, minor injuries take longer to heal and this particularly applies to the feet. Treat cuts and sores promptly with a simple antiseptic cream and if they don't heal within a few days, consult your doctor. If you're a diabetic, consult your doctor immediately if you have a break in the skin of your legs and feet. Feet become more prone to infections with age, so never soak them in hot water – this makes the skin soggy and is a perfect medium for bacteria. You should also avoid wearing tight trousers or panty hose on your legs, since this will worsen circulation and hinder blood returning to the heart via the veins.

Chilblains tend to become more of a problem as you get older. You can help to avoid them by keeping your feet warm and wearing thick, woollen socks or panty hose, and in cold weather, fleece-lined slippers and shoes. One way to discourage the development of chilblains is to start the day with a warm bath and massage your feet with lotion or oil, using circular movements, and then dry them with a rough towel. Never put your feet or legs near direct heat or hold them against a radiator.

Varicose veins are most often the result of deep vein thrombosis in the leg, and they run in families. See right for self-help measures if you suffer from them. Mild varicose veins can be injected so they shrink and eventually scar and shrivel. If they are extensive, they can be stripped out by a vascular surgeon. Modern surgery is less painful and requires less hospitalization than previously.

NAILS

Brittle and flaking nails can be a problem after the menopause because waning oestrogen levels result in poor quality collagen.

If your fingernails are brittle and flaky, avoid using nail varnish remover, as this can dry them out even more. Use an emery board rather than scissors and metal files, and massage hand and nail cream into your cuticles daily. When you cut your toenails, use good-quality clippers and cut the nails straight across the top to the edges – never cut them steeply at the sides, since this encourages ingrowing toenails. If your toenails are very thick, file them frequently and try to thin them down as well as shorten them. Trim both finger and toenails once a week to keep them in good condition. From the menopause onwards, it's wise to visit a chiropodist on a regular basis.

SKIN AND BLOOD VESSELS

Ageing causes skin to become thinner and appear more transparent. Gradual changes to connective tissue are most easily seen on the backs of the hands, but are widespread throughout the body, resulting in conditions such as arthritis, hardening of the arteries, reduced lung capacity and loss of skin tone.

CARING FOR VARICOSE VEINS

Try the following simple suggestions to make varicose veins more comfortable.

• *Wear support stockings or panty hose and avoid tight garters or bands.*

• *Keep your legs warm and moisturize them after washing.*

• *Try not to stand for long periods at a time.*

• *Rest the legs in an upright position whenever possible; if you can, lie on the floor and put your legs up against the wall for 30 minutes before putting on support hose.*

• *Treat abrasions, bruises or minor infections of the lower legs meticulously, and consult your doctor if necessary.*

CONTROLLING BLOOD PRESSURE

Follow the simple measures below to maintain your blood pressure at healthy levels.

• *Cut back on both smoking and alcohol.*

• *Control your weight.*

• *Try relaxation and meditation exercises to reduce stress; stress is another cause of high blood pressure.*

BLOOD PRESSURE

Some self-regulating mechanisms are lost as we age, such as the maintenance of blood pressure during changes in posture. This may result in dizziness, and a tendency to lose your balance when you have to get up suddenly, especially from a horizontal position. High blood pressure can, in fact, become an increasing hazard with age and can lead to serious health problems, such as stroke and heart disease. Try to keep your blood pressure at a sensible level by following the simple guidelines outlined on the left.

LUNGS AND KIDNEYS

Cells in the lungs may be affected by age or disease. There is a decrease in the surface area of the air sacs, which can account for the breathlessness you may experience on exertion. Medically supervised exercise can play an important part in combating this problem.

Kidneys are affected by the deterioration of the circulatory system. The rate at which blood is filtered slows down and valuable minerals are reabsorbed more slowly. To keep your kidneys functioning properly, drink plenty of water, follow a healthy diet and take reasonable exercise.

BRAIN AND MIND

Because brain cells do not reproduce themselves, their function and number decrease as we grow older. The result of this is most apparent when it comes to memory, particularly when committing new experiences to memory. Opinions and attitudes can also become more rigid, so that the acceptance of new ideas can become progressively more difficult. However, as long as mental skills are exercised continuously, they should not decline to any significant degree.

Although intellectual deterioration is considered to be a result of ageing, it is actually a physical process that begins around the age of 16. For most of our adult lives, we do not notice any deterioration, mainly because we gain new experiences and knowledge, which compensate. This is why an alert mind coupled with a willingness to embrace new ideas, opinions and situations will keep us mentally healthy. Just as an unused muscle wastes away, so does an unused mind.

5

NATURAL THERAPIES

Although many women seek medical help during their menopausal years, there are many strategies that you can adopt by yourself to manage your own treatment, including a range of natural therapies, from aromatherapy to yoga. All therapies have their strengths and weaknesses and most are better for some things than for others. Some you can practise yourself, while for others you will need to find a qualified practitioner in order to benefit from it. Knowledge is the key – and the information in this chapter will enable you to take the most appropriate course of action for yourself.

PRACTISING NATUROPATHY

Naturopaths consider nutrition to be the anchor of health, and treatment will usually involve fasting (one of the oldest therapeutic methods known). You will also be advised to:

• *Drink pure water.*

• *Eat organically grown, unprocessed and, as far as possible, uncooked food.*

• *Use food supplements from natural sources rather than vitamin supplements. Wheat-germ oil, kelp and royal jelly can be particularly beneficial during the menopause.*

• *Animal protein should not make up more than 25 percent of the diet.*

COMPLEMENTARY THERAPIES

Any medicine that heals or relieves discomfort without any harmful side effects is, in my opinion, good medicine. Although HRT is the major treatment advocated by the medical establishment, complementary medical practices offer many natural alternatives.

Traditional medicine is based on allopathy, a doctrine that follows the principle that when the working of the body goes wrong, the symptoms should be counter-acted. An example of this practice would be treating constipation with a laxative.

In contrast to this approach, the major branches of complementary medicine argue that each body has a life force that becomes disturbed when that body becomes diseased but reasserts itself if the body stops being abused and is nourished correctly.

Just like the best traditional medicine, the best complementary medicine is holistic – it treats the whole person, rather than an isolated symptom. The true naturopath is sceptical of symptomatic remedies because they fail to treat the root cause of the illness.

NATUROPATHY

Many types of complementary medicine are based on naturopathy. Its principles are as follows:
• The patient is treated, not the disease.
• The whole body is treated, not just a part of it.
• The underlying factors causing the disease must be removed.
• Disease is a disturbance of a life force, demonstrated by tension, rigidity or congestion somewhere in the body.
• The patient's own life force is the true healer.
• The body must have a "healing crisis" in which the life force cleanses the body by eliminating accumulated toxins. The use of drugs in orthodox medicine, while superficially curing the disease, drives it deep within the body, leaving behind a chronic condition for the future.
Naturopaths believe that health depends on adopting a well-balanced attitude of mind by practising relaxation, yoga, meditation and psychotherapy. Some also include hydrotherapy in their treatment programmes.

AROMATHERAPY

Although this is a fairly new addition to complementary medicine, its roots go back several centuries. Human beings have a highly developed sense of smell and we can react to an odour within a split second. Babies bond with their mothers through scent, and lovers are attracted by each other's pheromones, or chemical secretions. Smells can be mood-enhancing and they may relieve pain and illness. Massage using essential oils is relaxing and enjoyable, and beneficial in reducing many stress-related conditions.

The oil essences that are used in aromatherapy are pure distillations from plants, and are very concentrated. In a dilute form, they can be inhaled and absorbed through the lining of the air passages. Essential oils can be used singly or blended, and they have different properties: some are antiviral, some affect blood pressure and some are general healers.

Essential oils are absorbed through the skin during massage or bathing, and through the lungs when they are inhaled. Oral doses are not generally recommended except in the case of garlic, which may be taken in capsule form. The emphasis in aromatherapy is on the treatment of relatively minor ailments and the promotion of health and well-being, both physical and mental. For this reason, the use of essential oils has achieved a wide popularity in recent years.

USING ESSENTIAL OILS

Essential oils are very strong, so take care when using them. Try these simple tips.

• *Inhale as a vapour. Add three drops of essential oil to a bowl of steaming water, cover your head and breathe in.*

• *Add a few drops to a warm bath. Spend at least 15 minutes in it to derive the full benefit.*

• *Apply to the skin as massage oil. Dilute with a base, such as sweet almond oil or soya oil. Add about 20 drops to 100 ml (3.3 fl oz) of base oil.*

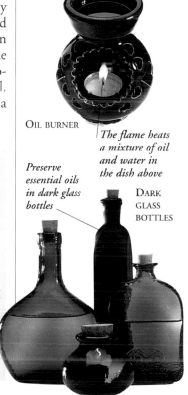

OIL BURNER

The flame heats a mixture of oil and water in the dish above

Preserve essential oils in dark glass bottles

DARK GLASS BOTTLES

MENOPAUSAL REMEDIES

ESSENTIAL OIL	SYMPTOM
Avocado, wheatgerm	Dry skin
Juniper, lavender, rosemary	Muscle and joint pain
Lavender, peppermint	Headaches
Basil	Fatigue
Neroli, lavender	Insomnia
Clary sage, rose	Depressed mood

USING HOMEOPATHIC REMEDIES

It's best to have a consultation to determine your constitutional "type", but if you treat yourself, bear in mind the following.

• *Increase the potency or seek medical advice if your symptoms are not relieved after six doses.*

• *Avoid substances such as coffee, peppermint, menthol and camphor, which can counteract the effects of homeopathic remedies.*

• *Avoid homeopathic pills coated in lactose if you are allergic to milk.*

• *Take a remedy hourly if your symptoms are very acute. For longer-term problems, remedies can be taken in the morning and at night.*

• *Stop taking a remedy as soon as your symptoms start to improve.*

• *Preserve remedies by storing them in a cool, dark place away from smells.*

HOMEOPATHY

This form of natural healing is based on the principle that a substance that produces the same symptoms as an illness will, in a very dilute form, help to cure it. The venom of the bushmaster snake, lachesis, for instance, is very poisonous, but because it is used in such a dilute form, it is not toxic. The potency of remedies affects the efficacy of treatment – the more dilute the remedy, the greater the potency. Homeopathic remedies have a number after them that indicates how dilute they are. For instance, *pulsatilla 30* is more dilute and therefore more potent than *pulsatilla 6*.

The homeopathic view of menopausal problems is that they reflect existing imbalances that can only be treated in relation to the mental and physical makeup of the individual. Women are encouraged to prepare for the menopause by looking at their overall health and developing a positive attitude of self before its onset.

The emphasis upon the individual and her physical and emotional history, rather than the illness she is suffering from, is fundamental to homeopathy. When consulting a homeopathic practitioner, your symptoms are assessed along with your personality and constitution, and likes and dislikes, to form the basis of your treatment. For example, the remedy *sepia* is suited to someone who is irritable, moody or dejected.

If you would like to treat your symptoms homeopathically, it is very important to consult a qualified homeopathic practitioner.

MENOPAUSAL REMEDIES

REMEDY	SYMPTOM
Lachesis	Hot flushes
Pulsatilla	Insomnia, PMS, joint pain
Sepia	Dry vagina, prolapse, flushes, thinning hair
Sulphur	Dry, itchy vulva and skin
Belladonna	Hot flushes and night sweats

HERBALISM

Some of the oldest methods of healing the sick are based on herbalism. Over the centuries, developments in orthodox medicine began to cast doubt on the efficacy of natural remedies, but since the 1950s herbalism has enjoyed renewed popularity and can sometimes be compared favourably with modern drugs, which may create allergies or spread resistant strains of bacteria.

Like homeopathy, the aims behind herbal treatment are to remove the cause of the symptoms rather than merely the symptoms themselves, and to improve the patient's general standard of health and well-being. A disadvantage of herbalism is that agreement over which remedies should be used for particular disorders is still surprisingly limited. However, it does offer an attractive alternative to other forms of conventional treatment in that it is based on natural principles and ingredients. Herbal remedies can also work as a complement to orthodox medicine.

Modern herbalism aims to correct what is wrong with the body by strengthening its natural functions so that it may heal itself. Herbs can be very effective in relieving menopausal symptoms, but although there is valuable anecdotal information about their benefits, few remedies have been subjected to tightly controlled clinical trials.

There are many herbs that can help to relieve both the physical and emotional symptoms of the menopause, but there are three in particular that are associated with it: sage, agnus castus and black cohosh.

Sage may help to alleviate hot flushes, and you can take it in tea form, made from fresh or dried sage. Simply pour boiling water on to two teaspoonfuls of leaves, infuse for ten minutes and strain. Sage tea has quite a strong taste, and although some women find it calming, others find it unpalatable – if you don't like the taste, buy the herb in tablet form from a herbalist.

The herb agnus castus (also known as chaste tree) has long been associated with menopausal disorders, and it may help to normalize hormone levels, acting as a natural type of HRT. Some herbalists recommend the following combination of herbs to treat hot flushes: blackcurrant leaves, hawthorn tops, sage and agnus castus. This may be drunk in an infusion three times

USING HERBS

Follow these simple guidelines for effective herbal treatment.

- *Consult a qualified herbalist before taking herbs, especially if you have heart disease, high blood pressure or glaucoma.*

- *Always use herbs in moderation and, if possible, discuss dosage with a qualified herbalist before treatment.*

- *Discontinue use if you start to experience side effects.*

- *Give each herb a week or two to assess its efficacy.*

- *Don't take herbs for longer than a few months without a break.*

- *Check with your doctor before you take a herbal remedy if you are already taking medication.*

- *Don't put off seeking medical advice because you are taking a herbal remedy.*

- *Buy herbs from a reputable supplier because it is very easy to make mistakes in identification.*

daily for six weeks. Black cohosh has oestrogenic properties and can be of assistance if you are feeling weak and tense. It also has antispasmodic and sedative properties and will help to alleviate premenstrual tension, pains and bloating. Black cohosh works well in combination with agnus castus.

ACUPUNCTURE

The word acupuncture comes from the Latin and means "to pierce with a needle". The use of acupuncture in China has been widespread for 5,000 years, but it has only been acknowledged and practised in the West during this century.

The theory behind acupuncture is that a life or energy force flows through the body along channels called meridians, which are quite distinct from the lines followed by nerves. This life force must flow unimpeded if bodily health is to be maintained. When we get sick, the energy flowing along a particular meridian may be affected at a site considerably distant from the sick part of the body. The acupuncturist tries to restore the flow of energy in the affected meridian by using copper, silver or gold needles inserted a small way into the flesh at specific points along the meridian. These needles are so fine that they can hardly be felt as they enter the skin. Depending on the position of the selected point, the needles may be inserted vertically, at an angle or sometimes almost horizontally. The needle is then rotated, moved up and down or used to conduct heat or a mild electric current. This is thought to set up some kind of current along the meridian line. It passes to the central nervous system and has an effect on the organ or area that is malfunctioning by re-establishing the flow of energy through the meridian.

Acupuncture is one of the few Eastern medical practices that is widely accepted and used in the West, although its applications are not nearly so widespread here. In China, even major operations, including heart transplants and brain surgery, may be performed using acupuncture as the only form of general anaesthetic.

The meridians
Acupuncture and acupressure are based on the theory that our life force flows along channels called meridians. When the flow of energy is disturbed, we get sick.

Acupressure points

Meridians

Electrical acupressure device
This hand-held device is used to locate and apply pressure to the acupressure points.

ACUPRESSURE

This technique follows the same principles as acupuncture, but pressure, rather than needles, is applied to the energy meridians. Massaging the acupoints with the thumbs and fingers helps to restore interrupted energy flow along the meridians. Pressure is applied to specific points, with the aim of stimulating the nerves that supply the affected organ.

Acupressure is claimed to help specific organs by releasing blocked energy. Unlike acupuncture, you can practise acupressure on yourself, although you may find it hard to locate the right pressure points at first. It can be used to alleviate pain, improve your general well-being or target specific symptoms, such as joint stiffness.

HYDROTHERAPY

Hydrotherapy aims to increase the blood flow to the skin and eliminate toxins (this should be viewed with scepticism as they cannot be expelled through the skin – we have a liver to do that). It also draws blood and nourishment to internal organs then flushes it out again.

Most forms use hot and cold water alternately. The hot water dilates the blood vessels, increasing blood flow to the skin. This part of the treatment may last five, ten or fifteen minutes, according to the severity of the condition and the patient's frailty. It should be avoided if you have any kind of heart condition since hydrotherapy can put an enormous strain on the heart. The second stage of therapy involves douching, sluicing or showering in cold water, which causes the blood vessels to constrict, reducing blood flow and driving blood back to the heart and the purifying organs, such as the liver. Never take any of the treatments listed on the right without checking with your doctor first.

MASSAGE

Many claims are made about the virtues of massage – some are false, some plausible and some indisputable. For example, massage does not help to break down fat, but it may relieve emotional tension, and it definitely speeds up local circulation and improves nourishment of tissues. During a massage, parts of the body are treated in a specific order. The direction of massage strokes is

WATER TREATMENTS

The following are the major therapeutic water treatments.

Sauna *Sitting in intense dry heat, is followed by a cold shower, then a second, shorter period in the sauna, followed by a scrub-down. It is said to improve circulation, tone up muscles, cleanse the skin and create well-being.*

Scotch douche *Hot and cold water is sprayed alternately up and down the spine to stimulate the nerves. It is thought to relieve migraine.*

Sitz Bath *This is a two-section bath, one for hot water and one for cold. Your buttocks and hips sit in hot water for five to ten minutes while your feet are immersed in cold. You then switch round, with your feet in hot, body in cold. It flushes blood into the pelvic area to nourish it, then out again to carry off waste material.*

Steam Cabinets *This is like a traditional Turkish bath, except the head is outside the steam area. The heat is wet rather than dry, so it produces sweat faster. It is said to clear the skin of waste materials very efficiently. The body will feel very hot and some people may find it debilitating. After 15 minutes, the bather takes a cold shower to restore skin to normal. Treatment should be followed by rest.*

always towards the heart, assisting the return of blood to the heart to be oxygenated in the lungs. The patient lies down and the masseur massages each foot and leg in turn. Next comes the abdomen, followed by the arms, wrists, hands and fingers, then the back of the body.

Swedish massage involves vigorous strokes, such as beating with the sides of the hands from the base of the spine to the neck and back again. Although it is usually a safe therapy, avoid vigorous massage if you have any sort of skin disease, or if your skin has been injured.

Neuromuscular massage consists of pressing with the fingertips. Specific motor points in the muscles are deeply massaged in an attempt to diminish the output to the

TYPES OF MASSAGE STROKE

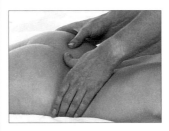

Pressing
Localized pressure can be given using the thumbs either in static form, pressing in one position, or circular, moving the thumbs in small circles.

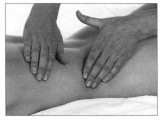

Circling
This is a very simple stroke, in which you use the fingers and palms of both hands to massage the skin in firm, circular movements.

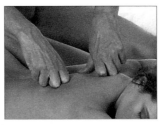

Knuckling
Here, the knuckles are used to exert pressure below the shoulder blades. This is good for getting rid of tension in painfully knotted muscles.

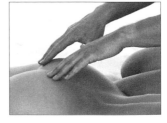

Feathering
This playful and gentle massage stroke involves lightly skimming the fingertips and fingernails across the surface of the skin.

sensory nerves to the area, and break the vicious circle of pain and muscle spasm from which we can suffer from time to time. Once muscular tension has been relieved using this technique, the muscle will be less likely to spring back into its previous tense position.

OSTEOPATHY

Modern osteopathy is based on the theory that our bodies have the ability to regulate and heal themselves, provided that they are structurally sound and nerve impulses and blood are able to move freely.

Harmful structural changes to the body may result from several things, including poor posture. Osteopathic stimulation tries to rectify these problems by manipulating the spinal vertebrae. Osteopaths also believe that relief of muscle spasm cures illnesses stemming from muscular strain.

The two basic techniques of osteopathy are the massage of muscles in spasm and the manipulative correction of misaligned bones in the spinal column. This involves gentle leverage of one part of the body against another, for example, the chin against the neck to adjust the position of the vertebrae at the base of the skull. Cranial osteopathy tries to make minute adjustments to the bones of the skull by delicately manipulating the bones of the cranium and the spine. Cranial osteopathy may be used to treat the same conditions as osteopathy itself. Osteopathy can claim many well-documented cures and is rapidly gaining acceptance by the medical profession. Before you have osteopathic treatment, you should request X-rays to exclude the possibility that you have osteoporosis.

CHIROPRACTIC

Chiropractic focuses on the anatomy of the spinal cord and on the nerves that branch out from it. Nerves run through each vertebra to the skin, bone, muscles, blood vessels and organs. The theory is that manipulating a particular vertebra will influence the health of a specific organ. For example, because the liver is supplied by nerves from the middle thoracic (chest) vertebrae, manipulating them will affect liver function. Even

Vicious circle of pain
Massage can relax the muscles and break the vicious circle of muscle tension and pain.

PRACTISING YOGA

Follow the guidelines below to make the most of this therapy.

• *Breathe deeply and rhythmically through your nose.*

• *Don't force yourself into a difficult position – some yoga positions can feel very uncomfortable at first.*

• *Work slowly towards becoming supple.*

• *Hold a posture only for as long as it is comfortable. Aim for about 30 seconds initially in standing and sitting postures.*

• *Wear comfortable, loose clothing and keep your feet bare to stop yourself slipping.*

• *Don't practise yoga for at least four hours after eating a large meal.*

relatively minor deviations of the anatomy of the spinal cord caused by conditions such as bad posture or inflammation, for instance, can impair the working of a nerve and the body part it supplies.

Vertebrae are manipulated using short, sharp thrusts designed to spring a bone back into place. This procedure demands great precision in placing the adjusting hand, and timing and directing the thrust.

Symptoms that respond best to chiropractic techniques are neck, muscle, shoulder and joint pain. As with osteopathy, chiropractic should be used with caution on any menopausal women who might be suffering from osteoporosis or who exhibit any signs of having very low bone mass.

YOGA

This is probably the best known of all the meditation and movement therapies. Its holistic approach, encompassing stretching movements, mental relaxation and deep breathing, can help you deal very effectively with menopausal symptoms.

The aim of yoga postures, called *asanas*, is to encourage a healthy mind to exist in a healthy body and bring both into harmony. Anyone can take up yoga, whatever her age: you simply do as much as you find comfortable. Many people find that it helps them to overcome specific health problems, such as smoking or excessive drinking, high blood pressure and menstrual problems.

Yoga must be learned slowly, avoiding all strain. It is simple and inexpensive to do – no equipment is needed, except perhaps a mat, a quiet room and loose, comfortable clothing. You may find it easiest to have some training to start with to help you master the breathing techniques. *Asanas* seem to be a very static way of conditioning the body. If you achieve the correct posture, however, each limb and muscle is stretching. After a series of *asanas*, allow yourself a period of relaxation in order to discipline and focus the mind and create a calm mood, before you resume your daily tasks.

It is generally felt that yoga promotes good posture and mental tranquillity, which may alleviate backache, mild depression and sleeping problems. Consult your doctor before taking up yoga, however, if you suffer from any existing medical condition.

6

SEXUALITY AND RELATIONSHIPS

If you had an enjoyable and fulfilling sex life before the menopause, you almost certainly will continue to have one afterwards. In fact, there are many advantages to postmenopausal sex, one important one being that you no longer have to worry about contraception and pregnancy. Understanding the changes that are taking place in both your and your partner's body will help to maintain and enhance your sex life together. Following the simple guidance and suggestions in this chapter will enable you to continue enjoying a fulfilling physical relationship with your partner for the rest of your life.

NATURAL VAGINAL HEALTH

Try the following suggestions for good vaginal health.

• *Apply yoghurt containing live bacteria,* Lactobacillus acidophilus, *to the vagina; there is anecdotal evidence that it helps to prevent infections. The yoghurt should remain in the vagina for at least two hours after application – wearing a tampon can keep it from leaking out.*

• *Douche with a solution of one tablespoon of white vinegar in a pint of water. This will keep the vagina acidic. (Too much sugar in your urine can make your vagina alkaline and prone to infections, such as thrush.)*

• *Add a cup of vinegar to bath water or use a tampon soaked in the solution.*

• *Consult a qualified herbalist for herbal remedies – there are many available.*

If any treatment causes soreness, stop using it immediately.

NATURAL SATISFACTION

One benefit of growing older with a partner is that you know how to strike a balance between shared interests and privacy. A well-kept secret is that many of us lose our inhibitions as we get older. We feel free to enjoy sexual pleasure, to express ourselves in ways that we kept hidden when we were younger.

The saying "if you don't use it, you lose it" is particularly applicable to sex during the menopause. Regular sexual activity can keep your sex organs healthy, and if you take care of yourself, you can remain sexually active for the rest of your life. There are, however, changes in your body, and often in your partner's body, that require adjustments to your familiar sexual routine. Once you know about these changes, you can begin to adapt your life accordingly to keep sex satisfying.

Factors that help sex after the menopause
• A rewarding relationship before the menopause.
• Positive attitudes towards sex and ageing.
• A good relationship with your partner.
• Physical and emotional fitness, and an accepting attitude towards your body.

Factors that inhibit sex after the menopause
• A history of unsatisfying sex.
• An unsupportive partner or an unhappy relationship.
• Problems such as vaginal dryness or soreness.
• Attitudes that equate sex with youthfulness or having children.
• Surgical removal of the ovaries.

VAGINAL CHANGES

During and after the menopause, the walls of the vagina become drier and less elastic. Even the shape changes – it becomes shorter and narrower (although it always remains big enough to accommodate an erect penis). The clitoris becomes slightly smaller, and the lips of the vagina become thinner and flatter. The covering of the clitoris may also become thinner and pull back, leaving it more exposed. This can make it extremely sensitive to touch, and you may find that you need quite a bit of lubrication before it can be stimulated with the fingers.

In young women, one of the first signs of arousal is the wetness produced by the walls of the vagina. Droplets of fluid form a slippery coat in the vagina and on the vulva, making penetration easy and pleasurable for both partners. Falling oestrogen levels mean that vaginal cells may not be able to lubricate as quickly as before. You may feel very aroused but it takes several minutes for your vagina to "catch up". If this is the case, explain to your partner that you need to take things slowly, and spend more time on foreplay.

In young women, thick vaginal walls serve as a cushion during intercourse, protecting the bladder and the urethra from friction. At the menopause, the vaginal walls become thinner, and it is common to feel a strong urge to urinate after sex. If this is the case, empty your bladder promptly. Some menopausal women also complain of a burning sensation during urination that can persist for several days. Drinking plenty of water can relieve this feeling.

Although vaginal dryness is common during the menopause, a small number of women still lubricate rapidly when aroused. The likely reason for this is that these women continue to have sex once or twice a week throughout their adult lives. This supports the belief that regular sex can promote vaginal health.

The vicious circle of vaginal dryness
The vagina and vulva become thin and prone to dryness after the menopause, and this can make sex painful. Ironically, if you abstain from sex, the problem may get worse.

HORMONAL CHANGES

Sex drive is hormonally related, and many studies have shown that women experience heightened sexual desire around the middle of the menstrual cycle, which is the time when they usually ovulate.

Oestrogen levels reach their peak at ovulation. However, ovulation is also marked by high levels of the male sex hormones, testosterone and androstenedione, and high levels of testosterone are known to create a high sex drive in both men and women. After the menopause, the ratio of testosterone to oestrogen becomes greater because oestrogen levels fall while testosterone remains the same (or increases). Contrary to the myth of sexual decline, some women – about one in six – report increased sexual desire after the menopause, which may be attributable to the relative excess of male hormones.

Research carried out on women who had undergone hysterectomies, including the removal of their ovaries, confirmed the role of testosterone in sexual arousal. The women were asked to rate the intensity of their sexual desire before and after their operations, and after surgery the women were given one of the following treatments: oestrogen; testosterone; oestrogen and testosterone; and a placebo. The study's conclusions were that only in those women taking testosterone or a mixture of oestrogen and testosterone was sexual interest restored to pre-menopausal levels, and that male sex hormones do therefore stimulate women's sexual interest.

For this reason, the quantity of testosterone your menopausal ovaries produce is likely to have a significant effect on your sex drive. Hormone levels vary considerably from woman to woman: in some, blood levels of male hormones actually increase after the menopause; in others, they decrease by 50 percent or more.

If you've noticed a decrease in sexual desire that seems to coincide with your menopause – particularly if you have had a hysterectomy with your ovaries removed – it could be due to decreased levels of male sex hormones. Even if testosterone replacement therapy would seem to be an answer, it is not; there are two major problems. First, the ideal level of testosterone for women has not been determined, and doctors can only use blood tests as a guideline to determine how your level compares with what is normal for your age. Second, male sex hormones have potent side effects and can cause lowering of the voice and hirsutism (hairiness) to occur.

Rather than agree to use a therapy whose benefits can be mixed, therefore, it makes more sense to concentrate on simple, natural measures to sustain your interest in sex and in your partner. Kegel exercises and the suggestions on page 284 could both be helpful.

CHANGES IN YOUR PARTNER

An interested partner is the most important factor for good sex at any age, and the influence of declining hormones on desire may have a modest effect in comparison to the importance of a fulfilling relationship. Menopausal women usually have partners who are experiencing changes in their own sexual behaviour, so it's helpful to be aware of male physiology, particularly if you have a partner over 50.

Changes in your partner's sexual behaviour are easier to understand if you realize that there are changes in his hormones. As men age, testosterone-inhibiting factors increase, causing a decline in the frequency of erection. Replacing hormones in men is not as beneficial as it is in women. Men need a minimum amount of testosterone, and if they already have it, testosterone replacement therapy will not usually help.

Most young men can have an erection within seconds of being stimulated. For men over 50, it may take longer, and more direct stimulation of the penis may well be necessary. Some men find that they cannot maintain their erections for as long as they used to. This is not a problem, it just means that you have to adjust your timing where sex is concerned, so that you are fully aroused at the same time that he is ready for penetration. Mutual masturbation as part of foreplay can be helpful.

As a man ages, his penis becomes flaccid faster, and it may take longer for him to have another erection. For a man over 50, the waiting period may be 12 hours; for men in their 60s and 70s, it can take several days. Older men don't necessarily ejaculate during sex. If your partner doesn't ejaculate on one occasion, it doesn't mean that he will never ejaculate again. Each man is different and follows his own timetable.

There is a popular fallacy that ageing robs a man of his capacity for sexual pleasure. It is not true, but many men are anxious about their sexual performance deteriorating. If your partner does not achieve an erection on more than one occasion, he may be afraid he is impotent and start avoiding sex altogether. This can lead to all sorts of misunderstandings: he may blame you, and you may feel guilty, or he may blame himself. It is therefore essential that you communicate frankly about your feelings.

SEEKING MEDICAL HELP

If your partner has severe problems getting or maintaining an erection, he should seek medical advice. Difficulties may well be physical in origin, particularly if he is taking certain medications. For instance, betablockers, which can be prescribed for high blood pressure, can affect sexual function, and so can antihistamines. In addition diabetes can cause damage to the nerves that stimulate erection and ejaculation.

MAXIMIZE LOVEMAKING

One of the most important things you can do to nurture your sex life is to make the time to create a relaxing, sensual environment. Pay attention to mood and atmosphere, have a drink together, play your favourite music and take turns at undressing each other. Using fragrant massage oil, gently stroke your partner all over, working your way slowly down his body from his head to his toes. When it's your turn, show your pleasure at what feels good, and be explicit about your preferences. Slowly move on to touching your partner's penis, and when he touches you, tell him what you would like him to do.

EVALUATING YOUR SEX LIFE

Take stock of your sex life by answering the following questions, which should help you assess your sex life and identify any areas that you would like to change. It may be useful for you and your partner to answer the questions together.

Your body
• Are you happy with your body?
• If you're not, are you prepared to improve your body by changing your diet and by exercising more?
• Are you inhibited about any one part of your body?
• Do you feel relaxed about undressing and being naked in front of your partner?

Your feelings
• Do you feel close to your partner?
• Do you think you and your partner are well matched sexually?
• Do you find it easy to talk about sex?
• Can you ask for what you want sexually?

The setting
• Where do you make love?
• Do you ever try to create a sexy atmosphere with soft lights, candles or mood music?
• Do you always make love in the same place?
• Do you have complete privacy?

The build-up to sex
• How do you initiate sex?
• Do you give conflicting signals?
• If your partner misunderstands you, how can you communicate better?
• Do you spend enough time on foreplay so that you are fully aroused when you have sex?

Intercourse
• Do you ever find penetration difficult or painful?
• What do you do to overcome this?
• Do you reach orgasm and, if so, how?
• If you don't reach orgasm during intercourse, do you ask your partner to stimulate you in other ways?

Answering all of these questions could give you a better idea of what, if anything, you might want to change or improve about your sex life. For example, you may feel that making love has become routine and predictable. Suggestions about how to inject variety into your lovemaking are given in the pages that follow.

Genital touching can progress to penetration or can bring you both to orgasm. If you choose mutual masturbation, lubricate your hands with oil or a water-based jelly (don't use fragrant massage oil if you are going to use a condom because it destroys the rubber). Although some women may be inhibited about giving or receiving oral sex, it is another good way to extend fore-play, or it can be used as an end in itself.

Some couples like to increase their arousal by sharing their sexual fantasies or by looking at erotic material. Arousal begins in the brain, and if you are mentally stimulated, genital stimulation will usually follow.

Don't assume that because you have been making love to your partner for years, you know everything about him sexually. The secret of satisfying sex is to keep communicating with each other, asking your partner what he wants, telling him what you like and sharing your sexual thoughts, dreams and fantasies. Break away from your normal sexual routine – make love in a new position, in a new place, at a different time.

SENSUAL MASSAGE

The power of touch and its importance in our lives never diminishes. Even in very old age, the importance of physical intimacy and touch is high – being hugged and petted is necessary for our physical and mental well-being. A massage is an excellent way to relax: you can explore your partner's erogenous zones and set the scene for sex. Use fragranced massage oil or cream to lubricate his skin – apply it to your hands first to make it warm, then follow the tips on the right. Pay attention to parts of the body that are usually neglected, such as the feet.

EXTENDED FOREPLAY

The main reason for extending foreplay is that you and your partner may have slower sexual responses than you once had. Build up to sex gradually by stroking each other gently, and prolong the moment when you touch your partner's genitals by massaging him with fragranced oil. Other possibilities include having a bath or shower to-gether and exploring your partner's erogenous zones by lightly nibbling them. When you touch your partner's genitals, spend time caressing him slowly until you both feel completely ready and eager for penetration.

SENSUAL MASSAGING

Try the following simple steps to help maximize your sensual experiences.

• *Lie your partner face down, sit astride his buttocks and run your fingertips lightly up and down his back.*

• *Progress to firmer strokes, using the thumbs, paying special attention to muscles between the shoulder blades and at the base of the neck.*

• *Roll him on to his back and massage his abdomen and chest. Use your fingertips to circle his nipples with light strokes.*

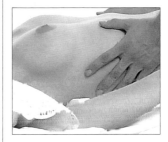

Erotic touching
Tell your partner where you'd like to be touched, or demon-strate by guiding his hand.

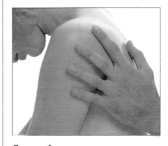

Sensual caresses
Spend time being stroked and caressed by your partner before you begin to make love.

MASTURBATING TECHNIQUES

If you have never masturbated, choose a time when you will be totally undisturbed, and a place where you feel relaxed.

• *Start by stroking the whole of your body, then focus on your genital area. Some women stroke or press their entire vulva, others concentrate on stimulating the clitoral area.*

• *Stroke or rub with the fingers to provide intense stimulation; some women use a vibrator. Or climax by pressing your thighs together.*

• *Fantasizing may enhance arousal.*

Vibrators
You can use a vibrator to bring yourself to orgasm, or your partner can use it on you as a means of enhancing foreplay.

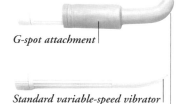

G-spot attachment

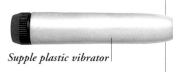

Standard variable-speed vibrator

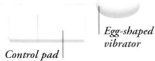

Supple plastic vibrator

Egg-shaped vibrator

Control pad

MASTURBATION

Self-stimulation is not only a safe form of sexual enjoyment, it is also an ideal way to explore your body and release sexual tension. If you don't have a partner, masturbation can provide vital sexual release – this can be a positive choice for many women. Even if you have a partner, you can use masturbation to complement intercourse. If you become aroused very slowly, your partner can spend time stimulating you manually. Alternatively, you can masturbate alone for pleasure. There are several different ways in which you can masturbate; see those listed on the left. Basically, however, whatever brings you satisfaction is absolutely fine, and you should never be afraid to experiment.

OVERCOMING PROBLEMS

Problems such as a low sex drive may be due to relationship problems or stress. Occasionally, there is a physiological basis, and you should always see a doctor to eliminate this possibility.

PROBLEMS ACHIEVING ERECTION

The first rule in achieving an erection is for your partner to learn to relax. Most sexual problems are psychological rather than physical in origin, and if your partner is anxious and afraid that he won't be able to achieve an erection, then he probably won't. If you feel your problems are particularly deep-rooted and that they are having a serious impact on your relationship, it may be useful to receive counselling.

Don't set out specifically to have intercourse, because this may put pressure on your partner. Spend a long time touching and stroking each other, and if he is aroused, concentrate on stimulating his genital area with your hands or mouth. If you use your hands to do this, lubricate the penis with a water-based jelly and massage the shaft firmly.

If your partner's problems result from medication he is taking, he should ask his doctor about alternatives. In severe cases of impotence, a penile implant consisting of two inflatable rods can be surgically installed in the penis. A pump in the scrotum inflates the rods, causing the penis to become erect.

LONG-TERM ILLNESS

Serious illness can be a major inhibiting factor in sex. This is particularly true if you or your partner have had heart problems. Because you are afraid of putting any extra pressure on your heart, you may abstain altogether. Fortunately, doctors agree that a normal sex life can greatly benefit people who have suffered heart attacks and other heart problems, and they encourage a return to normal sexual activity as soon as possible.

Arthritis can make intercourse uncomfortable, but pain can often be alleviated by some simple measures, such as having a hot bath to mobilize your joints, adopting a restful position during lovemaking and taking painkilling drugs an hour or so before you have sex. The spoons position is gentle and relaxing. The woman lies on her side with her knee raised, while the man penetrates her from behind. This gives him access to her breasts and upper body, while she can stimulate herself manually. Always remember that sex does not have to be penetrative every time – alternatives such as oral sex, mutual masturbation or stroking can also be stimulating.

Diabetes is another medical condition that can cause sexual problems. In women these include a dry, itchy vulva and yeast infections; in men they include difficulty in achieving an erection and problems ejaculating. Some diabetes drugs can cause impotence, so check this with your doctor and ask about alternative medications. If diabetes is treated early, all these problems may be lessened.

VAGINISMUS (VAGINAL SPASM)

Fear of penetration, which is sometimes referred to as vaginismus, can make sex very painful, and often impossible. The cause of vaginismus is almost always psychological and may stem from deep-rooted fears about sex. Some women develop it after menopause as a result of vaginal pain and dryness. They may become acutely sensitive to the stretching sensation that occurs during penetration and learn to anticipate pain, which triggers muscular contractions. If this is the case, there are effective self-help measures to alleviate postmenopausal sexual problems. If you had vaginismus before your menopause, it may be a defensive reaction to sexual situations that you cannot control.

VAGINISMUS EXERCISES

Try the following simple techniques to ease penetration.

• *Using a mirror, touch the vaginal entrance with your fingers.*

• *Relax by breathing deeply, and when you feel ready, insert the tip of one finger into your vagina. Use a lubricant, such as oil, lubricating jelly or saliva.*

• *Now insert your finger further into the vagina – if you feel your vaginal muscles contracting, stop, wait until you feel relaxed, and try again. Using this technique, try to get to the point where you can insert two or three fingers into the vagina.*

• *When making love, experiment with woman-on-top positions, which allow you to control the depth of penetration.*

BIRTH CONTROL

Although the menopause signals the end of fertility, women should continue to use birth control for at least one or two years after their last menstrual period. A common method of contraception chosen by women who have completed their families is the intrauterine device or IUD, but other methods, such as the pill or condoms, are convenient and highly effective.

Condoms are made from latex rubber or plastic

Spermicidal jelly

This is designed for use with a cap or a diaphragm. The jelly is squeezed into the diaphragm, which is then inserted into the vagina so that it covers the entrance to the cervix. Spermicidal creams and jellies are not effective contraceptives on their own.

Contraceptive jelly containing vaginal spermicide

Male condom

This is the most widely used contraceptive in the world and it works by preventing sperm from entering the woman's body. It is rolled on to the erect penis before penetration and should be removed immediately after intercourse.

The diaphragm prevents sperm from entering the uterus

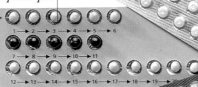

Triphasic pill

Mini-pill

Combination pill

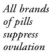

All brands of pills suppress ovulation

The pill

Combination pills contain oestrogen and progestogen; triphasic pills contain three different doses of oestrogen and progestogen; mini-pills contain progestogen only.

Diaphragm

The diaphragm is a soft rubber device with a flexible metal rim, designed to fit diagonally over the cervix. It is used with spermicidal jelly.

Intrauterine device (IUD)

This small plastic device is inserted into the uterus and can remain in place for several years. It works by preventing a fertilized egg from inplanting in the uterus.

The thread hangs down into the vagina

Vaginal sponge

This is impregnated with spermicide and should be put in water until it becomes foamy. It is then inserted deep into the vagina, where it will remain effective for up to 24 hours.

The sponge fits snugly over the cervix

Female condom

This is inserted into the vagina before sexual intercourse and removed immediately afterwards. The open end of the female condom sits outside the body on the vulva.

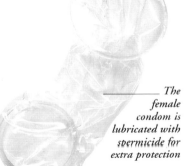

The female condom is lubricated with spermicide for extra protection

TYPES OF CONTRACEPTION

TYPES	ADVANTAGES	DISADVANTAGES
Diaphragm and spermicide	The spermicide can act as a lubricant. Can be inserted before lovemaking, and does not interfere with sex.	Difficult to see if you have a slight prolapse. May make urinary infections more likely, since the front rim of the diaphragm can press on the urethra.
Condoms (male and female)	Widely available without the need for a prescription. Protects against sexually transmitted diseases, such as the HIV virus.	Effectiveness is lower than that of the pill or the IUD. Condoms may sometimes interfere with a man's erection as he gets older.
Vaginal sponge	Easily available and can be self-fitted before intercourse.	Has the highest failure rate of all barrier contraceptives.
IUD	Very effective as a contraceptive. After insertion you can forget about it.	Requires insertion by a doctor. Some IUDs have to be removed due to irregular bleeding or infection.
Combined pill	High success rate. Offers protection against the risk of endometrial and ovarian cancer.	Carries more risk than barrier methods, e.g. thrombosis. Disguises the menopause by regulating menstrual periods.
Progestogen only mini-pill	Suitable if you are advised not to take oestrogen.	Has a slightly higher failure rate than the combined pill.

POSTMENOPAUSAL RELATIONSHIPS

Retirement can put a strain on marriages. Couples who live together quite happily in the evenings and at weekends find it can be hard to tolerate each other all the time. You might encounter problems that you never anticipated: your partner might compensate for his loss of power at work by demanding excessive attention, and you might respond by nagging. The suggestions that follow may help alleviate stressful situations.

• Plan separate, as well as joint, activities.
• Try to arrange your home so that each of you has a room to escape to.
• Respect each other's friends, conversations, interests and routines.
• Develop a common interest, such as a shared hobby, a small business venture or an evening class.
• Keep talking to each other. Your partner can be your closest friend.
• Maintain a wide circle of friends; you'll need to plan not only for today, but for the future, when one of you may be alone.
• Plan your finances together.

If a marriage has never been good and problems have never been resolved, the situation will be dramatically intensified when two people are thrown together for most of the time. Emotional strain at this time can be great, but preventable, if you tackle problems early on.

A full life includes physical love. If the frequency with which you and your partner make love declines, try to examine the reasons why. Some people believe that sex is dirty, indecent or at the very least aesthetically undesirable for older people. This attitude may spring from the traditional religious belief that sex for enjoyment only is wrong. These days, however, intercourse takes place more often for pleasure than for procreation. We know from many recent surveys that people in their 70s and beyond need and, indeed, have active sex lives. Sadly this is often kept secret. We must realize that, as we become older, we still have the same capacity for physical love as we did 20 or 30 years ago, and this is the ideal time to cast aside taboos and inhibitions.

Many older couples find that sex is better in the morning, when they are refreshed, than in the evening, when they are more likely to be tired. In fact, a man's highest sexual hormone level occurs between four o'clock in the morning and noon, and his lowest around eight o'clock in the evening.

Masturbation should be encouraged, particularly for single women and women whose partners are infirm. No matter how frequently it is practised, masturbation has no harmful effects.

DIVORCE

Marriage break-up gets harder as people get older. In the aftermath of divorce, many women fear that no one will desire them again. Some dislike going alone to social events after years of being accompanied by a partner, and some are bitter because they are left alone after 20 or more years of marriage. Financially, women may be very dependent on maintenance payments, particularly if they haven't been trained for a job.

Pessimism can lead women to believe that divorce is the end of their lives. But having lived through the despair, pain, self-pity and even self-hatred, many of us find that life improves. Some women get their first full-time job; others feel self-confident enough to go out with other men; yet others even enjoy sex for the first time in years after leaving a claustrophobic marriage, and finding fulfilment with a new, more sympathetic partner.

If you go through a divorce in midlife, remember that there are many years ahead in which to enjoy yourself. If you are postmenopausal, you don't need to worry about getting pregnant, and if you have children, they are likely to be grown up and able to take care of themselves. Your biggest concern should be how best to maximize the potential of the years ahead.

SINGLE LIFE

If you are on your own, you have a variety of lifestyles open to you. You can live alone, sublet a room of your house, rent a flat and let your home to tenants. You could even set up a commune: some 60-year-olds in Florida have gathered together and live in four homes as families, paying a younger couple to manage the homes and do the domestic work.

WHAT IS HRT?

HRT (hormone replacement therapy) aims to correct the deficit of the female hormones, oestrogen and progesterone, that occurs at the menopause. Doctors prescribe these two hormones in a variety of combinations, tailored to suit the individual, to alleviate symptoms such as hot flushes, and to prevent serious health problems, like ostcoporosis, that may occur when oestrogen levels decline. This chapter explores the medical issues connected with HRT and describes the methods and types of medication available, including tablets, patchcs, gcls, pessaries and creams. It explains the benefits and disadvantages of each method and helps you to make an informed choice about what is right for you.

WHO CAN USE HRT?

The mainstay of orthodox medical treatment of the menopause is hormone replacement therapy (HRT). This treats the menopause as a hormone deficiency state that can be alleviated by replacing the oestrogen and progesterone that a woman's ageing ovaries no longer secrete in sufficient quantities.

Because of the diverse range of HRT products, and the number of ways in which they can be administered, most women can find an HRT regime that matches their needs and produces few side-effects. However, for women who don't wish to take HRT or have a contraindication to its use, alternative medications are available.

IT'S YOUR DECISION

Understanding the benefits of HRT means that you have the knowledge to make an intelligent and informed choice. Only you have the final responsibility for your own health care.

It is important to gather as much information as you can and maintain the motivation to keep yourself in the best possible health. On average, women taking HRT live three to four years longer than their contemporaries. So on balance, not taking HRT seems riskier than taking it.

EXPLAINING HORMONAL MEDICATION

The basis of all HRT regimes is oestrogen; progestogens are added solely to induce a uterine bleed with shedding of the endometrium, or uterine lining. Although the main way of treating menopausal symptoms is to prescribe natural oestrogen and progestogen in the form of HRT, other hormonal treatments are available, such as medroxyprogesterone acetate or norgestrel (usually used as a contraceptive). These are both progestogens and may alleviate hot flushes.

HORMONAL MEDICATION

HRT is a substitute for the female sex hormones oestrogen and progesterone; it is prescribed when the body's levels of female hormones are low, most usually at or after the menopause. Oestrogen is given to maintain the health of the whole female body. Progestogen is generally given because it causes the uterine lining to shed, which prevents over-thickening of the lining and cancer of the uterus.

The main oestrogens used in HRT are natural, from plant sources, and are similar to oestradiol, which is produced by the ovaries. Some HRT products contain conjugated equine oestrogen, which is harvested from the urine of pregnant mares. Progestogen is the synthetic form of progesterone. Because natural progesterone is rapidly metabolized by the body, it does not produce a sustained effect when taken in tablet form.

The normal menstrual cycle depends on the sequential production of oestrogen and progesterone, so it makes good sense to include these ingredients in menopausal hormone replacement therapy. Another vital hormone is testosterone, which is also manufactured by the ovaries; if you have your ovaries removed, there will be 50 percent less testosterone in your bloodstream. High levels of oestrogen in HRT can neutralize available testosterone. Much of the female sex drive is attributed to this male hormone, and if you are taking HRT and suffering from a lack of libido, you can discuss with your doctor or gynaecologist the possibility of taking low-dose testosterone supplements.

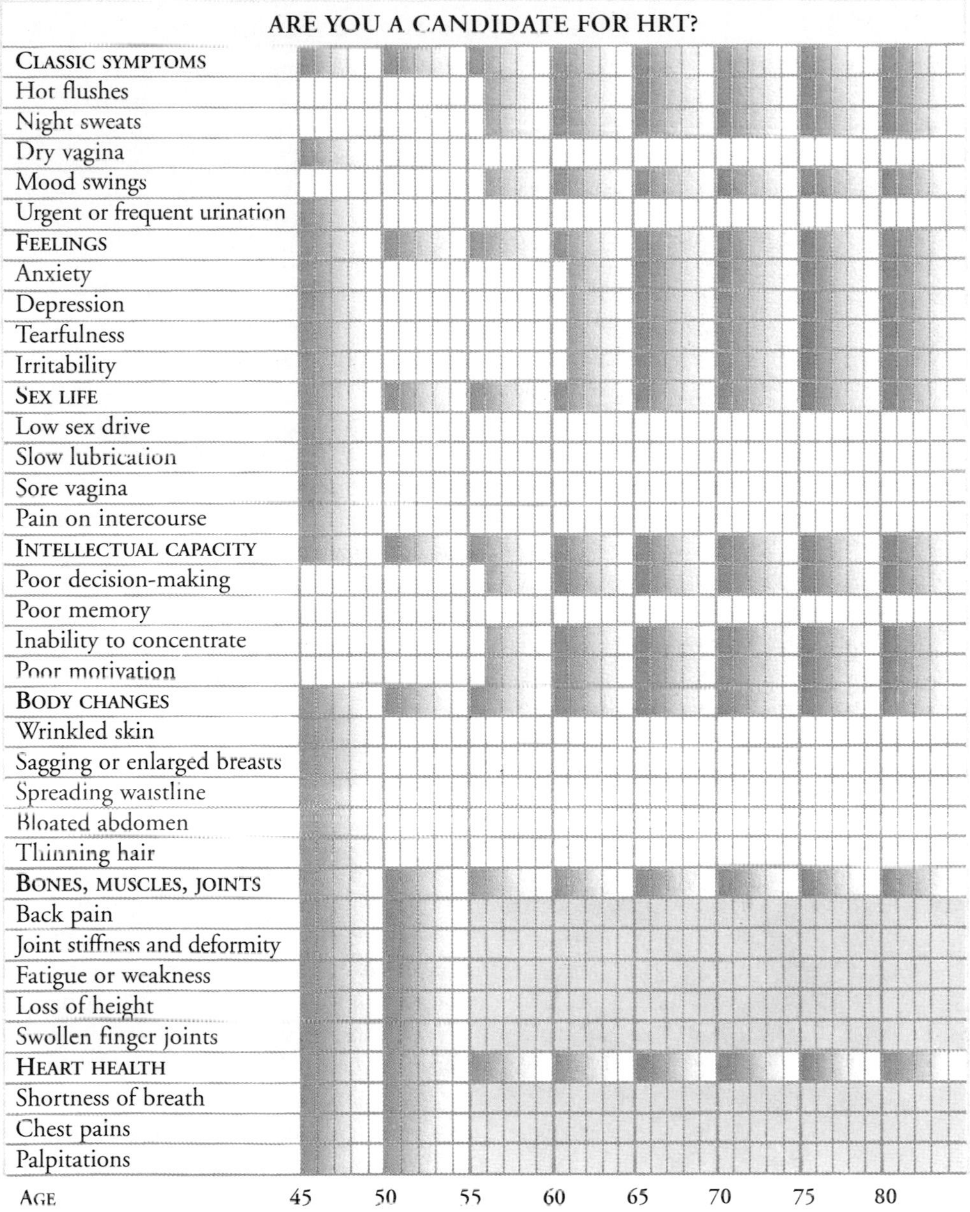
ARE YOU A CANDIDATE FOR HRT?
CLASSIC SYMPTOMS
Hot flushes
Night sweats
Dry vagina
Mood swings
Urgent or frequent urination
FEELINGS
Anxiety
Depression
Tearfulness
Irritability
SEX LIFE
Low sex drive
Slow lubrication
Sore vagina
Pain on intercourse
INTELLECTUAL CAPACITY
Poor decision-making
Poor memory
Inability to concentrate
Poor motivation
BODY CHANGES
Wrinkled skin
Sagging or enlarged breasts
Spreading waistline
Bloated abdomen
Thinning hair
BONES, MUSCLES, JOINTS
Back pain
Joint stiffness and deformity
Fatigue or weakness
Loss of height
Swollen finger joints
HEART HEALTH
Shortness of breath
Chest pains
Palpitations
AGE
45
50
55
60
65
70
75
80

Assessing your candidacy

The orange and yellow panels in this table indicate the maximum number of symptoms you may experience during the menopause and beyond. Find your age along the bottom of the table and look in the list above it to see which symptoms may occur in women of that age.

If you are experiencing two or more of the symptoms marked for your age, then you are highly eligible for HRT. If you have any of the symptoms shown in the orange area, then HRT may protect you against future heart disease and a decline in bone mass.

ABOUT OESTROGEN

Both natural and synthetic forms of oestrogen are available, as are other chemicals that have an oestrogenic effect, but are not, strictly speaking, oestrogens.

Natural oestrogens, derived from human or animal metabolism, are absorbed and excreted by the body more easily than synthetic ones.

Synthetic oestrogens are much more potent than naturally occurring ones and may have some unwanted effects on the body, for example increasing the risk of thrombosis. However, most oestrogens used in HRT are natural and have minimal effects on the body's metabolism. Also, with the wide range of products and potencies available, there is great scope for adjusting the treatment and for finding a product that is suitable for each individual woman.

BENEFITS OF HRT

In this age of preventive medicine, HRT should be hailed as one of the most effective treatments for counteracting long-term disease. Our whole orientation in medicine should be towards prevention rather than cure, and any regime that can cut down on expensive treatments, hospital admissions, and serious disease should be embraced enthusiastically by the medical profession.

Prevention of heart attacks Acute coronary artery disease kills one woman in every four aged over 50. Taking oestrogen in HRT has been shown to reduce the risk of acute coronary artery disease by up to 50 percent.

Maintenance of healthy organs, bones and muscles HRT has also proved successful in maintaining the health of all the female reproductive organs. In addition to keeping the tissues of the vagina supple and moist, it can prevent atrophy and thinning of the urinary tract and associated infections and incontinence. Oestrogen contributes to the health, strength and functioning of the bones, muscles and joints and can help to prevent backache – a problem that is common in menopausal women due to osteoporosis of the spine. The general toning effect of HRT on the musculo-skeletal system means a return of strength, stamina and energy.

Improvement in shape There are three ways in which menopausal women can change shape. First, by loss of muscle and ligament strength, second, by the tendency towards male fat distribution on the waist and abdomen, and third, by the loss of height due to osteoporosis. HRT can prevent these changes, which may be partly why some people perceive hormonal medication as youth-promoting. Don't make the mistake of thinking that oestrogen is a dietary or weight-control product – it is not a substitute for good nutrition and exercise.

Increased well-being Beta-endorphins are chemicals from the central nervous system that are associated with a general sense of well-being and euphoria. Reduced beta-endorphins are associated with depression, and it is thought that HRT will increase beta-endorphin levels.

Taking hormones during and after the menopause can directly raise your mood and feelings of self-worth, and alleviate anxiety. Your sense of emotional well-being is likely to improve – the so-called "mental tonic" effect of HRT. You may be able to work better and feel revitalized. Although HRT may alleviate depressed moods, it should not be considered an antidepressant drug.

Relief of menopausal symptoms Women who have hot flushes and night sweats find relief when they take oestrogen, regardless of how they take it. For 98 percent of women, HRT alleviates their symptoms and in over 90 percent, symptoms disappear completely. Very heavy periods can be experienced by women in their late 40s and early 50s. This can be helped by HRT, although severely abnormal bleeding may need the addition of a low-dose contraceptive. Vaginal dryness, soreness and painful intercourse may also be soothed by taking oestrogen. Headaches can become more frequent at the menopause and oestrogen can bring relief.

Your skin will respond to oestrogen by showing increased tone and suppleness. Your hair will be stronger and less prone to dryness and brittleness. Similarly, nails that were brittle and prone to splitting become stronger. Gum recession around the time of menopause can also be alleviated by HRT.

Intellectual problems, for example, an inability to concentrate and difficulty making decisions, tend to disappear within a month or so of taking HRT. In one study, women found relief from panic attacks when they took HRT and received psychotherapy.

The response of the libido to HRT is different for every woman. You may notice an increase in sexual enjoyment, but not necessarily an increase in sex drive. There are low-dose testosterone products that, if taken daily, can bring about a subtle return to sexual vitality without side-effects such as facial hair or lowering of the voice.

Studies from sleep laboratories show that oestrogen changes the proportion of sleep time spent in the rapid eye movement (REM) stage that is characteristic of dreaming. Women may dream more when they take oestrogen and dream less when they are oestrogen deficient. As REM sleep increases, your general state of peacefulness improves and you feel more rested after sleep.

ABOUT PROGESTERONE

The synthetic forms of this naturally occurring hormone are progestin and progestogen.

Originally, HRT consisted only of oestrogen. Progestogen was added when it was found to lower the rate of endometrial (uterine) cancer, and HRT then became the norm for women with a uterus.

Taking progestogen has the disadvantage of a monthly withdrawal bleed. Moreover, a small number of women (about 10–15 percent) experience side-effects, similar to premenstrual syndrome. Fortunately, these side-effects subside in about four months for half of all women who take HRT. Your progestogen intake can be reduced by taking it as part of your regime only once every three months.

IF SIDE-EFFECTS PUT YOU OFF...

Only a sixth of the women who start taking HRT continue to take it for one year. Women who drop out are usually anxious about side-effects like weight gain, have read panic stories in the press, or have misconceptions about their treatments.

It is worth remembering that certain side-effects, such as headaches, indigestion and tender breasts, can occur whether you're taking hormones or not.

In several well-controlled studies, women who were told they were taking HRT, but were actually taking a placebo, had as many symptoms as women taking HRT. The important factor seems to be how well informed you are about the side-effects; women who are warned of potential minor problems seem to cope with them better than women who are not so well informed.

YOU AND YOUR DOCTOR

The best doctor–patient relationships are those in which you receive full attention and satisfactory answers. You should be able to visit your doctor with a complete list of questions to which you require answers.

Unfortunately, although this kind of easy relationship should be the norm, some women encounter entrenched conservative opinion that dismisses the menopause as a woman's legacy, requiring neither help nor treatment. If your doctor espouses these attitudes, my advice is to change to a more sympathetic doctor as soon as possible. Don't continue with a doctor with whom you have little rapport. Some of the symptoms you may experience will require you to be open and confident enough to discuss them in intimate detail. If you feel at all inhibited, that doctor is not for you. Remember, doctors are there to help you and provide a service. Shop around until you can find a doctor who really suits you. He or she must be able to tailor your treatment to your individual needs in the light of your medical and gynaecological history. Your doctor should be aware of the possible side-effects of taking hormone replacement therapy, be responsive to your comments about a particular HRT regime, and be able to implement changes in regime or dose until you are happy with your treatment. A doctor who is not well versed in menopausal medicine may not be able to provide quite such an individual service, in which case you should seek specialist advice from menopause or well-woman clinics, or from a gynaecologist.

MANAGING YOUR TREATMENT

Not all women who should get HRT do get it, and many women who are prescribed HRT do not take it for a sufficiently long period to prevent their bone mass declining and to protect them against heart disease. In my opinion, more women should consider trying HRT and more doctors should be prepared to prescribe medication for a four-month trial period. Within four months your doctor can adapt the treatment so that you are able to find the regime that suits your body most. It is worth embarking on the search for the right dose and type of HRT because it can greatly affect your physical and emotional well-being.

A MONTHLY BLEED

The first decision for you and your doctor to make when you are contemplating taking HRT is whether or not to have a withdrawal bleed. The consensus of medical opinion is that if you have an intact uterus, you should have a menstrual bleed at regular intervals. Two new approaches – combined continuous therapy and a progestogenic drug called tibolone – have allowed some women to avoid bleeding altogether, and various menopause experts have been researching three-monthly, rather than monthly withdrawal bleeding (see right). At one time (and I was involved in this research more than 25 years ago), it was thought that the HRT cycle should be similar to the natural menstrual cycle in that a bleed should take place every month. This was achieved by giving women progestogen for 11–13 days in the second half of the cycle. The current thinking is that this may be unnecessary for quite a number of women – your doctor may be able to carry out a progestogen challenge test on you to be absolutely certain that it is safe for you to bleed as infrequently as once every three months.

There is also another way of taking HRT, which allows you to take progestogen "on demand". A study in the Netherlands found that the sensitivity of the menopausal endometrium to oestrogens and progestogens is unique to each woman. Research shows that it is possible to monitor growth – induced by oestrogen – of the endometrium, or lining of the uterus, with a technique called vaginosonography, in which an ultrasound picture is used to show the thickness of the uterine lining. This technique can also monitor endometrial shedding after the addition of progestogen to the HRT regime. Vaginosonography enables doctors to find out which type and dose of oestrogen causes the lowest endometrial growth for you, and which type and dose of progestogen causes the best endometrial shedding, with minimal withdrawal bleeding.

Another remarkable and important discovery was that the endometrium could shed itself without withdrawal bleeding after the addition of progestogen; also certain progestogens cause shedding of the endometrium without withdrawal bleeding more often than others. Vaginosonography is available at most specialist centres.

RESEARCH

Doctors involved in research at the Medical Care Programme in Oakland, California, hypothesized that the addition of progestogen every three months instead of every month would be safe.

To evaluate the acceptability of this regime 200 women, who had previously been taking progestogen on a monthly basis, were asked to complete a daily diary and, at the end of the study, to complete a preference questionnaire about which HRT regime they felt suited them best. On the three-monthly regime, the average duration of menstruation was two days longer than it had been formerly. The safety of the treatment was checked by performing a physical examination and carrying out biopsies on the uterine lining at the beginning of treatment and after one year.

The results of the preference questionnaire showed that women preferred the three-monthly progestogen regime to the monthly one, despite the fact that their periods were longer and heavier than before. In addition, a reduction in blood pressure occurred over the year of the study and biopsies of the uterine lining did not reveal any abnormalities, suggesting that a three-monthly progestogen regime is as safe as a monthly one.

This method of taking HRT is available in most parts of the world, so you could discuss it with your doctor.

CHANGING THE DOSE OF HORMONES

Side-effects can occur if you are taking more hormones than your body needs. As a woman's body gets older, it becomes more and more sensitive to female hormones, and a much lower dose is needed for HRT than is needed for contraception.

The aim of HRT is to be effective at the lowest possible dose. For instance, if you are taking conjugated equine oestrogen, it is possible to halve the dose from 1.25 micrograms of oestrogen per day to 0.625 micrograms. Similarly, progestogen could be reduced from 500 micrograms of norethisterone acetate per day to 300 micrograms. Make sure that these changes in your dose of hormones are handled by your doctor in sequence rather than in parallel.

CONTROLLING THE SIDE-EFFECTS OF HRT

If you experience side-effects while you are taking HRT, there are several ways that you and your doctor can bring them under control. With time and patience you can adapt your regime by changing the type of hormones, the dose, the route of administration or the medication regime.

Oestrogens can be divided into synthetic types, such as mestranol and ethinyl oestradiol, and natural types like conjugated equine oestrogens and oestradiol varieties. Synthetic oestrogens in higher dosages than those normally used in HRT may increase the risk of thromboembolism (potentially fatal blood clot). Natural oestrogens are usually prescribed in HRT, but you should find out which of these two types you are taking and suggest to your doctor that you switch from a synthetic hormone to a natural one, or, if you are already taking a natural oestrogen, that you try a different brand.

The main progestogens used in HRT vary quite markedly in their effects, and if you have side-effects, lowering the dose or switching to another type of progestogen may help. A drug called tibolone has few progestogenic side-effects.

TAKING HRT

Most doctors start women off on HRT tablets. However, this method of taking HRT does not suit all women. For example, high oral oestrogen can cause nausea (if you are affected in this way, try taking your tablet at night so that you sleep through any nausea).

As with any drug taken by mouth (rather than being absorbed through the skin or implanted in the fat layer), a larger dose than necessary is given because after absorption much of the drug is removed from the bloodstream by the liver. The tablet form of HRT therefore contains more hormone than is necessary to alleviate symptoms and this may explain why you experience side-effects.

If you cut your dosage of oral medication and you still have problems, try switching to a patch form of HRT, which contains much less hormone than oral HRT, or ask your doctor about an implant, which is formulated to release oestrogen slowly and consistently over a period of four to six months.

If you find that your menopausal symptoms affect your urogenital tract more than any other part of your body, and you have symptoms such as a dry vagina, pain during sex and frequent, urgent urination, then vaginal pessaries or cream may be sufficient to relieve your symptoms. Because these are applied locally, they prevent your whole body from being exposed to hormones. However, creams and pessaries will not have the protective qualities of oral HRT on your heart and bones.

Some women who experience progestogenic side-effects such as mood changes respond well to progesterone taken in a suppository form. This may be advantageous in that suppositories contain natural progesterone instead of its synthetic counterpart, progestogen. Some women find that they can tolerate the natural hormone better than synthetic progestogen. However, bigger doses of natural progesterone are needed to control the HRT cycle than if synthetic progestogens are used (this is why progesterone is not widely prescribed). A combination of an oestrogen skin patch and a progesterone suppository may be the best way for you to take HRT.

CHANGING YOUR REGIME

Most women will take continuous oestrogen and 10–14 days of progestogen a month. However, there are several variations in how HRT can be taken, one of which is sure to suit you. If you are taking oestrogen tablets you can begin to leave a space between medications. With your doctor's supervision, you could try taking your tablet two days out of three, three days out of four, or every other day, and see how you feel. Skin patches can be left on for four days at a time instead of three to four, or they can be left off for a day. This may be particularly helpful in relieving mastalgia (breast pain) and weight gain.

You could ask your doctor if you can try the very latest regime, "combined continuous HRT", on which you'll stop bleeding in a few months. If you have progestogenic side-effects and you are taking HRT in which progestogen and oestrogen are combined, ask your doctor to prescribe different products in which the hormones are separate. For example, you could take

INDIVIDUAL TREATMENT

The essence of success in HRT is matching the treatment to each individual woman.

You and your doctor should work together to find the hormone combination that suits you best. In a survey of 100 women, it was found that only 17 percent had stayed on their first treatment over many years, and all the others had made one or two adjustments. If something does not seem right, discuss with your doctor whether the dose or the method is suitable for you. If you're experiencing premenstrual symptoms or have troublesome bleeding, modification of the progestogen may help.

To compensate for the low levels of oestrogen in your bloodstream, you can boost your own internal oestrogen production in two ways.

The first is exercise, which can be almost as good as HRT in the postmenopausal years when your body needs relatively little oestrogen to thrive.

Your second source of internal oestrogen comes from fat cells, which is why it is dangerous for peri- and postmenopausal women to diet excessively and become underweight. Thin women generally have an earlier menopause than those who are overweight, because fat cells all over your body manufacture oestrogen, and in their absence hormone levels can fall very low.

If you don't wish to take HRT, but are having symptoms of oestrogen deficiency, make sure that you keep your weight up slightly. Whatever you do, don't lose so much weight that you are left with very little body fat, since you will be depriving yourself of an important source of natural oestrogen.

oestrogen in a skin patch form and progestogen in tablet form. This way you and your doctor can juggle the dose of the progestogen so that you have a withdrawal bleed without troublesome side-effects.

FINDING THE RIGHT DOSE

Many people believe that if something is doing you good, taking more will be even better for you. This is not a maxim to which doctors subscribe. As a general principle, doctors prefer you to take the lowest possible dose of any medication for the maximum effect and for the fewest side-effects. As a rule of thumb, medication should be taken for the shortest possible time – HRT is a rare exception to this rule.

It may take a little time to find your optimum dose, and you and your doctor may have to experiment a little because there is no way of anticipating how each individual woman will respond to the many different oestrogens that are available. When you begin to take HRT, it is wise to have a minimum of a four-month trial because it takes that long for your body to settle down. If necessary, your doctor can assess whether your hormone dose is correct by measuring the amount of oestrogen in your bloodstream. Even in low doses, hormones are powerful substances and it is unwise to change your dose without consulting your doctor first.

MONITORING HRT

As you approach the menopause you should be seeing your doctor for annual blood pressure checks, regular cervical smear tests and mammography. Your doctor should also check your weight and carry out a pelvic and breast examination before you take HRT. Once you're taking hormones, you should have these examinations annually, and your weight and blood pressure should be checked every six months. Bone density scans to check on the health of your bones may also be appropriate.

SIDE-EFFECTS AND RISKS

Women are much more likely to give up HRT if their doctors have given them insufficient information. Those who are given a sympathetic hearing and have the opportunity to discuss side-effects have a more realistic view of HRT and tolerate minor side-effects.

The main reasons why women give up HRT are the side-effects of progestogen, the inconvenience of monthly bleeds and a fear of breast cancer. As far as the latter is concerned, the consensus of medical opinion is that there is no added risk as long as your HRT regime includes progestogen. Indeed, the progestogen may help to prevent breast cancer.

For about 10–15 percent of women, the progestogen is what's so troublesome. To varying degrees, women complain of symptoms such as weight gain, fluid retention, abdominal cramps, backache, acne, greasy skin, irritability, aggressiveness, moodiness, tearfulness and loss of libido. Your doctor can prescribe an alternative form of progestogen or a smaller dose of the one you're taking to alleviate symptoms.

Hypertension (high blood pressure) As hypertension is known to increase the risk of heart attack and strokes, it is a condition that should be taken very seriously in postmenopausal women. Oestrogen will not alter your blood pressure unless you are specifically sensitive to it, which is a very rare phenomenon. This means that you can take HRT even if you do have raised blood pressure, but you should make sure that your blood pressure is checked shortly after starting HRT. If the reading is high, switch from tablets to the patch because taking HRT orally occasionally causes the liver to produce chemicals that raise blood pressure.

Breast pain HRT may cause the type of breast swelling and tenderness that is characteristic of the week prior to menstruation. In the first half of the month, the oestrogen in HRT stimulates growth of milk glands and ducts. In the second half of the cycle the progestogen may cause fluid retention within the breast. At this point, the breast may feel as though it is full of orange pips – these are swollen milk glands.

Breast swelling and tenderness may lessen if you cut down your intake of salt, coffee and chocolate, which will also benefit your general health. Taking 100 mg of vitamin B^6 daily for up to five days can also reduce breast pain, and modifying the progestogen dose may help. Breast pain that occurs throughout the HRT cycle is usually due to a dose of oestrogen that is too high.

IRREGULAR BLEEDING

Occasionally, HRT can lead to irregular bleeding, and your doctor will need to take a sample of the uterine lining by dilatation and curettage to check and make sure that there are no abnormalities.

You may consider a D & C an inconvenient procedure, but it is best to have an early examination to clear up any possible medical complaints.

DILATATION AND CURETTAGE

This procedure, often called simply a D & C, is used to determine the contents of the uterine cavity. It can diagnose the many causes of irregular bleeding, or bleeding after the menopause.

A D & C may be performed under anaesthetic in a doctor's surgery or at a hospital. A speculum is inserted into the vagina and the cervical canal is dilated using progressively bigger metal rods. The next step is to introduce either a metal curette (a spoon-shaped instrument) or catheter (plastic tube) into the uterus.

The uterine lining is removed either using an up-and-down scraping motion of the curette or by suctioning out the tissue through the catheter. A sample of the tissue is examined under the microscope to determine the cause of the bleeding.

Fibroids Benign lumps in the uterine lining may become more widespread if you take HRT. However, if your menopausal symptoms are severe, fibroids should not deter you from taking HRT. Women of any age should have fibroids monitored or removed.

Diabetes If you are diabetic, it's essential to discuss your health with your doctor before embarking on a course of HRT. This is because carbohydrate metabolism is altered by HRT. If you are prescribed HRT, you should check your blood sugar and urine frequently.

Gallstones Between the ages of 50 and 75, three women in 100,000 are estimated to die from complications of gallbladder disease. This rises to six in 100,000 among women taking HRT because oestrogen therapy increases the concentration of the bile in the gallbladder. Obesity is also associated with an increase in gallbladder disease and so it is important to reduce the amount of cholesterol in your diet and to take HRT in a form that does not pass through the liver. The skin patch will be better than a tablet at reducing the possibility of gallstones.

Migraine The response of migraine to HRT is unpredictable. Some women find that their migraines disappear completely while others experience worse attacks. The usual complaint is that migraines occur during the progestogen phase or just after the progestogen is completed. These migraines can often be alleviated by changing the type or dose of progestogen. Migraines that occur at other times during the cycle may be due to an oestrogen dose that is too low.

Cancer The possibility of a link between HRT and uterine and breast cancer is a major concern to women. Fortunately, we now know that the use of progestogen may protect against the risk of uterine cancer. However, the debate surrounding HRT and breast cancer is complicated, since experts do not agree. A persuasive body of evidence indicates that in almost all cases of breast disease, HRT is not the cause. If you are not obese, you don't smoke and breast cancer does not run in your family, then the evidence seems to weigh in favour of taking HRT.

TYPES OF MEDICATION

A combined form is the usual way for women with an intact uterus to take HRT; this means that you take both oestrogen and progestogen. Doctors often prescribe these two hormones in tablet form, so that you take oestrogen every day, and progestogen for around 12 days in each month or cycle. The latter induces a withdrawal bleed. However, your doctor may also prescribe a patch, an implant or an oestrogen cream. These different forms of HRT are known as routes of administration, and each one has its own advantages and disadvantages. They are all very effective at relieving menopausal symptoms, with the exception of oestrogen creams and pessaries, which treat only local urogenital symptoms, for example dryness, soreness or itchiness. These will not help symptoms such as hot flushes or night sweats, and they will not prevent a decline in bone density as other routes of administration can.

The skin patch contains a reservoir of oestrogen that is released transdermally (across the skin) into the body. This means that, unlike HRT taken in tablet form, hormones do not have to pass through the liver – this is advantageous for some women. You may be prescribed progestogen tablets with your patch, or you may be prescribed a combined patch that already contains progestogen. Patches need to be changed every three or four days.

Oestrogen implants also avoid oestrogen having to pass through the liver, and once they are inserted by a doctor into the fatty tissue underneath the skin of the abdomen or buttock, they last for up to six months. Progestogen tablets are prescribed with this form of oestrogen therapy.

A new product is a gel containing a synthetic form of oestradiol that is rubbed into the skin. Other products that may come on the market are vaginal rings containing oestrogen and an intrauterine device (IUD) that delivers progestogen or progesterone directly into the uterus.

Pessaries and creams
These forms of HRT deliver oestrogen directly into the vagina but the low dose does not offer protection against heart disease or osteoporosis.

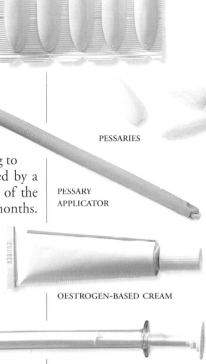

PESSARIES

PESSARY APPLICATOR

OESTROGEN-BASED CREAM

VAGINAL CREAM APPLICATOR

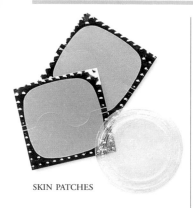

SKIN PATCHES

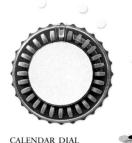

CALENDAR DIAL
OF OESTROGEN

APPLICATOR AND
PHIAL CONTAINING
OESTROGEN PELLET
FOR IMPLANT

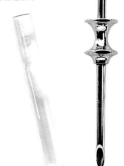

Patches, pills and implants

These forms of HRT deliver oestrogen directly into the body. They protect against osteoporosis and heart disease and effectively treat most menopausal symptoms.

TYPES OF HORMONE REPLACEMENT THERAPY

TYPE	ADVANTAGES	DISADVANTAGES
Tablets	• Highly effective in combating physical and emotional symptoms. • Contain oestrogen and/or progestogen. Protect against osteoporosis.	• You may experience side-effects such as breast tenderness and nausea. • You may experience breakthrough bleeding if you forget to take a tablet.
Creams and pessaries	• Help to alleviate urinary incontinence. • Relieve vaginal dryness and itchiness.	• Do not protect against osteoporosis. • Not effective in combating hot flushes and night sweats.
Skin patches or gel	• Equally effective as oral HRT in treating most menopausal symptoms, and preserves bone density in 85–95 percent of women. • Easily changed and simple to stop using.	• A very few women develop red, itchy skin at the site of the patch. This may get worse in a hot climate.
Implants	• Excellent relief from physical symptoms. Protects against osteoporosis. Some women find that problems, such as depression and irritability, disappear more readily than with other forms of HRT. • You can forget you are on HRT. • Testosterone can also be given as an implant.	• Implants are inserted under the skin by your doctor. • Wrong doses cannot be easily modified. • If you decide to stop using HRT, implants are difficult to remove.

TAKING HRT

The three main ways in which HRT medication can be administered are described in the regimes below. The main difference is in the bleeding pattern that results.

Continuous therapy Continuous oestrogen therapy with added progestogen medication has now become the most common way to take HRT. You can take a daily tablet of oestrogen or wear a skin patch twice a week. Progestogen is taken either in pill form or in a combination skin patch for 12–14 days. Over 90 percent of women will have a monthly bleed on this regime if the uterus is intact. Take notice of your bleeding pattern, which should occur after you stop taking progestogen. If bleeding begins before this, the dose of progestogen may be too low for you and should be adjusted.

Cyclical therapy A less common HRT regime is to take oestrogen and progestogen cyclically. Oestrogen is taken from the first day of the cycle to the 21st, and progestogen is added for the last 12 or 13 days of the cycle. Both medications are stopped on the 21st day and a withdrawal bleed will occur between days 22 and 28; the patch- or pill-free days. Over 90 percent of women who have not had a hysterectomy will experience a withdrawal bleed in the interval between ending one treatment and beginning the next. However, bleeding usually lessens over time and may disappear altogether.

The most up-to-date way to take cyclical therapy is to take progestogen once every three months. This means that you go two months without a bleed, then bleed in the third month, so that you have four menstrual periods a year. To find out if this regime is suitable for you, have a chat with your gynaecologist.

Combined continuous therapy (No-bleed HRT) This method of taking HRT involves taking continuous daily doses of both oestrogen and progestogen. The aim of this continuous therapy is to avoid periods, and even if you do have withdrawal bleeding at first, it will probably stop within a few months. No-bleed HRT is popular among women on long-term treatment. Between 50 and 70 percent of women find this regime successful.

PROGESTOGEN IUD

Women who do not wish to bleed and find continuous progestogen by mouth unsatisfactory can have an IUD impregnated with progestogen inserted.

Progestogen is released in tiny amounts sufficient to prevent thickening of the endometrium, but the effects are entirely local and therefore unwanted side-effects are minimal. Oestrogen is taken continuously. This method is the latest way of taking progestogen.

CONTRA-INDICATIONS

If you have experienced any of the conditions listed below, see the chart on page 377 to identify whether or not HRT is right for you.

- *Any type of abnormal vaginal bleeding.*

- *Breast cancer.*

- *Ovarian cancer.*

- *Uterine cancer.*

- *Recent stroke.*

- *Pancreatic disease.*

- *Recent heart attack.*

- *Recent liver disease.*

- *Recent venous thrombosis (clot in the veins).*

- *Recent pulmonary embolus (clot in the lung).*

WHEN HRT MAY NOT BE THE ANSWER

The term "contraindication" refers to a medical condition that may be exacerbated by a particular drug. In the case of HRT, there are some conditions that are thought to be "absolute contraindications", such as breast cancer or uterine cancer. However, some doctors now believe that there is no such thing as an absolute contraindication, and that only "relative" contraindications exist, provided that the dose and route of administration is individually tailored. Other doctors subscribe to the theory that certain medical conditions (see left) make it risky to take HRT. The items in this list are still frequently quoted as contraindications, but when they are scrutinized, the dangers diminish (and in some instances disappear). This is partly because of increased medical understanding, but mainly because theoretical disadvantages of HRT can be overcome by careful adjustments to therapy and tailoring the HRT regime to suit each patient.

In older lists of this kind, angina and a family history of heart attacks, strokes and venous thrombosis may have been included. Now, these conditions are regarded as positive indications for HRT, since HRT will protect you against them.

CONTRAINDICATIONS IN PERSPECTIVE

The first warnings about contraindications were based on the oral contraceptive pill (which contains a much higher dose of hormones than HRT), and they are therefore not directly referable to HRT. Lists of contraindications for HRT are usually supplied by drug companies who have special reasons (for example avoidance of litigation) for including a wide range of conditions that do not necessarily reflect medical thinking or practice.

You need to evaluate the pros and cons of taking HRT. Although it treats your menopausal symptoms, if you have had a condition such as breast cancer your doctor may be reluctant to prescribe HRT. These decisions should be negotiable. If you can't cope with hot flushes and night sweats, and your doctor is unsympathetic, go to a gynaecologist or a menopause clinic who may try to find a suitable form of HRT for you.

HRT AND YOUR MEDICAL HISTORY

Do you have, or have you ever had, any of the following?	Can you take HRT if you have, or have had, this condition?	Take note of these comments that reflect the latest thinking of experts in the field of HRT·
Unexplained abnormal vaginal bleeding	No	Any unusual bleeding must be thoroughly investigated by your doctor.
Breast cancer	Possibly not. Must be discussed fully with your doctor.	Prescribing HRT to women with these conditions is very controversial, but some doctors and gynaecologists believe that as long as the form and dose of HRT is carefully chosen, HRT is safe.
Ovarian cancer		
Uterine cancer		
Stroke		
Pancreatic disease		
Angina	Yes	
Gallstones	Yes	
Heart attack	Yes	If you have had a recent heart attack you should not take HRT. However, if you have had a heart attack in the past then you can take HRT, provided you have three-monthly cardiovascular tests.
Liver disease	Yes	If you have had liver disease in the past you can take HRT. If a liver function test is abnormal at any time you should avoid HRT.
Deep vein thrombosis	No	If you have had a thrombosis, you should not take HRT.
Pulmonary embolus	No	If you have had a pulmonary embolism, you should not take HRT.
Diabetes mellitus	Yes	Have your blood sugar and urine checked frequently.
Corticosteroid therapy	Yes	Corticosteroids (which are used to treat rheumatoid arthritis) have a detrimental effect on bone health. Taking HRT will compensate.
Ovarian cysts, fibroids, endometriosis, migraine	Yes	Use the skin patch method of HRT.
Varicose veins	Yes	If your veins become inflamed, consult your doctor.

IT'S NEVER TOO LATE TO START

A woman is never too old to start taking HRT, either for menopausal symptoms, which don't necessarily decline when periods cease and may re-emerge during their 60s and 70s, and for purely medical reasons when HRT can be life-saving.

More than a few women experience hot flushes and night sweats that are troublesome enough to merit treatment for the first time in their middle 60s and even later or after having stopped HRT. I receive hundreds of letters from these women who find that their doctors are reluctant to treat them with HRT and who say that the symptoms aren't related to the menopause. They are wrong. We know that the symptoms are menopausal and respond well to HRT. An older woman whose doctor won't prescribe HRT should ask for a referral to a gynaecologist who certainly will.

There are many medical reasons for prescribing HRT, in addition to helping classical menopausal symptoms. Having a heart attack or a stroke is a strong medical indication for taking HRT because it will cut your risk of having a second one by 80 percent. So after such an event, talk to your doctor about whether or not HRT is advisable for you. Symptoms of osteoporosis, such as severe bone pain, decrease in height, collapsed vertebrae or fracture, are strong reasons for taking HRT because it can rebuild bone to its former strength in little more than two years and so will prevent further problems. If you have brittle bones, you should stay on HRT for life.

HRT prevents blood clots and lowers the cholesterol, so it's crucial for anyone with heart disease, and very importantly, it does not alter blood pressure.

If you're a high-risk woman for heart attack, a stroke or osteoporosis you're a candidate for starting HRT at the menopause to lower your risk. HRT lowers the risk of a heart attack by 50 percent, so if you have a family history of heart attack, stroke or osteoporosis, you should take HRT early for your health's sake. It's never too late to start taking HRT and there's no age when you need to stop taking it. Indeed there's no reason to stop taking HRT at all, if you don't want to.

HEALTH CHECKS

Monitoring your health is the key to continuing a healthy and active life. Observing and reading the messages your body sends, then responding to them, brings a great sense of satisfaction and well-being. Being aware of your health gives you control over your body, and helps you to spot potential medical conditions early, when they may be more easily and successfully treated. Far and away the most important health checks for menopausal women are breast self-examination and mammography – which you should have at least every two years.

Doctors can monitor your physical health during the menopause with a range of medical procedures. Here are the most common ones.

- *Eye test.*

- *Blood test for hormone levels and thyroid function.*

- *Mammogram.*

- *Blood pressure test.*

- *Blood test for high cholesterol.*

- *Urine test for diabetes.*

- *Cervical smear test.*

- *Bone density scan.*

- *Electrocardiogram.*

MONITORING YOUR HEALTH

As you reach the menopause you will need to have a variety of health checks done regularly. Certain tests that you have had in the past will be carried out more frequently, while new tests may need to be done because of your changed status as a menopausal woman. There are also procedures such as colposcopy that may need to be done if routine checks reveal any abnormalities. Ideally, there will be a large team of people to help monitor your health, of whom you are the first member. The others would include your doctor and gynaecologist, the radiologist who interprets your mammogram, the cytologist who reads your smear and so on. Think of them as a supportive team with whom you can interact, discuss and make informed decisions.

Doctors have a responsibility to women on hormone replacement therapy, and, before HRT is prescribed, your doctor should carry out an examination of your pelvis and breasts, take a cervical smear and check your weight and blood pressure. Ideally, you should have a mammogram to assess the health of your breasts and a bone density test to predict your likelihood of developing osteoporosis. Once you are taking HRT, you should have six-monthly consultations with your doctor in which you discuss any side-effects and bleeding, and have your weight and blood pressure checked.

SELF-CHECKS

There are several checks you can do to monitor your health. For example, excess weight at 55 is much more difficult to lose than at 35, so it's worth keeping a weekly check on your weight. This way you should never have more than a few kilograms or pounds to shed and can take immediate steps to lose them over a few weeks.

You can also assess what stage of the menopause you have reached by keeping a detailed diary of your menstrual periods, physical symptoms and mood changes. This information will lead to increased self-awareness and may help you to develop strategies, including taking HRT, to cope with menopausal symptoms.

BREASTS

In some women the menopause can bring with it an enormous increase in the size of the breasts, and they may be tender and even painful. A possible explanation for this is the increase with age of menstrual cycles in which we don't ovulate. This means that there is no progesterone to control the effect of oestrogen. The breasts are therefore exposed to prolonged periods of unopposed oestrogen stimulation and swell as a result.

BREAST SELF-EXAMINATION

It is important to examine your breasts once a month. If you are still menstruating, the best time is at the end of your period when your breasts are not swollen or tender. You can do a breast examination at any time of the month if you are postmenopausal.

How to feel your breasts

Lie on your back with your head on a pillow and your shoulders slightly raised. Keep the arm you are not using by your side and with your fingers flat, examine each section of the breast using gentle circular movements. Finish by extending the arm you are not using behind your head and checking for lumps along the collar bone and in your armpits.

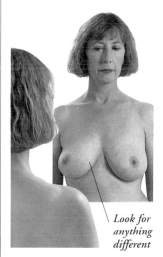

Look for anything different

What to look for

Stand naked in front of a mirror. Observe your breasts with your arms at your sides, then raised with your hands behind your head. Look for differences in the shape or texture of your breasts and nipples, and for swellings or lumps, a dimpled, puckered appearance or a newly inverted nipple.

Check for swollen lymph nodes in your armpits

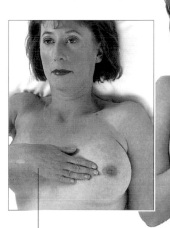

Use the right hand to feel the left breast and vice versa

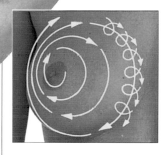

Feeling pattern

Move your hand in towards the nipple, using a clockwise circular direction on the left breast and an anti clockwise direction on the right breast.

RECOMMENDED TIMING

If you have not had a mammogram performed in the last year, and you are planning to take HRT, your doctor may suggest you have one done before you start treatment. Every time you ask for your HRT prescription to be repeated, you can ask your doctor to perform a manual examination of your breasts in addition to the one you carry out yourself.

If your mammogram reveals a lump you will probably be advised not to take HRT until the cause of the lump has been diagnosed. This is because some doctors regard breast cancer as a reason not to take HRT. However, some gynaecologists will tailor the dose and method of giving you HRT to suit your individual needs, placing you at minimal risk.

MAMMOGRAPHY

This is a type of X-ray, known as a "soft" X-ray, that reveals changes in the consistency of breast tissue, including cysts and tumours. Mammograms penetrate only a few centimetres and are harmless. A radiologist uses them to locate any areas of increased density in the breast, possibly even calcification, which may indicate abnormalities or cancer.

HOW IS A MAMMOGRAM DONE?

To have a mammogram, you will need to be naked from the waist upwards and stand in different positions so that your breasts can be X-rayed from various angles. In order to photograph every angle, the breasts may sometimes have to be gently compressed between two X-ray plates; although you may find this uncomfortable, it is not usually painful, unless your breasts are tender.

Mammography is a particularly reliable technique for the examination of large breasts, since accurate pictures are obtained and there is a high degree of contrast between normal tissue and abnormal structures. A radiologist will be able to use a mammogram to discern extremely small cysts and tiny tumours that you would not be able to feel or notice yourself during your monthly breast examination.

Mammograms are likely to be less revealing if you have had breast implants, since these can obscure the view of the breast tissue. Mammograms also tend to be less accurate on small-breasted women.

FREQUENCY OF PROCEDURE

You should have a mammogram every two years from the age of 45, or earlier if you have a family history of breast cancer, particularly if your mother or sister had the disease. Because mammography can detect minute tumours before they have the chance to spread, it is the most important procedure for the early detection of breast cancer. Research data shows that almost 90 percent of breast cancers detected by mammography emerge in the first "baseline" reading. If your baseline reading is clear, it is less likely that any tumours will be found in subsequent mammograms. The procedure will, however, show up any later changes.

BONE DENSITY

In the first few years after oestrogen levels decline, many women go through a phase of rapid bone density loss. Oestrogen is crucial in maintaining bone repair, a process called remodelling, and without sufficient oestrogen you lose more bone than you build up, resulting in fragile bones and osteoporosis. Within a few years of the menopause, the rate of bone loss slows down, but by that time, the damage could be irreparable.

BONE DENSITY SCANS

A bone density scan provides a window on your skeleton. It's based on the principle that X-rays cannot penetrate hard structures such as bone; the whiter your bone X-rays are, the more dense and healthy your bone. The darker the X-ray, the less dense your bones are, and the more brittle they are likely to be.

A bone density scan is useful both as a diagnostic tool, to reveal osteoporosis for the first time, and as a way of monitoring progress after treatment for osteoporosis has begun. Experts in this field suggest that one bone density measurement around the time of the menopause can predict your future risk of osteoporotic fractures. Women can be divided into two risk groups: those with low bone mass and high risk of future fracture, and those with high bone mass and low risk of fracture.

HOW IS THE SCAN DONE?

Dual energy X-ray absorptiometry (DEXA) is currently the most precise and widely used method of assessing bone density. This non-invasive procedure can be carried out in hospital X-ray departments, menopause clinics, well-woman clinics and consultants' surgeries. Your bone density is assessed by a radiologist.

To have the scan, you lie on a table and a radiation beam is passed over you. The density of the spine and the thigh bone usually provide a good indication of bone health throughout the body. In a similar technique, called single photon absorptiometry, the bones in your wrist are measured. You place your arm between a beam of low-level radiation and a detector. Your X-rays will be rated on a specially devised scale, which correlates the appearance of bone X-rays with bone health.

WHO NEEDS A BONE DENSITY SCAN?

In my opinion, all women with menopausal symptoms, but particularly those suffering from bone, muscle, back and joint pain, should have a bone density scan.

The best time to have the scan done is when your symptoms first start, but any time during the menopause is sufficient.

BLOOD TEST FOR OVARIAN CANCER

Recent experimental research has revealed that the presence of a hormone called inhibin may be a forewarning of ovarian cancer.

Inhibin can be identified with a simple blood test, which is a more straightforward and less traumatic procedure than a laparoscopy (inserting a tube through the abdominal wall).

Inhibin appears very early in the course of the disease – as much as 20 months before the actual cancer shows – making early diagnosis possible. This is a potentially great advance in the management of ovarian cancer, because tumours can grow quite large and spread before they cause symptoms.

Cure rates are directly related to early diagnosis, so this test could increase survival rates significantly. Monitoring inhibin levels also reveals whether treatment is working, but this test is likely to be available at only a few specialized centres.

TESTS ON THE UTERUS AND OVARIES

Between the ages of 55 and 65, the incidence of uterine cancer more than doubles. Malignant ovarian growths are also most common after the age of 50.

CERVICAL SMEAR TEST

Although cervical cancer is comparatively rare in postmenopausal women, the cervical smear test is so effective in the prevention of cervical cancer it is an important gynaecological test for women of all ages. Before cancer develops there is a precancerous stage that is symptomless and does not produce signs that are visible to the naked eye. However, there are cellular changes in the cervix and by taking a sample of cervical cells, staining them and examining them under a microscope, doctors can identify any abnormalities and decide upon the appropriate treatment.

If abnormal cervical cells are discovered as the result of a smear test, the changes are classified as mild, moderate or severe (see Test Results, right). In the first case, a repeat smear test will be recommended in three to six months' time, since sometimes abnormalities can simply disappear. If the cell changes are moderate or severe, a procedure known as a colposcopy (see right), which allows your doctor to see a microscopic level of detail on your cervix, is likely to be recommended. Occasionally, women may be called back for a repeat smear – not because there are any abnormalities, but because the smear is "unreadable". This may be because either blood or inflammatory cells were present (you should not have a smear test while you are menstruating or if you have a gynaecological infection), or because the cells were collected from the wrong part of the cervix.

The area of the cervix that is affected by abnormal cell growth is called the transformation zone, and its exact location depends on a woman's age. In postmenopausal women the transformation zone moves up into the cervical canal, making the zone less accessible during a smear test. This is remedied by the use of an endocervical brush, which can be gently inserted into the cervical canal to gather the sample of cells.

A common reason for abnormal changes in the cervix is the genital wart or human papilloma virus (HPV). Some types of HPV can cause changes that show up in a smear test, but as many as a third of these abnormalities can disappear spontaneously. For this reason, if you have a history of genital warts, you should make sure that you have a smear test annually. Other women should have a smear test every two or three years.

HOW IS A CERVICAL SMEAR DONE?

A smear test entails an internal examination in which a speculum is inserted into the vagina. The speculum holds open the vagina and allows your doctor to gain access to the cervix and note any abnormal changes. A thin layer of cells from the cervix and some mucus are collected. A smear test is carried out when you are lying down with your knees apart. Although you may feel a mild scraping sensation, the procedure should be painless.

TEST RESULTS AND RECOMMENDATIONS

The results of a smear test are classified into four or five categories. Negative gives you the all-clear; no follow-up is needed. Your next smear should be in three years' time. The mildest inflammation is known as mild dysplasia (called CIN I); this means you have some infection and should be tested again in six months' time. A positive smear test means there is a detectable change in the cells necessitating further investigation. For moderate dysplasia (called CIN II), this will be a colposcopy; for severe dysplasia with or without invasive cancer (called CIN III), this will be a colposcopy with or without cone biopsy (see column, right).

COLPOSCOPY

If a smear test reveals any abnormal cells, this is a further non-invasive procedure that a specialist will use to decide on an appropriate treatment. Using apparatus resembling a pair of binoculars on a stand, a microscopic level of detail can be seen on the surface of the cervix. Expert colposcopists can recognize chronic inflammation, infection, polyps and areas of pre-invasive cancer. If your colposcopist finds something that appears abnormal to the eye, he or she may recommend laser treatment, a cone biopsy or loop excision (see column, right).

CONE BIOPSY

This procedure is done if a colposcopy (see left) shows the presence of cancerous cells in the cervix, or if a colposcopy is inconclusive. The latter is likely to be the case for women over 35, because less of their cervical tissue can be seen due to retraction of the cervix caused by age.

Under general anaesthetic, a piece of the cervix in the shape of a cone is removed using a laser or scalpel. The base of the cone is on the outside of the cervix and the apex is deep in the cervical tissue. This cone is then finely dissected so that the exact extent of disease can be determined. The area will be stitched to reduce bleeding, although diathermy (electrical stimulation) or freezing is also effective as an alternative.

LOOP EXCISION

The most recent procedure for removing abnormal cervical cells is loop excision.

This straightforward technique involves the removal of tissue using a heated wire loop. Its great advantage is that it can be performed in the outpatient department of a hospital without the need for a general anaesthetic. Loop excision also removes a smaller amount of tissue than a cone biopsy.

CARDIOVASCULAR (HEART) TESTS

If you have no symptoms, you exercise several times a week, you are not overweight and don't smoke, it's very unlikely that you have any heart disease, and occasional check-ups will be sufficient.

Heart checks include listening to your heart, measuring your blood pressure, and possibly having an electrocardiogram (ECG) and a blood test. If you have raised blood pressure or high blood cholesterol, a family history of heart disease, you are overweight, you smoke or you rarely exercise, you should have annual heart check-ups from the age of 35. You should not need an ECG unless your doctor finds an abnormality.

An ECG can be done in a doctor's office, at home or in a hospital. Electrodes connected to a recording machine are applied to your chest, wrists and ankles. Electrical signals, which record the contractions of the heart muscle, are charted and displayed as a trace on a moving graph or screen. To an expert, this reveals detailed information about the health and functioning of your heart. Minute changes on the tracing reflect potentially dangerous changes in your heart function.

In conjunction with an ECG, you may be given an exercise tolerance test. You will be asked to perform a set exercise, such as walking on a motorized treadmill, and a reading will be taken to record your heart's response to the extra strain.

OTHER TESTS

With the first symptom of the menopause, your doctor may suggest checking on your level of oestrogen and, since heart disease is the greatest killer of postmenopausal women, checking your heart, too.

HORMONE LEVEL TEST

Specialized hormone tests are more likely to be carried out by gynaecologists than by doctors, although you may find that hospital clinics adapt some procedures slightly.

Profound changes happen to your sex hormones at the menopause (and then again in your 70s and 80s). The two major oestrogen hormones, oestradiol and oestrone, plummet after the menopause, and oestradiol stays low for the rest of your life unless HRT is taken. Oestrone follows a slightly different pattern. During a woman's 50s, 60s and 70s, levels decline, but after that oestrone begins to increase. Low levels of oestrone or oestradiol in midlife mean that the menopause is imminent. This shows up in a blood test as high levels of follicle stimulating hormone (FSH) and luteinizing hormone (LH).

If you go to see your doctor when you are symptomless, before the onset of the menopause, it's unlikely that you'll convince him or her of the need to carry out hormone tests. If, however, you have early symptoms of the menopause, such as the occasional hot flush, back pain or slight dryness of the vagina, it could be that you're on the rising part of the curve, and this could easily be confirmed by performing a blood test for FSH or LH.

RECOMMENDATIONS

I feel that information about hormone depletion is crucial for women who are approaching or going through the menopause. It gives you knowledge about what's going on internally, which can help you to understand the symptoms that you may be experiencing. It also means you can plan ways of dealing with the menopause. For example, you can argue your case for HRT if, having read the table on page 363, you feel you are a candidate for it and would benefit from it. If you have a family history of heart disease or brittle bones, low blood hormone levels of FSH and LH will support the case for your taking HRT before the onset of the menopause.

LONG-TERM HEALTH AND HRT

The falling level of oestrogen during the menopause together with the natural ageing process in the postmenopausal years means that women can become increasingly susceptible to illness and disease. One of the most painful conditions is osteoporosis, which is the single most important health hazard for women past the menopause – it is more common than heart disease, stroke, diabetes or breast cancer. Other more minor conditions, for example cystitis, urinary incontinence and pelvic prolapse, are not life-threatening but may still cause women considerable distress. These can be overcome with a combination of preventive, medical and self-help measures.

WHY IT HAPPENS

As oestrogen and progesterone levels fall, bones begin to lose mass by 0.5–3 percent a year. An 80-year-old woman can easily have lost 40 percent of the bone mass in her body.

Healthy bone has blood vessels and nerves and a very efficient system for maintenance and repair. There are special cells called osteoblasts, that renew, repair and lay down new bone. The activity of these cells is controlled mainly by hormones, including oestrogen, which is thought to increase the repair and renewal rate of bone. If oestrogen levels fall, bone is not replaced as efficiently.

Bone that is healthy is rich in calcium. Oestrogen facilitates the uptake of calcium from the blood into the bone and inhibits calcium loss. A fall in oestrogen levels therefore leads to bone disintegration.

When tiny holes form within the bone, two things happen. First, the overall structure and supporting tissue of the bone is thinned out and, second, there is less of the inner, spongy bone matrix in which calcium can be deposited. Eventually the tiny craters in bone expand to look like holes in Swiss cheese. Bones lose their thickness and density and become brittle and break with relative ease. For a woman with severe osteoporosis of the spine, minor knocks, jolts or falls can cause the spinal bones to fracture.

BRITTLE BONES (OSTEOPOROSIS)

A painful, crippling and life-threatening condition, osteoporosis is the single most important health hazard for women past the menopause – it is more common than heart disease, stroke, diabetes or breast cancer. In its early stages, osteoporosis has no obvious symptoms, so many women may be unaware that they have it. Because of its life-threatening nature, it is vital that all women be told the facts about this disease, and take measures to prevent osteoporosis from destroying their lives.

The word "osteoporosis" is derived from the Greek and means "bone that has many holes". A clinical definition of osteoporosis is "a condition where there is less normal bone than expected for a woman's age, with an increased risk of fracture". However, some experts restrict the term "osteoporosis" to describe low bone density where fractures have already occurred, and use the term "osteopenia" to describe women who have bones with low density, but have not suffered fractures. Osteoporosis is commonly called "brittle bone disease".

RISK FACTORS

Ageing is the main cause of osteoporosis, but it can also be the result of malignant disease, chronic liver disorder or rheumatoid arthritis. Black women, who have greater bone density, have a lower risk of developing osteoporosis than white women. Certain conditions, situations and habits are also contributory factors. The most significant of these is impaired peak bone density.

LOW BONE DENSITY

From infancy, your bones grow in size until peak bone mass or density is achieved between the ages 25 and 35. After this point bone mass no longer increases. The amount of bone in your skeleton as you approach the menopause will depend on three things: the peak level of bone mass you achieved, the time at which your bone loss begins and the rate at which bone loss proceeds. If your peak bone mass is low to begin with, you have a much greater chance of developing severe osteoporosis after the menopause.

AMENORRHOEA

Osteoporosis occurs in some women with premenopausal amenorrhoea (lack of menstrual periods), and is related to low oestrogen levels. Two examples of high risk categories are young women with anorexia nervosa and young sportswomen who exercise excessively while living on a restricted diet. When the body receives so little food that the fat-to-muscle ratio drops, it responds by switching off oestrogen production in the ovaries.

HYPERTHYROIDISM

Women who have an overactive thyroid gland or who take high doses of thyroxine for thyroid deficiency are at risk of developing osteoporosis. Women overtreated with thyroxine may lose bone mass at seven times the normal rate. If you are taking thyroxine, ask your doctor to check your thyroid function and dosage requirements periodically, and ask about a bone density test.

PREMATURE MENOPAUSE

The earlier the age of the menopause, with its depletion of oestrogen, the greater the risk of osteoporosis. The National Osteoporosis Society reports that a very high number of women aged between 60 and 69 who have osteoporosis had a premature menopause. While most doctors would offer hormone replacement therapy to treat the more obvious and immediate menopausal symptoms, such as hot flushes and night sweats, they often neglect prescribing it for the full length of time needed to protect against osteoporosis.

HYSTERECTOMY AND OVARIAN REMOVAL

The ovaries are a woman's main source of oestrogen, so it is not surprising that their removal leads to loss of bone mass. Most women show early signs of osteoporosis within four years of removal of the ovaries if HRT is not given. Even women who have had hysterectomies without having the ovaries removed are more prone to bone loss than women who retain their uterus.

The National Osteoporosis Society produced statistics showing that only two women out of 100 who had undergone hysterectomies and removal of the ovaries had been offered HRT.

FACTORS AFFECTING PEAK BONE MASS

How much tissue your bones contain when they are at their most dense is the best determinant of how much will be present when you're older. The density of bone is affected by the following:

- *Adequate amounts of both calcium and vitamin D. They are essential for bone health.*

- *Little or no exercise in your 20s will lower peak bone mass; too much exercise, causing amenorrhoea (lack of menstrual periods), is also unhealthy.*

- *The early onset of menstrual periods, a late menopause, taking hormonal contraceptives and multiple pregnancies have a positive effect on bone mass.*

- *Traits inherited from parents. If your parents have thick or heavy bones, generally you will have a similar bone structure.*

"DOWAGER'S HUMP"

This debilitating condition has four characteristics: loss of height, hunched posture, a protruding abdomen and a shuffling gait.

As the bones of the spine gradually lose density, the collapse of the vertebrae causes the ribcage to tilt downwards towards the hips. A curvature in the upper spine creates a second curve in the lower spinal column, pushing the internal organs outwards.

Because the spinal column is compressed, up to 20 cm (8 in) in height can be lost. Internal functions are impaired as the compressed organs shift position and obstruct other organs and systems. Constipation can be a problem; breathing may become laboured; and aches and pains in the lower back and throughout the body may arise from pressure on the nerves emanating from the collapsed vertebrae. Managing life day-to-day can become increasingly difficult.

SMOKING

The menopause may start up to five years early in heavy smokers. Smoking severely reduces the benefits of HRT to bone health, and limits the amount of oxygen your body can take in. When oxygen consumption is low, bones tend to be weak. Passive smokers are also at risk. Blood tests have shown that a passive smoker inhales one-fifteenth of the nicotine that is inhaled by a smoker in the same room. Female passive smokers, on average, reach the menopause about three years earlier than women in non-smoking households. The golden rules are to stop smoking well before the menopause and to avoid spending time in a smoke-filled environment.

CORTICOSTEROIDS

Some of the most dangerous drugs that cause bones to become osteoporotic are steroids, such as cortisone or prednisone. These drugs treat a number of conditions, including severe cases of rheumatoid arthritis. When prescribed over long periods of time in high doses, corticosteroid usage can lead to osteoporosis. If you are taking these drugs, ask your doctor to prescribe the lowest effective dose, in order to minimize bone damage.

DIAGNOSING OSTEOPOROSIS

Successful treatment and possible prevention of osteoporosis depend on early detection of bone changes. Both sufferers and potential sufferers need to be identified. Your mobility and self-esteem may be severely affected if you allow osteoporosis to progress to the point where it causes severe medical problems, particularly spinal and hip fractures (see right) – a third of women over 65 will suffer a fracture of the spine, and by the age of 90, a third of women will have had a hip fracture. Both can be extremely painful and can make you housebound. These physical problems may be compounded by feelings of awkwardness or a loss in confidence. Take matters into your own hands and make sure you are given the treatments you need to keep your bones strong and healthy.

If you are 50 or over, any curvature of the spine (called kyphosis) and loss of height deserve particular attention. Other common symptoms of osteoporosis include pain, breathlessness, indigestion, acid reflux and urinary incontinence. If you suddenly begin to suffer low-back pain, you should ask your doctor to carry out a test for spinal osteoporosis, and consider the possibility of spinal fracture. No one can tell with complete certainty whether you will develop osteoporosis, although bone density scans, which measure the density of high-risk areas such as the wrist, can provide the most accurate predictions.

FRACTURES

Osteoporosis usually stays undetected in the early stages, and most osteoporotic fractures caused by minor trauma are still not diagnosed as being due to osteoporosis. The working rule is that if you sustain a fracture after minor trauma, osteoporosis is present. Therefore, if you are over 40 and you fracture your wrist or hip after a minor fall, you are likely to have osteoporosis. Fractures of the wrist are known as Colles' fractures and usually result from attempting to break a fall with the hand. Hip fractures are one of the most serious types of fracture, since they are very painful and can severely impair mobility. Compression fractures of the vertebrae are also common, and if you don't receive treatment, you may experience further fractures. Don't leave it too late: 30 percent of your bone mass may have been lost by the time you have a hip fracture.

BACKACHE

Constant pain in the lower back should be taken as a sign for you to seek treatment from a menopause clinic, well-woman clinic, doctor or gynaecologist. (Another common cause of backache in menopausal women is prolapse.)

On average, women who develop spinal osteoporosis begin to notice an increase in the occurrence of severe backache about nine to ten years after their final menstrual period, or sooner if they have had a surgically induced menopause (as a result of surgical removal of the ovaries or hysterectomy).

Sufferer may feel housebound

Lack of exercise and vitamin D

Loss of self-esteem

Painful vertebral fractures

Clothes don't fit properly

Immobility leads to further bone loss and fractures

Pain on movement

Fear of being pushed in crowds

The vicious circle of vertebral collapse
Women who suffer from osteoporosis can find themselves trapped in a vicious circle that gradually erodes both their health and their sense of self-esteem.

MEDICAL TREATMENT

The aim of prescription drugs is to halt bone loss, prevent further fractures and replace or repair bone whenever possible. Once fractures occur, at least a third of bone mass has already been lost; in some cases as much as 60 percent is gone.

Over two million people in the UK have already suffered osteoporotic fractures, and although there are some treatments that can reverse osteoporosis, broken joints or bones that have been severely damaged are not likely to respond to treatment. Fortunately, there are several methods that can be effective in halting bone loss, the most potent treatment being HRT.

HORMONE REPLACEMENT THERAPY (HRT)

If you have low bone mass, it is highly recommended that you take HRT. Even if you have high bone mass, your future risk of fracture will be reduced with HRT. Calcium loss can be reduced by taking very low doses of oestrogen, and several studies have suggested that when progestogen (the synthetic version of progesterone) is taken with oestrogen, bone metabolism responds favourably. The progestogen appears to stimulate a small amount of bone formation, while the oestrogen halts further loss of bone.

Studies have also demonstrated that oestrogen therapy helps bone to maintain its mineral strength and mass. The oestrogen effect here appears to be dose-dependent. With high dosage, oestrogen can increase bone mass in the spine, but a low dose merely slows down the natural ageing loss. It is interesting to note that menopausal women who used oral contraceptives (containing oestrogen) for long periods of time have been found to have heavier and stronger bones than women who have never taken oral contraceptives.

NON-HORMONAL TREATMENT

The first line of defence against osteoporosis is increasing calcium intake through diet. Eat plenty of calcium-rich foods, including dairy products and canned fish with bones, such as sardines, and ask your doctor about calcium supplements. To maximize benefits, calcium should be taken with other treatments, such as HRT.

The drug etidronate has been shown to be effective in treating established spinal osteoporosis. It works by inhibiting the bone-resorbing cells (the osteoclasts) and allowing the bone-rebuilding cells (the osteoblasts) to work more efficiently. This results in a small net gain in the amount of bone in the vertebrae. However, research studies have not yet given us conclusive evidence of etidronate's effectiveness against hip fractures.

Sodium fluoride (available only at specialist treatment centres and not on prescription) can stimulate bone formation and may be given to women with severe vertebral osteoporosis. It is given in daily doses and must be taken with calcium supplements. A low, controlled dose can increase bone density and may reduce fracture rate. However, in higher doses, it can be associated with an increase in hip fractures. Careful monitoring is required when taking sodium fluoride because there may be side-effects of indigestion and nausea.

PAIN RELIEF

Women with vertebral osteoporosis can suffer intense back pain, especially after a new fracture. If pain is very acute, a strong pain-reliever, such as morphine, will be prescribed. This produces rapid relief and may make a journey to hospital more comfortable. Curvature of the spine (called kyphosis) produces ongoing muscular and ligament pain, but this can be treated with painkillers, such as paracetamol or codeine. Paracetamol is a safe, non-addictive drug, although you should be careful not to exceed the recommended dose or frequency of use; codeine may cause constipation.

Physiotherapists may also use various forms of electrotherapy or ultrasound to help relieve pain. Some now also use complementary techniques, for example acupuncture, and recommend the use of heat pads, hot-water bottles or ice packs at home. TENS (Transcutaneous Electrical Nerve Stimulation) machines are available in most treatment centres for pain relief.

If you have back pain, an occupational therapist can advise you on how to organize your home and work environment. You should sit in chairs with high backs that give support to the whole spine, and your bed should be firm, but not so hard that it cannot accommodate the altered shape of your spine.

PHYSIOTHERAPY

Increased muscle strength, improved spinal power and posture, maintenance of bone strength, relief of pain and toning of pelvic floor muscles to cope with stress incontinence are all benefits of physiotherapy.

Special exercises can also help with breathing difficulties that are exacerbated if the head falls forward, causing compression of the chest. Physiotherapy is often overlooked, but it should be an important part of your treatment for osteoporosis. A home exercise programme can be established to continue the treatment.

One of the most basic lessons taught by physiotherapists is how to breathe correctly. You don't need to go to a class to learn, but it is helpful initially to have a teacher's supervision to make sure you are learning the techniques correctly. People who keep themselves supple with exercise and special physiotherapy regimes are less likely to fall over, and they do less damage to themselves when they do fall than people who don't take regular exercise.

Hydrotherapy is another form of physiotherapy. It involves exercising in a pool of water at body temperature, 37°C (98°F), allowing you to move easily while the water supports you. The warmth relaxes the muscles and joints, relieves pain and increases mobility. Buoyancy makes exercise easier, while the water resistance strengthens muscles.

Since the greatest danger of osteoporosis is fracture, it is vital that you help yourself prevent its occurrence.

As women get older, falls can be related to poor coordination and blackouts, so you should ask your doctor to check your heart and blood pressure. It is also important to maintain good vision by having your eyes tested regularly, particularly for a condition known as glaucoma, which becomes more common with age. Avoid sedatives and other drugs that might reduce your alertness, such as antihistamines, and try to limit your alcohol intake.

Reduce hazards at home by removing any trailing electrical flexes and loose carpets. Make sure that stairs have a firm handrail and be particularly on guard when walking on slippery or uneven surfaces.

Many women with painful spinal fractures suffer severe loss of confidence and self-esteem in a vicious circle of physical and emotional distress. In some women, loss of self-esteem may lead to problems that are as serious as their physical discomfort.

Counselling, emotional support from friends and family and talking to other menopausal women with similar problems can do much to give a woman a more positive attitude to life and help her become more outgoing and confident.

PREVENTING OSTEOPOROSIS

Since all of us are at risk of developing osteoporosis, it is important that we adopt self-help measures in order to build up our natural resistance to this life-threatening disease. Fortunately, there are a number of ways in which we can change our lifestyles to help maintain healthy bones. Regular exercise, a balanced diet and mental alertness can help to maintain overall fitness. You should also have regular health checks with your doctor and consider taking HRT.

TAKE REGULAR EXERCISE

Investigators studying the relationship between bone density, prevention of bone fractures and exercise found that the amount of weight-bearing exercise, such as jogging, relates directly to increased bone mass. Women who take exercise twice a week have denser bones than those who take exercise once a week, who, in turn, have denser bones than those who never take exercise at all. It is never too late to improve your body. Bones can be strengthened to resist the effect of oestrogen depletion during the postmenopausal years.

If you are not physically active, ask your doctor about the best exercise programme for your level of fitness. Brisk walking will help to strengthen your bones. Try to exercise daily for 20–30 minutes, enough to moderately accelerate your pulse rate.

EAT A CALCIUM-RICH DIET

The most important dietary advice for the early prevention of osteoporosis is to eat calcium-rich foods. Calcium is lost from the body in sweat, urine and faeces, and maintenance of the correct amount is dependent on our dietary intake of calcium, combined with the presence of oestrogen and vitamin D. The bone deterioration that ends in osteoporosis begins a long time before the first fractures and the longer you wait to take action, the smaller your chances of recovery. In brief, to prevent your bones from becoming brittle, you need calcium for bone mass, vitamin D to absorb the calcium from your blood into your body and oestrogen to maintain the calcium inside your bones. For good food sources of vitamin D and calcium, see pp. 316 and 318.

BREAST CANCER

This is the most common type of cancer in women, and the leading cause of death in women who are aged between 35 and 50. In the UK, women have about a one in 12 chance of developing breast cancer.

Despite great advances in the technology used to treat breast cancer, the mortality rate has hardly changed this century. We do know, however, that the cure rate for breast cancer depends on the stage at which it is detected, and whether it has spread. The earlier any abnormality is discovered, the more likely it is to be cured.

Although there is no equivalent of the cervical smear test, which detects precancerous changes in the cervix, an X-ray procedure called mammography exists, which is able to detect very small breast tumours that cannot be felt manually. However, sometimes early and curable breast tumours can be found by routine monthly examination, and all women should learn how to examine their breasts).

SYMPTOMS

A small tumour may be detected during a routine self-examination of the breasts. The most common site for a malignant breast tumour is on the upper and outer part of the breast, where a lump can usually be felt rather than seen. A tumour is rarely painful. Signs to look out for include nipple discharge, a newly inverted nipple, lumps or swellings in the breasts, armpits or along the collar bone and a puckered or dimpled appearance of the breast.

MEDICAL TREATMENT

Radical treatments, for example partial or extended mastectomy, do not necessarily improve survival rates. Many surgeons now recommend lumpectomy combined with radiotherapy or anti-cancer drugs (chemotherapy).

Sometimes, before you undergo breast surgery, you may be asked to sign a form that will allow your surgeon to carry out treatment during an exploratory operation. Think carefully about this – you should always be an active participant in all decisions regarding your treatment. If there are signs that a tumour has spread to the lymph nodes in the armpit, you will need more extensive

RISK FACTORS

Certain dietary habits can put you in a higher risk group than average. There is a documented link between breast cancer and a high intake of animal protein, saturated animal fats and dairy products. Other risk factors are listed below.

Medium to high risk factors for breast cancer are:
- *Having a family history of breast cancer (especially close female relatives, for example, mother or sister).*

- *Early onset of menstruation and a late menopause.*

- *Being over the age of 40.*

- *Having children later than average.*

- *Being Caucasian.*

- *Being obese or having a diet high in animal dairy fat.*

Low risk factors for breast cancer are:
- *Having several children.*

- *Breast-feeding.*

- *Being short and thin.*

- *Late onset of menstruation and an early menopause.*

At one time, women taking oral contraceptives were thought to be at greater risk of breast cancer than women who did not take the pill. However, recent studies now suggest that there is no correlation.

DIAGNOSIS OF BREAST CANCER

The majority of doctors will refer a woman with a breast lump to a hospital so that further tests can be made.

If you have a cyst, the fluid can be removed and examined, so that a clear-cut diagnosis can be made. This procedure, called a needle biopsy, is a painless technique in which, under anaesthetic, a fine needle is inserted into the lump and some of the cells are drawn out. In 85 percent of cancerous tumours, malignant cells will be detected by a needle biopsy.

If a lump is small and shallow (not deep in the tissue of the breast), it is possible to have an outpatient lumpectomy. The lump is removed with some surrounding tissue and examined in the laboratory. If cancer is discovered, blood tests, X-rays and bone scans will be carried out to help decide upon the appropriate treatment.

treatment in order to prevent any further spread. If your tumour is of a type that is sensitive to hormones, an anti-oestrogen drug may be prescribed.

Tamoxifen is a drug used in the treatment of certain types of breast cancer. It works by blocking the oestrogen hormone receptors in the breast cells and has fewer adverse effects than other anti-cancer drugs. Side-effects may include hot flushes, nausea, vomiting, swollen ankles and irregular vaginal bleeding. Women at high risk of developing breast cancer, for example with a family history of the disease, may be prescribed tamoxifen to help prevent any cancer from developing.

BREAST CANCER AND HRT

The use of HRT in women with breast cancer (past or present), as well as other female cancers, is controversial. Although many doctors regard breast and other cancers as a reason not to give HRT, some doctors will still prescribe it. Where appropriate, I have tried to reflect current medical thinking on HRT, but ultimately your doctor should decide your eligibility.

OUTLOOK

If a very small tumour is treated early, a complete cure is likely. All women who have had breast cancer will be asked to attend regular check-ups to detect any recurrence of the cancer or spread to the rest of the body. It is very important that regular breast self-examinations and yearly mammograms are carried out. Even if the cancer recurs, it can be controlled for many years with surgery, drugs and radiotherapy.

Comparative death rates from common cancers
Women become more susceptible to many types of cancer after the menopause. Breast cancer is the most prevalent cancer in women.

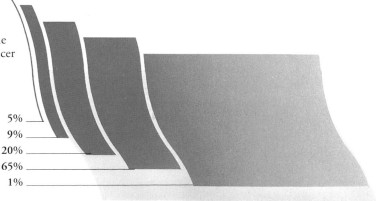

OVARIAN CANCER	5%
COLO-RECTAL CANCER	9%
BREAST CANCER	20%
OTHER CANCERS	65%
UTERINE CANCER	1%

THE UTERUS AND OVARIES

It's just good health management to have checks on all your reproductive organs at the time of the menopause when the hormones that keep them healthy start to wane.

OVARIAN CANCER

Malignant ovarian growths are most common after the age of 50; approximately 5,000 cases are diagnosed each year in the UK. Ovarian cancer is three times more common in women who have never had children, but less common in those who have taken the contraceptive pill. It may remain symptomless for some time and may be advanced by the time of diagnosis.

DIAGNOSIS

To determine whether a tumour is malignant or benign a laparoscopy will be carried out. This is an examination of the abdominal cavity through a fine fibre-optic viewing instrument. It is done through a tiny incision in the abdominal wall under general anaesthetic. If the tumour is very large, you may need an exploratory operation.

UTERINE CANCER

Unlike cervical cancer, which is most common in young women, uterine or endometrial cancer is most common in older women: three-quarters of all sufferers are over the age of 50, and very few are under 40. Between the ages of 55 and 65, the incidence of uterine cancer more than doubles. As the proportion of older women in the population increases, this upward trend is likely to continue. In the UK, there are nearly 3,500 new cases every year. Although cancer of the uterus is the third most common cancer of the female reproductive organs, it has a much better survival rate than cancer of the ovary.

SYMPTOMS

The earliest, most common sign of uterine cancer is abnormal vaginal bleeding, especially if you are postmenopausal. If you are still menstruating, any bleeding between periods, slight spotting, heavy and

TREATMENT OF OVARIAN CANCER

All tumours will be surgically removed, and microscopic examination of the cells will identify malignancy.

As much of the cancerous growth as possible will be removed, which may mean taking away part of the bowel, the Fallopian tube, the ovary and the uterus. Surgery is usually followed by radiotherapy and anti-cancer drugs.

OUTLOOK

If the growth is confined to the ovary, two-thirds of patients will probably survive for more than five years.

If the growth has spread, only one in five women will survive for more than five years. New techniques and drugs for detecting and treating ovarian cancer are improving survival rates. However, an annual pelvic examination by your doctor is the most important detection tool.

RISK FACTORS FOR UTERINE CANCER

Uterine cancer is more likely to occur among women who have never had children, and women of low fertility.

There is also thought to be an association between cancer of the uterus and oestrogen replacement therapy when it is taken without progestogen. However, nowadays HRT is prescribed in its combined form and this may actually protect women against uterine cancer.

Women who are obese (being overweight results in high blood levels of oestrogen), have a family history of uterine cancer, suffer from high blood pressure, diabetes, fibroids or disturbed menstrual patterns with long intervals between periods are all at a higher risk of developing uterine cancer.

TREATMENT OF UTERINE CANCER

A complete hysterectomy, with removal of the ovaries, Fallopian tubes and uterus, is the usual treatment.

In nearly all parts of the world this procedure, combined with radiotherapy in selected cases, before or after the operation, has vastly improved cure rates.

The overall cure rate is as high as 90 percent when the cancer is localized to the lining of the uterus and has not spread.

prolonged bleeding, or bleeding after intercourse are all symptoms that should be investigated. Advanced cancers may give rise to menstrual cramps, pelvic bloating and distension, with pressure in the lower abdomen. Symptoms affecting the bladder include frequent and urgent urination.

HYSTERECTOMY

This is the surgical removal of the uterus with or without other reproductive organs. In developed countries it is one of the most frequently performed operations, second only to episiotomy (surgical enlargement of the vagina during childbirth). You should always question your doctor's reasons for wanting to perform a hysterectomy.

WHY IS IT DONE?

• To remove cancer in the vagina, cervix, uterus, Fallopian tubes or ovaries.
• To treat severe and uncontrollable pelvic infection.
• To stop acute haemorrhage.
• When certain life-threatening conditions affect the organs lying close to the uterus, and it is technically impossible to deal with the primary problem without removing the uterus.
• To treat extensive and very painful endometriosis.
• To remove large or multiple fibroids.
• After injury to the pelvic musculature during childbirth, which is severe enough to interfere with bowel or bladder function.
• To treat heavy vaginal bleeding that doesn't respond to treatment and results in anaemia.

Although these conditions are all debilitating, there are some serious but poorly publicized side-effects associated with having a hysterectomy. Loss of sexual desire is quite common even if your ovaries are intact. A significant number of women experience a decline in their sexual desire after having their uterus removed, and taking HRT doesn't seem to help. Indeed, several studies show that HRT eliminates a dry vagina and pain on intercourse, but it does not influence sex drive.

There is also data from Scandinavia that suggests sexual activity is greater, and the incidence of painful intercourse lower, in women who do not have their cervix removed. Some women who had had a complete hysterectomy (involving the removal of the cervix) claimed there was a significant loss in their capacity for orgasm, and they experienced orgasm in intercourse less than one in four times. The presence of sensitive nerve endings in the cervix may play a crucial role in your post-operative ability to have an orgasm.

We know that the ovaries, even after they stop secreting oestrogen, continue to secrete androgens, and these hormones are very important in maintaining libido in women. Removing the ovaries during a hysterectomy denies a woman this sexual stimulant. However, if testosterone therapy is taken after the operation, some women notice that their sex drive returns to normal.

There are other important health reasons for retaining the ovaries. They are our main source of oestrogen, and we know that oestrogen deprivation results in an earlier onset of heart disease and osteoporosis.

All of these are indisputable reasons for discussing with your doctor exactly which reproductive organs will be removed. Do not make a decision without such prior discussion and ensure you have the power to make the final decision. Your partner will almost certainly support you in your decision. Make sure that he is involved in all discussions about treatment.

OUTLOOK

Many women are concerned that they will gain weight after a hysterectomy. Fortunately, this is a myth. A diet that rich in fresh vegetables, fruit, fish and poultry will help you regain your strength and give you sufficient energy to start exercising and restore tone to flabby muscles.

Some women experience a psychological reaction after a hysterectomy. The following statistics have been compiled from various studies:
• Women who have their ovaries removed may blame the operation for hot flushes, lethargy and other menopausal symptoms.
• Women who have had hysterectomies are four times more likely to become depressed in the three years after surgery than other women.
• Depressed women who have had hysterectomies are likely to remain depressed for twice as long – on average two years – as women who have not.

WHY HAVE A HYSTERECTOMY?

A hysterectomy should be a comparatively rare operation. However, 30 percent of all women aged 50 and over in the United States have had hysterectomies, often when it was not absolutely necessary.

The removal of small fibroids, for instance, hardly warrants such a radical operation. Some doctors even advocate routine hysterectomy once childbearing is over. They argue that a hysterectomy forestalls the risk of cancers. Fortunately, this view is not widespread.

You should make certain that you and your partner are fully informed of the consequences of a hysterectomy, and have no reservations about such an irrevocable step. Remember, it is you who decides whether or not you wish to spend the rest of your life without your uterus.

Most medical conditions will respond to treatment without surgery if a doctor is positive and determined. I personally would never consider having a hysterectomy without obtaining a second opinion, regardless of persuasive arguments.

If your ovaries are removed as well as your uterus, you will experience menopausal symptoms after the operation. These can, and should, be alleviated by long-term HRT.

TREATMENT OF FIBROIDS

Small symptomless fibroids, which are often discovered during a routine pelvic examination, usually need no treatment except monitoring.

Surgery is required only for fibroids that cause symptoms such as pain or heavy bleeding. A hysterectomy may be considered if there are a large number of fibroids or if you are experiencing significant pain or pressure.

Myomectomy, which involves shelling the fibroid out of its capsule, saves the uterus and is an alternative.

If you are experiencing hot flushes and other menopausal symptoms, you should not necessarily be deterred from using HRT because you have fibroids. However, your doctor will want to carry out regular abdominal or internal examinations. Both the uterus and fibroids tend to shrink at the menopause, and the benefits of HRT in promoting good bones, a sense of well-being and improved sexual function need to be weighed against the inconvenience of symptoms due to fibroids.

- Women who have had hysterectomies are five times more likely to seek psychiatric help for the first time than women who have not.
- The majority of women who seek psychiatric help following a hysterectomy are those who were not suffering from a life-threatening condition. This suggests that if a woman believes her hysterectomy was performed unnecessarily, she may become depressed as a result.
- Women grow more dissatisfied with the effects of their hysterectomies as time passes.

FIBROIDS

These benign tumours grow slowly in or on the uterine wall, and their exact cause is unknown. Women who are below the age of 20 rarely suffer from fibroids, but they affect a fifth of women between the ages of 35 and 45, and a quarter of women over 80.

Progesterone production declines as women near the menopause, and the relatively unopposed oestrogen of the perimenopausal years may be responsible for the increasing number of fibroid tumours. Decreased levels of oestrogen after the menopause usually causes fibroids to shrink. When fibroids do increase rapidly in postmenopausal women, there are grounds for concern since these tumours have the greatest potential for becoming cancerous. Current dosages of HRT are not thought to be sufficiently high to affect postmenopausal fibroids one way or the other.

SYMPTOMS

Small fibroids may be symptomless. However, if a fibroid distorts the size or shape of the uterus, it may cause heavy or prolonged periods and anaemia. Large fibroids may press on the bladder, causing discomfort or frequent and urgent urination. Pressure on the bowel causes backache or constipation. Occasionally, a fibroid attached to the uterine wall becomes twisted on its stalk and can cause sudden pain in the lower abdomen.

DIAGNOSIS

Fibroids can cause the uterine wall to become lumpy and bumpy. If your doctor notices abdominal swelling he or she may recommend an ultrasound scan to confirm whether fibroids are present.

ATHEROSCLEROSIS

This is a disease of the arterial wall in which the inner layer thickens, causing narrowing of the channel, reduced blood flow and increased blood pressure (hypertension). The thickening is due to the development of raised patches called plaques inside the artery. These plaques consist of a fatty substance known as atheroma, and they tend to form in regions of turbulent blood flow, such as the junction of two arteries.

Atheroma worsens with age, causing irregularities in the smooth lining of the blood vessels and encouraging thrombus (abnormal blood clot) formation. Sometimes, a fragment of thrombus breaks off and forms an embolus, which travels in the bloodstream and blocks smaller blood vessels.

Atherosclerosis is a leading cause of death in the UK and atherosclerotic heart disease of the coronary arteries is the single most common cause of death. Strokes resulting from interference in the blood supply to the brain are the third most common cause of death (cancer is the second most common).

Atherosclerosis can also cause serious illness by impeding blood flow in other major arteries, such as those that supply the kidneys, legs and intestines. Before the menopause, women are protected from atherosclerosis by the body's production of oestrogen, so it tends to affect men and postmenopausal women. As most of the research on atherosclerosis and heart disease has been carried out on men, all statistics I have quoted relate to men, not women, unless otherwise stated.

SYMPTOMS

Until the damage to the arteries is severe enough to restrict blood flow, atherosclerosis is symptomless. When blood flow becomes impeded – generally after a number of years – you may experience angina, which is pain in the chest on exertion. Another symptom is intermittent claudication, which is leg pain brought on by walking and alleviated by rest. If blood flow is restricted in the arteries supplying the brain, you may experience temporary stroke symptoms, dizziness and fainting attacks. Kidney failure is also possible if the renal artery becomes narrowed.

RISK FACTORS

Obesity, smoking, high blood pressure, being menopausal and postmenopausal, lack of exercise, a high cholesterol level, poorly controlled diabetes and a family history of arterial disease all increase your chances of suffering from atherosclerosis.

A personality type known as type A, characterized by aggression and competitiveness, may also be a risk factor.

The incidence of atherosclerosis in women increases with age. In the 35–44 age group, coronary artery disease kills six times as many men as women. In the 55–70 age group, death due to atherosclerosis is nearly equal in men and women. This is due almost entirely to the decline of oestrogen levels during the menopause.

Women who develop heart disease after the menopause are more likely to have had excess body hair when they were younger (this occurs in women with high levels of testosterone). They should pay particular attention to the cardiovascular risk factors that are under their control, such as smoking, diet and stress levels. They should also discuss with their doctors the possibility of taking oestrogen in HRT to balance testosterone production.

SURGERY FOR ATHEROSCLEROSIS

People who don't respond to treatment, or who are likely to suffer complications, may need surgery.

A common surgical technique used to treat atherosclerosis is balloon angioplasty. This opens up narrowed blood vessels and restores blood flow. Coronary artery bypass surgery can restore blood flow to the heart, and a technique called endarterectomy can replace diseased blood vessels with woven plastic tubes.

DIAGNOSIS AND MEDICAL TREATMENT

Atherosclerosis can be diagnosed by angiography, a procedure in which a radio-opaque substance is injected into the blood vessels, enabling X-rays to show up the blood flow in an artery. Other techniques include Doppler ultrasound scanning (plethysmography), which produces a tracing of the pulse pattern.

Treating atherosclerosis with drugs is difficult, since by the time symptoms appear, the damage to the arteries has already been done. Although anticoagulant drugs can be used to stop further damage by preventing secondary clotting and embolus formation, they do not provide a cure. Vasodilator drugs will open up the arteries of the legs, and help to relieve symptoms.

PREVENTION

Lowering risk factors, especially in early adulthood and midlife, can help prevent atherosclerosis developing. If you smoke, you should try to give it up. You should have your blood pressure checked regularly and get treatment for high blood pressure. Lose any excess weight, keep your diet low in saturated fats, and if your cholesterol levels still remain high, you may need medication. Meticulous control of diabetes mellitus is important, and regular exercise is essential.

HRT may prevent coronary heart disease in that oestrogen has a beneficial effect on fat deposits in the blood, blood coagulation, blood glucose and insulin levels, and blood pressure. Women receiving HRT have half the risk of heart disease of non-users. This may be because they have higher levels of the healthy HDL cholesterol and lower levels of the dangerous LDL cholesterol that leads to hardening of the arteries.

Other new findings show that when oestrogen and progestogen are combined in HRT, blood glucose and insulin are lower and healthier in users than in non-users. Although high blood pressure is sometimes regarded as a reason not to give HRT, studies carried out in 1993 showed no rise in blood pressure in women taking HRT.

There is also a lower level of fibrinogen (a coagulation factor) in the blood of HRT users. This means that the blood is thinner and the likelihood of forming clots that might lead to a heart attack or a stroke is diminished.

UROGENITAL PROBLEMS

Hardly a woman beyond the menopause escapes some urinary symptoms because oestrogen is crucial in keeping the bladder and urethra healthy. Local oestrogen cream relieves many symptoms.

UROGENITAL AGEING

Oestrogen receptors are found in abundance in the genital organs, the lower urinary tract and the bladder, so the genital and the urinary organs can be treated as one system. When oestrogen is plentiful, the receptors keep this system healthy and resistant to infection. When hormone levels fall during the menopause, the receptors can no longer bind with oestrogen, and, as a result, are unable to keep organs strong and healthy. The urogenital system thins and becomes susceptible to infection.

SYMPTOMS

Signs of genital atrophy include a dry, itchy vagina and vulva, which causes pain during sex. These symptoms are often combined with the frequent, urgent desire to urinate and incontinence. This combination of symptoms is the most common reason for women over the age of 55 to visit a gynaecologist.

CYSTITIS

Oestrogen is so crucial to the health of the urinary tract that after the menopause the bladder is far more susceptible to bacterial infection. Cystitis is much more common in women than men anyway, because women have a shorter urethra (the tube leading from the bladder to the outside of the body). Nearly all infections that reach the bladder are due to bacteria entering the urethra from outside and then spreading upwards and inflaming the lining of the urethra and bladder. You should treat cystitis promptly because if it is allowed to recur it can become chronic, making it very difficult to eradicate.

SYMPTOMS

Only a woman who has suffered from cystitis knows how agonizing the following symptoms can be:
• The urgent need to pass urine frequently. You may start to pass urine involuntarily, and then find there

DIAGNOSIS AND TREATMENT

A bladder pressure reading will show if the bladder muscle contracts spontaneously causing urine to dribble away, leading to the symptoms of urgency and sometimes (but not always) incontinence.

A smear test will determine whether the vaginal lining has atrophied, with a loss of the protective acid vaginal secretions.

The first line of treatment should be oestrogen therapy. Research shows that oestrogen creams applied to the vagina diffuse through the urethra and the bladder and relieve symptoms in days. Oestrogen pessaries and rings are almost 100 percent effective. Oral and skin patch HRT also eliminate symptoms.

CYSTITIS SELF-HELP

Right at the beginning of an attack, you should drink lots of water or diluted fruit juice.

Infection from the bacterium E. coli is the most common cause of cystitis. E. coli cannot multiply in alkaline urine, and you can make your urine alkaline by taking a teaspoonful of bicarbonate of soda in a glass of water. Drink this three times within five hours of the first twinge. Soluble aspirin and a hot-water bottle can help to relieve pain.

Each time you pass urine, pay attention to hygiene and wash your hands carefully before and afterwards. You should also wipe your perineum (the area between your vagina and anus) from front to back once with damp cotton wool. Soap and water can dry out the vagina and perineum and make you more prone to infection. When you dry yourself, pat gently – don't irritate the urethra by rubbing briskly.

If your cystitis is provoked by intercourse, it is probably best to refrain from sex until you are feeling more comfortable. Otherwise, reduce friction with a lubricating jelly and experiment to find the most comfortable sexual position. You should also wash carefully and pass urine after sex.

is very little urine to pass. This irritability of the bladder muscle is due to inflammation of the bladder lining, caused by the presence of bacteria. Even a few drops of urine can stimulate the bladder to contract.

• Severe pain and a burning sensation when you pass urine. This pain may occur when the flow begins and the bladder muscle starts to contract down on the inflamed lining, it may be during urination or it may be at the end, when the muscle squeezes the last few drops of urine out of the bladder.

• A dragging pain in the lower abdomen that may radiate up into the back. (Severe pain in the lower back could mean that you have a kidney infection and you should see your doctor immediately.)

• Blood in the urine – whether obvious streaks of red or simply a pale-pink tinge to the urine – indicates severe inflammation of the bladder lining.

DIAGNOSIS AND MEDICAL TREATMENT

Your doctor will ask for a sample of your urine for analysis and for growing bacteria in a culture to see which particular bacterium is causing your symptoms. This will enable him or her to prescribe an antibiotic specifically to treat the bacterium.

Make an appointment to see your doctor as soon as possible, and take a specimen of urine in a clean receptacle with you. You will need a course of antibiotics and you should take the full course even though the symptoms may disappear within 36 hours. A minimum course for mild cystitis is five days, and in the case of a severe attack seven to ten days. With chronic infections, you may need to take antibiotics for three to six weeks.

Oestrogen cream, applied to the vagina by means of an applicator, will do a great deal to help prevent cystitis; oestrogen diffuses through the vaginal wall to reach the urethra where oestrogen receptors make the urethral lining healthy and resistant to infection.

PRURITIS VULVAE

Itching is a sign of oestrogen deficiency, and chronic, uncontrollable itching of the vaginal area is usually worst in hot weather or at night. Diabetes, vaginal yeast infections, such as thrush, and urinary tract infections, can all cause pruritis vulvae. However, it can be psychogenic in origin. Repeated scratching can become more and more pleasurable, even to the point of orgasm. Eventually, the sufferer will develop profound soreness and thickening of the skin in the vaginal area.

MEDICAL TREATMENT

Pruritis vulvae usually responds well to oestrogen cream. Your doctor can also prescribe an emollient cream that keeps the skin soft and well lubricated. You should apply these creams as directed. If there is excessive inflammation your doctor may give you a cream that contains hydrocortisone. If infection is suspected, he or she may give you a mild hydrocortisone cream containing an antibiotic. Oestrogen vaginal pessaries should also help.

If pruritis vulvae does not respond to treatment, your doctor can refer you to a dermatological specialist for further assessment of your condition.

INCONTINENCE

This occurs when the sphincter muscle at the base of your bladder becomes so weak (or the bladder muscle becomes overactive) that you have little or no control over the flow of urine. Although this condition is not life-threatening, it can be debilitating and embarrassing, and may make you housebound. Oestrogen helps to keep the sphincter muscle tight, and when oestrogen levels decline during the menopause, the muscle can become weak and flaccid, allowing leakage of urine.

The other probable causes of incontinence at or after the menopause are an irritable bladder, diabetes mellitus or local infections such as cystitis. The three types of incontinence are as follows:

• Stress incontinence is when a small amount of urine leaks and dribbles away. It is caused by an increase in pressure inside the abdomen when you sneeze, cough, laugh or lift a heavy object.

• Urge incontinence occurs if you wait to urinate until you need to do so urgently. The bladder starts to contract involuntarily and empties itself. This type of incontinence is often triggered by a sudden change in position, such as standing up.

• Mixed pattern incontinence is a combination of both urge and stress incontinence, and may be the result of two faults in bladder function.

PRURITIS VULVAE SELF-HELP

You can prevent pruritis vulvae from getting worse by trying not to scratch the vaginal area.

Consult your doctor if the condition persists for more than two days – if you don't, you may find yourself in an unbreakable itch-scratch-itch cycle. Pay particular attention to normal hygiene but, if possible, avoid the use of soap and detergents since they will strip the skin of oils and make it more sensitive.

Use only warm or cool water, and try applying an unscented silicone-based hand cream to the itchy area after each wash. Ice packs may help to numb the itch too. Don't use local anaesthetic creams and sprays, however tempting, since these may cause allergic reactions.

INCONTINENCE SELF-HELP

Mild incontinence is often due to weakened pelvic floor muscles, and you can improve your bladder control by doing Kegel exercises, also known as pelvic floor exercises.

These involve repeatedly contracting and relaxing the muscles of the urogenital tract. If you are suffering from urge incontinence, self-help measures include emptying your bladder every two hours, and avoiding diuretic drinks such as coffee, tea and chocolate.

Aids for incontinence sufferers include waterproof bed sheets, incontinence pads, female urinals and waterproof pants. However, you should consult your doctor long before these become necessary. If you suffer from stress incontinence when you exercise, try emptying your bladder beforehand. Wearing a tampon during exercise can act as a splint to the urethra.

MEDICAL TREATMENT

Sometimes all you need to combat stress incontinence is oestrogen cream. Other forms of HRT will also help, and you should try consulting your doctor about them. Treatment may also include anticholinergic drugs, which are effective for an irritable bladder, an operation for stress incontinence and bladder retraining.

PROLAPSE

Prolapse, or "pelvic relaxation", occurs when the pelvic musculature is unable to support the pelvic organs and allows them to drop out of position. The affected organs include the uterus, bladder, rectum and urethra. The uterus is the most likely to prolapse. Because of advanced age, childbirth and a decline in oestrogen levels, the uterine muscles become weak and sag. The pull of gravity is a contributing factor. Prolapse is especially noticeable when abdominal pressure is increased by coughing or straining during a bowel movement.

FOUR TYPES OF PROLAPSE

Uterine Prolapse This type of prolapse is caused by a weakening of supporting pelvic ligaments and muscles. The uterus may descend from the pelvic cavity down into the vagina, causing irritation to the vagina, slight backache, and sometimes a sensation that your insides are going to fall out. The dropped cervix will also prevent deep penile penetration during intercourse.

Mild or first degree prolapse is when the uterus begins to descend into the vagina. Second and third degree prolapse are more severe. In second degree prolapse, the cervix begins to protrude from the vagina, and third degree prolapse is when the cervix and uterus protrude outside the vaginal opening. This condition is extremely uncomfortable and debilitating.

Prolapse is often the result of childbearing, especially if the pelvic floor muscle or the cervix was injured during delivery of a baby. Occasionally, the same conditions that have produced hernias in men, such as strenuous physical or athletic activity, may produce prolapses in women. Obesity and complaints such as constipation and chronic coughing all aggravate the condition because they increase the intra-abdominal pressure and cause the pelvic muscles to become weak and slack. Increased pressure can also lead to stress incontinence, in which you leak small amounts of urine when you cough, laugh, sneeze or lift heavy objects.

Urethrocele In this type of prolapse, the urethra bulges into the lower front wall of the vagina. Irritation of the urethral lining can lead to frequent urination.

Rectocele In this type of prolapse, the front wall of the rectum bulges into the rear wall of the vagina. Extreme discomfort is experienced when you have a bowel movement. In fact, it may be bearable only if a finger is inserted into the vagina to support the rear wall.

Cystocele The bladder bulges into the upper front wall of the vagina. This type of prolapse is nearly always accompanied by bladder problems, such as recurrent cystitis. Sometimes the bladder sags below the level of the urethral outlet, which makes emptying the bladder extremely difficult. In such cases, it may be emptied by inserting a finger into the vagina and pushing up the sagging part.

MEDICAL TREATMENT

In the early stages of prolapse, HRT may help rebuild tissue structures that are inclined towards atrophy (thinning) because of low oestrogen levels. For older women, whose prolapse is not very severe, or where infirmity makes a general anaesthetic inadvisable, a ring or shelf pessary can be placed in the vagina where it supports the cervix and uterus. It should not be worn for very long periods because it may wear away the thin atrophied tissues by friction.

Surgery is needed for severe prolapse, when the cervix and uterus both protrude outside the vaginal opening. An operation is performed through the vagina and is tailored to the individual woman's problems. The anterior and posterior walls of the uterus can be repaired and the supports of the uterus shortened. If the uterus is severely prolapsed it can be removed. However, this is a major decision so discuss it thoroughly with your doctor or gynaecologist and seek a second opinion if necessary.

PROLAPSE SELF-HELP

These simple measures may help and are worth trying.

Wearing a girdle counteracts the dragging feeling that you may have and can relieve the discomfort to a certain extent.

Backache is one of the most common symptoms and it is very important not to stand for long periods, to maintain good posture and to rest with your feet up whenever you can.

You can protect yourself from prolapse by performing Kegel exercises, avoiding over-strenuous activity, losing weight if you need to and giving up smoking, especially if you have a cough. Eat plenty of fibre, fruit and vegetables to keep your bowels regular and the stools soft.

TREATING HYPOTHYROIDISM

Diagnosis is confirmed by tests that measure the level of thyroid hormones in the blood. Treatment consists of replacement therapy with the thyroid hormone thyroxine.

In most cases of hypothyroidism, hormone medication must be continued for life. However, if this treatment does not cure a goitre, surgery may be required.

SYMPTOMS OF DIABETES MELLITUS

Some women can suffer from a mild form of diabetes, which may be symptomless, although the condition can cause the following symptoms:

• *Damage to the back of the eye and blurred vision.*

• *Excessive thirst.*

• *Fatigue.*

• *Weight loss.*

• *Frequent urination.*

• *Itchiness of the vulva and vaginal infections.*

• *A tingling sensation in the hands and feet.*

OTHER HORMONAL CONDITIONS

All our hormone glands age as we get older and so the thyroid gland may underperform and a type of diabetes may emerge – both are easy to treat.

HYPOTHYROIDISM

The underproduction of thyroid hormones is caused by the body developing antibodies to its own thyroid gland, preventing the production of thyroid hormones. A condition called Hashimoto's thyroiditis is an example of this. More rarely, hypothyroidism may result from an operation to remove part of the thyroid gland, or from taking radioactive iodine as a treatment for a condition called hyperthyroidism (overactivity of the thyroid).

Hypothyroidism can occur at any age, but it is most common in elderly women. The condition affects one in 100 of the adult population.

SYMPTOMS

A deficiency of thyroid hormones can cause generalized tiredness and lethargy, muscle weakness, cramps, a slow heart rate, dry and flaky skin, hair loss, a deep and husky voice and weight gain.

A syndrome known as myxoedema may develop, in which the skin and other body tissues thicken. In some cases a goitre (an enlargement of the thyroid gland) develops, although not all goitres are caused by hypothyroidism. The severity of symptoms is dependent on the degree of thyroid deficiency. Mild deficiency may cause no symptoms, severe deficiency may produce the whole range of symptoms.

DIABETES MELLITUS

This is a deficiency of the hormone insulin. Sufferers whose bodies produce no insulin of their own and are dependent on insulin injections have type I diabetes. The type of diabetes that usually affects women over 40 is type II diabetes, in which insulin is still produced, but in insufficient quantities. This type of diabetes has a slow onset and may be discovered only during a routine medical examination.

Insulin, produced by the pancreas, controls the effective use of glucose in the body. Insufficient insulin makes the glucose level in your blood rise dramatically, and you start to excrete glucose in your urine instead of using it as energy, or storing it. The fact that you cannot utilize your most accessible form of energy has a detrimental effect on the body, and you may experience symptoms such as fatigue, weight loss, excessive thirst, the need to pass large amounts of urine, blurred vision and itchiness or redness of the vulva.

RISK FACTORS

Obesity is associated with diabetes. If you are overweight and have a high intake of carbohydrates, the amount of glucose in your blood will be high, and your pancreas may not be able to cope. Losing weight and changing your diet may be helpful. Other risk factors are heredity (a third of diabetics have a family history of the condition) and old age.

DIAGNOSIS

Your doctor will test your urine for glucose and a substance called ketones (a byproduct of fat breakdown). He or she may also take a sample of your blood after you have not eaten for a few hours. If both your urine and blood are found to contain significantly high levels of glucose and ketones, diabetes is likely.

MEDICAL TREATMENT

Serious cases of type II diabetes may need to be given hypoglycaemic drugs to lower blood glucose. Injections of insulin are not required since they are prescribed only for sufferers of diabetes mellitus type I.

The complications that can arise from severe diabetes mellitus include damage to the retina at the back of the eye (retinopathy), damage to nerve fibres (neuropathy), damage to the kidneys (nephropathy), atherosclerosis, hypertension and gangrene.

Both diabetes and HRT alter the way that you metabolise carbohydrates, and for this reason HRT may be relatively contraindicated for diabetics. However, if your diabetes is stable, if you test your urine regularly, and if you liaise closely with your doctor, it may be safe, particularly in the very low dose skin patch form.

DIABETES MELLITUS SELF-HELP

It is important to monitor the amount of glucose you are ingesting. Too much glucose in the blood (hyperglycaemia) will exacerbate your diabetic symptoms, and too little (hypoglycaemia) will cause dizziness, weakness, confusion and finally unconsciousness.

You can monitor your glucose levels with a kit, which your doctor will give you, by dipping an impregnated strip into a sample of your urine and then comparing the colour change against a chart.

Your doctor will advise you about how to control diabetes with diet, but, as a rule, you should avoid all sugar. Eat small amounts of carbohydrates at regular intervals so that you do not have drastic fluctuations in glucose levels, and eat plenty of fibre. In mild cases of diabetes that are due to obesity, simply cutting out sugar and reducing your weight will greatly improve your condition because your pancreas will be producing enough insulin to cope with your reduced body size.

ENJOYING LIFE BEYOND THE MENOPAUSE

As you grow older, you may go through a period of major reassessment. You may have a nagging feeling about something in your life you would like to change, but you may have deferred making changes because the time was never right. You may be dissatisfied with your job situation. You may feel that you don't spend enough time doing the things you want to do. You may want to make some changes in your relationship, or arrange some time away from your partner. If any of the above apply to you, confront your feelings and try to be honest with yourself. Talk over your thoughts with your partner, with friends, or perhaps even with a counsellor. If you let people know what you are looking for – whether it be a job or a new friendship – communicating your thoughts may open the door to new opportunities.

COMMIT YOURSELF TO ACTION

Once you've made up your mind about what you want to change and how to go about it, you must take the leap and commit yourself. This doesn't have to mean walking out of your job or filing for divorce, it just means taking a step in the right direction, whether it be registering with an employment agency or spending more leisure time away from your partner.

Try to avoid thinking of yourself as selfish – others close to you, such as your partner, can benefit from any changes that you decide to make. For instance, if you have spent most of your life at home bringing up a family, a new part-time job or a course could increase your sense of independence and make you feel more fulfilled, and this can have a positive effect on your relationship. You may have always wanted to follow a career and, as your husband approaches retirement, you could suggest swapping roles. Alternatively, you may be looking forward to a restful retirement.

Remember, you have already made many decisions and experienced many changes in your life and you're well equipped to cope with new experiences. Think of retirement as a period of self-renewal and it shouldn't be the crushing change that people often perceive it to be.

When asked what they miss most about working life, many people mention money and the social environment of work. However, there are very many advantages to retiring: you can follow your own body clock – eating, sleeping and studying when you feel like it; you no longer have to comply with authority; you have more time to spend on your family, friends and hobbies; and being out of the rat race can dramatically reduce your stress levels.

People usually start to prepare for retirement when they are in their 50s. You may start to reduce your job workload, seek financial advice or you may even decide to move to a smaller house. On a personal level, you may start to put more into your intimate relationships.

Whereas some people find retiring a natural transition, others, particularly women who have had fulfilling careers, may find it harder. We must prepare for this time since there may be little space for adjustment if we don't.

Retirement preparation is now a widely recognized need. Many firms, voluntary organizations and adult education centres give advice or run courses about financial planning, buying and dispersing personal property and assets, attending to health needs and organizing leisure time.

ORGANIZING YOUR TIME

Working fewer days in the week or less hours each day, taking longer holidays or working from home are just a few ways in which to make the move from paid work to retirement. If retirement could be less of a cut-off point and more of a transition, this might help to lessen its social stigma and improve emotional stability.

The loss of relationships at work following retirement, the departure of your children or even the death of your partner all mean that you may become more reliant on your friends and the younger members of your family. Friendships are important and likely to become more so as you grow older.

If you have time on your hands and feel at a loss, you are probably having problems making the emotional transition to retirement. Note times when your friends and relatives are free, and share your interests with them. Think up new projects and revive old hobbies. Sleep in late, meet a friend for lunch, read in the afternoon and put your feet up whenever you feel like it.

Useful Addresses

If you would like to receive information from any of the organizations listed below, please send a stamped, addressed envelope with your enquiry.

GENERAL

Age Concern
Astral House,
1268 London Road,
London,
SW16 4ER
Tel: 020 8679 8000

ARC (Arthritis & Rheumatism Council for Research)
Copeman House,
St Mary's Court,
St Mary's Gate,
Chesterfield, S41 7TD
Tel: 01246 558033

Association for Continence Advice
Winchester House,
Kennington Park,
Cranmer Road,
The Oval,
London, SW9 6EJ
Tel: 020 7820 8113

British Diabetic Association
10 Queen Anne Street,
London,
W1M 0BD
Tel: 020 7323 1531

British Heart Foundation
14 Fitzhardinge Street,
London,
W1H 4DH
Tel: 020 7935 0185

Migraine Trust
45 Great Ormond Street,
London,
WC1N 3HZ
Tel: 020 7831 4818

MIND (National Association for Mental Health)
Granta House,
15–19 Broadway,
Stratford,
London, E15 4BQ
Tel: 020 8519 2122

National Back Pain Association
The Old Office Block,
16 Elmtree Road,
Teddington,
Middlesex, TW11 8ST
Tel: 020 8977 5474

National (Breast) Screening Co-ordination Office
The Manor House,
260 Ecclesall Road South,
Sheffield,
S11 9PF
Tel: 0114 271 1060

National Endometriosis Society
50 Westminster Palace Gardens,
Artillery Row,
London,
SW1P 1RL
Tel: 020 7222 2781

National Osteoporosis Society
PO Box 10,
Radstock,
Bath, BA3 3YB
Tel: 01761 471771

Open University
PO Box 724,
Milton Keynes,
MK7 6ZS
Tel: 01908 653231

RAPE Crisis
PO Box 69,
London,
WC1X 9NJ
Tel: 020 7837 1600

Women's Health
52–54 Featherstone Street,
London,
EC1Y 8RT
Tel: 020 7251 6333
Helpline: 020 7251 6580

Women's Nutritional Advisory Service
PO Box 268,
Lewes,
East Sussex,
BN7 2QN
Tel: 01273 487366

CANCER

Action Against Breast Cancer
B363 Curie Avenue,
Harwell International
Business Centre,
Oxon,
OX11 ORA
Tel: 01235 820777

BACUP (British Association of Cancer Patients)
3 Bath Place,
Rivington Street,
London,
EC2A 3JR
Tel: 020 7696 9003
Freephone: 0808 800 1234

Breast Cancer Care
Kiln House,
210 New Kings Road,
London,
SW6 4NZ
Tel: 020 7384 2984
Freecall helpline: 0808 800 6000

Bristol Cancer Help Centre
Grove House,
Cornwallis Grove,
Clifton,
Bristol,
BS8 4PG
Tel: 01179 809500

Cancer Care Society
11 The Cornmarket,
Romsey,
SO51 6GB
Tel: 01794 830300

Cancer Link
11–21 Northdown Street,
London,
N1 9BN
Tel: 020 7833 2818

Cancer Relief Macmillan Fund
Anchor House,
15–19 Britten Street,
London, SW3 3TZ
Tel: 020 7351 7811

Cancer Research Campaign
Cambridge House,
6–10 Cambridge Terrace,
London,
NW1 4JL
Tel: 020 7224 1333

Cancer Research Campaign Trials Unit
CRC Institute for Cancer Research,
University of Birmingham,
Clinical Research Block,
Queen Elizabeth Hospital,
Edgbaston,
Birmingham, B15 2TT
Tel: 0121 414 3802

Imperial Cancer Research Fund
PO Box 123,
44 Lincoln's Inn Fields,
London,
WC2A 3PX
Tel: 020 7242 0200

Marie Curie Cancer Care
89 Albert Embankment,
London,
SE1 7TP
Tel: 020 7599 7777

Reach to Recovery Mastectomy Support/Advisory Service
Ulster Cancer Foundation,
40–42 Eglantine Avenue,
Belfast,
BT9 6DX
Tel: 01232 663281

Women's Nationwide Cancer Control Campaign
128–130 Suna House,
Curtain Road,
London,
EC2A 3AQ
Tel: 020 7729 1735

DEPENDENCY

Alcohol Concern
32–36 Loman Street,
London,
SE1 0EE
Tel: 020 7928 7377

Alcoholics Anonymous
2nd Floor, Jacob House,
3–5 Cynthia Street,
London,
N1 9JE
Tel: 020 7833 0022

ASH (Action on Smoking and Health)
102 Clifton Street,
London,
EC2A 4HW
Tel: 020 7739 5902

Alcohol Recovery Project
68 Newington Causeway,
Elephant and Castle,
London,
SE1 6DF
Tel: 020 7403 3369

WAC (Women's Alcohol Centre)
66A Drayton Park,
London, N5 1ND
Tel: 020 7226 4581

Westminster Drugs Project
470 Harrow Road,
London,
W9 3RU
Tel: 020 7286 3339

MENOPAUSE

The Amarant Trust
80 Lambeth Road,
London,
SE1 7PW
Tel: 020 7401 3855
Helpline: 01293 413000

Women's Health Concern
93–99 Upper Richmond Road,
London,
W15 2TG
Tel: 020 8780 3916
Helpline: 020 8780 3007

FERTILITY

AIMS (Association for Improvement in Maternity Services)
2 Bacon Lane,
Hayling Island,
Hampshire, PO11 0DN
Tel: 0175 3652781

Association for Post-Natal Illness
25 Jerdan Place,
London,
SW6 1BE
Tel: 020 7386 0868

British Pregnancy Advisory Service
Guildhall Buildings,
Navigation Street,
Birmingham,
B2 4BT
Tel: 0121 643 1461

Brooke Advisory Service
233 Tottenham Court Road,
London,
W1T 7QL
Tel: 020 7323 1522

413

Family Planning Association
2–12 Pentonville Road,
London,
N1 9FP
Tel: 020 7837 5432

Margaret Pyke Centre
73 Charlotte Street,
London,
W1P 1LB
Tel: 020 7530 3600

Maternity Alliance
45 Beech Street,
London,
EC2P 2LX
Tel: 020 7588 8582

NCT (National Childbirth Trust)
Alexandra House,
Oldham Terrace,
London,
W3 6NH
Tel: 020 8992 8637

SANDS (Stillbirth and Neonatal Deaths Society)
28 Portland Place,
London,
W1N 4DE
Tel: 020 7436 7940

SEXUAL HEALTH

Herpes Viruses Association
41 North Road,
London,
N7 9DP
Tel: 020 7609 9061

Terence Higgins Trust
52–54 Gray's Inn Road,
London,
WC1X 8JU
Tel: 020 7831 0330
Helpline: 020 7242 1010

SPOD (Association to Aid Sexual and Personal Relationships of People with a Disability)
286 Camden Road,
London, N7 0BJ
Tel: 020 7607 8851

Marie Stopes Clinics
108 Whitfield Street,
London, W1P 6BE
Tel: 020 7388 2585

COUNSELLING

British Association for Counselling
1 Regent Place,
Rugby,
Warwickshire, CV21 2PJ
Tel: 01788 578328

Divorce, Mediation and Counselling Service
9–13 St Andrew's Street,
London, EC4A 3AE
Tel: 020 7353 2323

Eating Disorder Association
First Floor, Wensum House,
103 Prince of Wales Road,
Norwich,
NR1 1DW
Tel: 01603 619090
Helpline: 01603 621414

Gingerbread
16–17 Clerkenwell Close,
London,
EC1R 0AN
Tel: 020 7336 8183

London Marriage Guidance Council
76A New Cavendish Street,
London,
W1M 7LB
Tel: 020 7580 1087

Relate
Herbert Grey College,
Little Church Street,
Rugby,
Warwickshire,
CV21 3AP
Tel: 01788 573241

Women's Therapy Centre
10 Manor Gardens,
London,
N7 6JS
Tel: 020 7263 6200

COMPLEMENTARY MEDICINE

Anglo-European College of Chiropractic
13–15 Parkwood Road,
Bournemouth,
BH5 2DF
Tel: 01202 436200

Homeopathic Trust
15 Clerkenwell Close,
London,
EC1R 0AA
Tel: 020 7566 7800

Institute for Complementary Medicine
PO Box 194,
London,
SE16 7QZ
Tel: 020 7237 5165

National Institute of Medical Herbalists
56 Longbrook Street,
Exeter,
Devon
EX4 6AH
Tel: 01392 426022

GLOSSARY

Acupuncture
A system of treatment in which needles are inserted into the skin and either left or manipulated for several minutes. Acupuncturists are not usually medical doctors.

Acute
A term used to describe an illness or pain that comes on suddenly. Acute attacks may tend to be brief but usually more severe.

Allergen
Any substance that is normally harmless but provokes an allergic reaction in susceptible individuals. Common allergens include types of food, animal fur, pollen or even specks of dust.

Allergy
A reaction to an allergen. Allergies occur as the result of an inappropriate response by the immune system to otherwise harmless substances. Allergic ailments include hayfever and asthma.

Anaesthetic
A drug or drugs used to produce a loss of sensation, during medical and surgical procedures. Anaesthetics can be *local*, where the numb sensation is confined to the area of the body being operated upon, or *general*, when it produces complete unconsciousness. The former is given for relatively minor procedures, while the latter is reserved for more major operations.

Analgesic
A painkilling drug. Aspirin and paracetamol are common analgesics.

Aneurysm
A swelling that occurs if a blood vessel or the heart wall becomes weakened and balloons outwards as a result of pressure of the blood within it.

Antibiotic
A drug used to treat bacterial infections. Penicillin is one of the most commonly used antibiotics.

Antibodies
Complex substances produced by special types of white blood cells to neutralize or destroy antigens ("foreign" proteins in the body). The formation of antibodies against these invading organisms is part of the body's defence against infection.

Antifungal
A drug that is prescribed to treat fungal infections, such as **thrush**.

Antigen
Any substance that can be detected by the body's immune system. Detection usually stimulates production of antibodies.

Antihistamine
A drug that is used to block the effects of *histamines*, chemicals released during an allergic reaction.

Antiseptic
Chemicals that destroy bacteria and other micro-organisms, thereby preventing *sepsis* (infection).

Aspiration
A surgical procedure in which fluid or other matter is sucked from a body cavity by means of an instrument such as a tube or syringe. Aspiration can be used to carry out early termination of pregnancy.

Benign
A term used to describe a mild form of a complaint or disease. A benign growth such as a cyst or polyp will neither spread to surrounding tissues nor recur after it has been removed. The opposite, a malignant or cancerous growth, may do both.

Biopsy
A medical procedure during which a small piece of tissue is removed from anywhere in the body for further miscroscopic analysis. Biopsies are usually carried out in order to determine whether or not a growth is malignant or benign. **Cone biopsy** and **endometrial biopsy** are examples.

Blood count
A diagnostic test of a specimen of blood in order to determine the numbers of the various cells (white, red and platelets) within a standard volume.

Carcinoma
The most common type of cancer. This malignant growth is composed of abnormally multiplying surface or gland tissue of any organ.

Catheter
A flexible tube used to inject liquid into the body or to drain liquid (urine, for example) from it.

Cauterization
The destruction of tissue (e.g. growths such as warts) by burning away with caustic chemical or a red-hot instrument, or by diathermy.

Chancre
An ulcerated, swollen, painless lump. Can be an early symptom of **syphilis**.

Chemotherapy
The treatment of a disease or cancer by a course of specially selected drugs.

Chronic
A term used to describe a condition that has been present for some time.

Congenital
A term used for a disease or condition present at birth.

Contagious
The term used to describe a disease, such as influenza or measles, that is spread by ordinary social contact.

Cyst
An abnormal growth filled with fluid or solid material, which can be located in any organ or tissue, such as the ovaries or cervix.

Cystology
Examining cells from a lump or cyst for any evidence of cancer.

Diathermy
A procedure that uses a high frequency hot electric current to destroy or heal body tissues. The electric current can burn away the tissue it touches without causing bleeding.

Diuretic
Any substance that increases urine production, thus reducing the fluid content of the body.

Drip
The non-medical term for an intravenous infusion. A fluid is injected into the body by letting it flow down into a vein from an elevated, sterile container. The rate of flow is measured by counting the rate of dripping.

Embryo
The term used to describe an unborn child up to eight weeks after conception. Thereafter, it is known as a fetus for the remainder of the pregnancy.

Endoscope
An instrument that enables a doctor to look into a body cavity. The basic instrument is a tube equipped with a lighting and lens system, to which various attachments, such as a camera or forceps, can be fixed. Different types of endoscopes designed for use in specific parts of the body have special names – for example, a laparoscope is used to examine the abdominal cavity.

Hormone
A chemical released directly into the blood stream by a gland or tissue. The body produces many different types of hormones, each one of which has a specific range of functions – for instance, oestrogen and progesterone control the menstrual cycle.

Immune system
A collection of cells and proteins that recognizes potentially harmful invading organisms, such as bacteria and viruses, and protects the body against them.

Infectious
A term used to describe an illness that is spread by disease-carrying organisms, such as bacteria and viruses. In practice, most sufferers catch infectious diseases through sexual contact, contaminated food or water or airborne droplets. Diseases such as **AIDS**, meningitis and chickenpox are infectious.

Keratin
A hard or horny substance present in skin, hair, nails and teeth.

Laser beam
An intensified, controlled beam of light powerful enough to cut or fuse body tissues. Laser beams can be precisely focused for use in delicate operations such as those carried out in eye surgery, and in treatment of cervical abnormalities.

Lymph
A diluted form of plasma that seeps from blood vessels into tissues and delivers nutrients to local cells. Lymph collects in thin-walled vessels and eventually drains back into the circulation, carrying with it waste products from the cells.

Lymph gland
A bean-shaped organ at the junction of several lymph vessels. Each of the many lymph glands in the human body contains thousands of white blood cells for combating invading organisms in the lymph as it passes through the gland.

Mammography
An X-ray procedure used to detect any breast abnormalities in women. All women are advised to have a mammogram at least once every three years in order to protect them from breast cancer.

Menarche
The onset of menstruation. Menarche usually occurs in the UK between the ages of about 12 and 15.

Oncology
The study of cancer. An oncologist is a specialist in cancer and cancer treatments.

Oophorectomy
The removal of one or both ovaries. This operation is now usually performed as part of a **hysterectomy**.

Pessary
A device placed in the vagina. Pessaries are used to treat genital complaints such as **thrush** and can also be used to help induce a **termination of pregnancy**.

Polyp
A swelling that grows, usually on a short stalk, from the wall of a cavity, such as the uterus, or from the skin.

Pus
A thick fluid, usually yellow or greenish, composed of dead white blood cells, decomposed tissue and bacteria. A collection of pus within solid tissue is called an abscess.

Radiotherapy
A course of treatment, which uses either radioactivity or X-rays. Radiotherapy is used to destroy malignant, cancerous growths and to slow down or stop the spread of abnormal cells.

Sarcoma
A malignant tumour composed of diseased connective tissue. Sarcomas originate in bones, cartilage, fibrous or muscular tissues. All types are rare and tend to be difficult to treat.

Secondary
A term applied to a condition, often a malignant growth, that develops as a result of spreading (metastasis) from an earlier (primary) tumour.

Tissue
A collection of cells specialized to perform a specific task in the body, for example connective tissue, where the cells are programmed to hold the body together.

Tumour
A new lump that can be benign or malignant.

Ulcer
An open sore on any external or internal surface of the body. The tissues of an ulcerous area rot away, and pus is likely to ooze from the sore.

Venereal
A term usually applied to disease caused by, or resulting from, some form of sexual contact.

Wart
A common, contagious, growth on the skin or mucous membranes. Warts affect only the topmost layer of skin. **Genital warts** are soft warts that grow in and around the entrance of the vagina and anus and on the penis. They are transmitted by sexual contact.

X-rays
Rays with a short wavelength that enables them to pass through body tissues. An X-ray photograph resembles the negative of an ordinary photograph, with dense tissues such as bones showing up as white shapes. X-rays with very short wavelengths, which can penetrate tissues deeply enough to destroy them, are used in radiotherapy.

ACKNOWLEDGMENTS

Dorling Kindersley would like to thank the following individuals and organizations for their contribution to this book.

PHOTOGRAPHY
All photographs by Ian Boddy, Paul Robinson, Julia Selmes, Debi Treloar except Mr. J. D, Frame, page 170; Eleanor Moskovic, The Royal Marsden NHS Trust, page 156; Science Photo Library/Chris Priest, page 106

ILLUSTRATIONS AND CHARTS
Dave Ashby, Joanna Cameron, Kuo Kang Chen, Tony Graham, Aziz Khan, John Lang, Joe Lawrence, Sue Linney, Andrew Macdonald, Kevin Marks, Annabel Milne, Coral Mula, Sheilagh Noble, Howard Pemberton, Jim Robins, Sue Smith, Sue Sharples, Emma Whiting, Paul Williams, Lydia Umney

PAPER SCULPTOR
Clive Stevens

EXERCISES
Juliette Kando devised and performed the movements on pages 326–329, Kando Studios, 88 Victoria Road, London, NW6 6QA

MEDICAL CONSULTANTS
Samir A. Alvi, MB, BS Lond.; Neil D. Cox, FBCO, FAAO; Sami Girling, MCSP, SRP, PGSDSP; C. J. Hilton, FRCS; Professor R. E. Mansel, MS, FRCS; Diana J. Mansour, MRCOG; Elizabeth Owen, MD, MRCOG; Nicolas Siddle, MB, ChB, MRCOG

ADVICE AND ASSISTANCE
Breast Cancer Care, Dr. Helena Earl, University Hospital, Birmingham; Mr. Ian Fentiman, Guy's Hosptial; Mr. J. D. Frame, FRCS, FRCS (Plast); Mr. Jerry Gilmore, MS, FRCS, FRCS (Ed.); Dr. Eleanor Moskovic, MRCP, FRCR, The Royal Marsden NHS Trust; National Screening Co-ordination Office; Angela O'Grady, King's College Hospital; Patricia Paniale, Royal Free Hampstead NHS Trust; Professor R. D. Rubens, MD, BSc, FRCP, Guy's Hospital; Professor John Sloane, University of Liverpool; Mr. Merion Thomas, The Royal Marsden NHS Trust; Dr. David Tong, Guy's Hospital

EDITORIAL AND DESIGN ASSISTANCE
Nicky Adamson, Claire Cross, Maureen Rissik, David Summers, Ruth Tomkins

EQUIPMENT
Ann Summers, Boots The Chemist, Braun UK, The Bullen Health Care Group, Manchester, Colourings by The Body Shop, Kays Shoes, Marie Stopes Health Clinics, Neal's Yard Remedies, Nicola Jane, Chichester, Rigby and Peller, St Bartholomew's Hospital

TEXT FILM
The Brightside Partnership, London